BEHAVIORAL SCIENCE & NURSING THEORY

POWHATAN J. WOOLDRIDGE, Ph.D.

Associate Professor, School of Nursing,
State University of New York at Buffalo,
Buffalo, New York

MADELINE H. SCHMITT, R.N., Ph.D.

Associate Professor, School of Nursing and
Department of Sociology, University of Rochester,
Rochester, New York

JAMES K. SKIPPER, Jr., Ph.D.

Professor, Department of Sociology,
Virginia Polytechnic Institute and State University,
Blacksburg, Virginia

ROBERT C. LEONARD, Ph.D.

Professor, Department of Sociology,
University of Arizona, Tucson, Arizona

The C. V. Mosby Company

ST. LOUIS · TORONTO · LONDON   1983

MOSBY

A TRADITION OF PUBLISHING EXCELLENCE

Editor: Alison Miller
Assistant editor: Susan R. Epstein
Manuscript editor: Timothy O'Brien
Book design: Jeanne Bush
Cover design: Diane Beasley
Production: Mary Stueck, Judy England, Kathleen L. Teal

The C.V. Mosby Company
11830 Westline Industrial Drive, St. Louis, Missouri 63141

Library of Congress Cataloging in Publication Data

Main entry under title:

Behavioral science and nursing theory.

Includes bibliographical references and index.
1. Nursing—Philosophy. 2. Nursing—Research.
3. Nursing—Psychological aspects. I. Wooldridge,
Powhatan J. [DNLM: 1. Behavioral sciences.
2. Nurse-patient relations. 3. Philosophy, Nursing.
WY 87 B4197]
RT84.5.B43 1983   610.73'01   82-14394
ISBN 0-8016-5623-0

GC/VH/VH   9   8   7   6   5   4   3   2   1   01/C/083

Contributors

JEANNE QUINT BENOLIEL, R.N., Ph.D.

Professor, School of Nursing, University of Washington, Seattle, Washington

JEAN E. JOHNSON, R.N., Ph.D.

Professor, School of Nursing, University of Rochester, Rochester, New York

HOWARD LEVENTHAL, Ph.D.

Professor, Department of Psychology, University of Wisconsin, Madison, Wisconsin

IDA M. MARTINSON, R.N., Ph.D.

Professor, School of Nursing, University of Minnesota, Minneapolis, Minnesota

PAUL V. MARTINSON

Associate Professor, Luther-Northwestern Theological Seminary, St. Paul, Minnesota

v

Preface

Nursing theory, nursing research, and nursing practice are often seen as discrete and perhaps even as opposed to one another. In point of fact, all three perspectives are integral and complementary parts of nursing science. For this reason, we have tried to write a nursing theory book that talks as much about nursing research and nursing practice as it does about theory in the abstract. This holistic approach may complicate an already complex topic, but it is absolutely necessary to achieving our goal—to contribute to the development of nursing theory that will be relevant to achieving excellence in nursing research and excellence in nursing practice. We have not attempted to be comprehensive in the sense of endorsing or discussing all conceptions of nursing theory, research, or practice. Instead we have chosen to focus on those orientations and perspectives that, in our judgment, have the greatest immediate potential for advancing nursing as a science and a profession. At the same time, we have tried to acknowledge other perspectives and to mention exceptions to our generalizations.

In order to maximize relevance to practice, nursing theory and research should be defined as focusing on areas in which the nursing profession has had the greatest autonomy to determine standards or guidelines for professional health practice. While the nurse-practitioner movement has led to greater autonomy of individual nurses in the use of chemical and physical means of intervention, medicine still has the dominant authority in determining standards of practice in these areas, and it is physicians (in collaboration with "natural" scientists) who have done and continue to do the great majority of the research that attempts to rationalize such practice. We believe that nursing can and will eventually develop a comparable dominance as the health profession that determines standards of practice for the use of social and psychological means of intervention. For nursing to achieve this potential will require nursing research (in collaboration with behavioral scientists) to develop both general theories and practice guidelines for the implementation of psychosocial means, and to document the effectiveness of the standards proposed in promoting patient welfare.

We originally took this position in our *Behavioral Science, Social Practice and the Nursing Profession* (1968). Since then, the Commission on Nursing Research (1975) has taken a very similar position, and most (although not all) of the major advances in knowledge about patient care based on nursing research have focused on "the human and behavioral questions that arise in the treatment of disease and the prevention of illness or maintenance of health" (as the Commission on Nursing Research defined the domain of nursing research). Our position should be understood as based on an objective analysis of the relative emphases of nursing and medicine and of their relative power to set standards of practice, not as a value statement of what ought to be or as a denial of the obvious fact that their spheres of influence and authority overlap.

The method of choice for establishing the effectiveness of clinical means has been and will remain the controlled experiment, in which outcomes for the patients receiving one means of intervention (or "treatment") are compared with outcomes for patients who do not receive the treatment (or who receive an alternate form of treatment). Even in the early stages of theoretical development, "exploratory" field experiments may provide a more direct route to practice theory development than questionnaire surveys or participant observation. We have presented this point of view in detail in *Methods of Clinical Experimentation to Improve Patient Care* (1978), which contains a detailed discussion of how a series of clinical experiments was used to develop and test a theory of stress prophylaxis through symbolic interaction between patient and nurse. Although we believe that clinical experimentation with randomized control groups should be viewed as the "prototype," or theoretically best design against which other designs should be compared, we do not believe that nursing research should be restricted to this one technique. We recognize that most nursing research is not experimental. The metatheoretical and methodological issues we discuss are even more important and relevant when applied to nonexperimental research, and Chapter 7 shows how they can be used to identify and analyze theoretical generalizations from non-experimental research.

This book is organized into four sections that serve separate but interrelated purposes. Section I presents a metatheoretical position on how to define and construct nursing practice theories, and how to develop them through collaboration between behavioral scientists and nurses by applying behavioral science theory and doing clinical research. Section II presents an analysis of selected nursing theorists from the metatheoretical perspective of Section I. In Section III, three nurse-scientists and two collaborating behavioral scientists present their clinical nursing research and discuss their use of theory to guide research and their use of research to develop theory. In the last section, the research studies presented in Section III are used as case study examples for a discussion of the relation between nursing theory, nursing research, and nursing practice.

The first section of this book, "Behavioral Science, Social Practice, and the Nursing Profession," is a revised and condensed version of our book of the same title, which was written in the mid-60s and published in 1968. Where necessary, references have been updated; and the definitions of nursing theory and social practice have been broadened. However, we have left virtually unchanged the basic positions that we took at that time, since they seem as useful today as they were then. The additional sections of the book represent new material that has been added to show how the paradigms provided in the first section can be applied to the analysis of selected nursing theorists and nursing research.

We have attempted to minimize the use of third person singular pronouns and possessives in those cases where subjects might be of either gender; where such pronouns are used, we have adopted the usual editorial convention of referring to nurses as "she" and to all others as "he." In Chapters 1 and 2, we use the term *client* when we wish to refer to the clients of social practitioners in general and the term *patient* where we wish to refer to the clients of health care practitioners in particular.

Powhatan J. Wooldridge
Madeline H. Schmitt
James K. Skipper, Jr.
Robert C. Leonard

Contents

SECTION FOUR

Nursing theory, nursing research, and nursing practice, 263

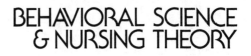

BEHAVIORAL SCIENCE
& NURSING THEORY

SECTION ONE

Behavioral science, social practice, and the nursing profession

IN MODERN SOCIETY the expansion of science and its related technology and philosophy permeates almost every phase of human life. Now as never before human actions are likely to be judged and evaluated from a pragmatic point of view rather than by traditional values or by intentions. The impact of scientifically based rationalism is most evident in professions that have developed theories of practice derived from such physical and life sciences as chemistry, physics, and biology. Less apparently, but no less significantly, practice theories based on such behavioral sciences as sociology, psychology, and anthropology have begun to play a major role in the rationalization of professional practice. In this section we will focus on (1) the way in which the accumulated theoretical and methodological knowledge of the behavioral sciences can be used to improve the effectiveness of nursing practice and (2) the way in which the empirical experience of social practitioners such as the nurse can be used to modify and improve behavioral science theory.

A problem of this breadth cannot be dealt with comprehensively in a single analysis. Our discussion will necessarily emphasize certain aspects of the problem at the expense of other, unquestionably important ones. We will attempt to single out those aspects of the problem that seem to us to have been either ignored or imperfectly understood by behavioral scientists and nurses alike.

Health professionals have often looked to the behavioral sciences for concepts and theories. Similarly, many behavioral scientists have come to value the theoretical insights and research opportunities provided by professional health practice. The result has been a great deal of education, research, and publication focused on behavioral science and its relationship to health practice.

In spite of efforts to develop the practical implications of behavioral science theory and the theoretical implications of professional experience, theoretical implications have been difficult to conceptualize, and practical implications have only recently begun to be demonstrated scientifically. This situation stands in contrast to the relationship between the physical sciences and the health professions, wherein mutual contributions have been many and apparent. There are a number of reasons for this difference. First, the collaboration between the physical sciences and the health professions has been more intensive, extensive, and of longer duration than that between the behavioral sciences and the health professions. Second, the physical sciences are presently more mature than the behavioral sciences; their body of theoretical knowledge is better integrated and tested, and its limitations are better understood. These considerations do not in any way imply that the potential benefits of collaboration between behavioral scientists and health care practitioners are less than those derived from collaboration between physical scientists and health care practitioners. They do imply a need to emphasize basic theory building and theory testing and a need to be cautious in drawing immediate implications for practice.

There are three major obstacles to the development of a productive give-and-take between the behavioral sciences and the health care professions. The first is the lack of a clear understanding of theories of practice and the way they relate to general theories of human behavior. The second obstacle, which grows out of the first, is the difficulty of designing research projects that will make simultaneous contributions to both kinds of theories. The third obstacle is the differences that typically exist between the motives, attitudes, and values of social practitioners and those of behavioral scientists.

The general characteristics of these problem areas are similar between any health care profession and any behavioral science, but specific details vary for different pairings of science and profession. In this book we intend to restrict our detailed comments almost entirely to the relationship between the social sciences and the profession of nursing. On the other hand, we will phrase many of our general comments in terms of the relationship between any behavioral science and any health care profession.

This section is based on our book *Behavioral Science, Social Practice, and the Nursing Profession*, which was published in 1968. We were all at Yale in the mid-1960s and the positions we have taken were developed while we taught graduate students, supervised master's theses, and collaborated on practice research with students and faculty at the Yale School of Nursing. The position we developed from this experience is in some respects similar to that of other nursing theorists who were at Yale at that time (most notably W. Dickoff, P. James, and E. Weidenbach). These similarities, particularly in some of the terminology, have led some nursing theorists to conclude mistakenly that practice theory as we define it means the same thing as prescriptive theory as defined by Dickoff, James, and Weidenbach (1968a, 1968b). There are in fact some major differences, which will become apparent on a careful reading of Chapter 1.

Most of the quotations and references in this section reflect the time at which the original manuscript was written. We feel that most of the metatheoretical positions we took at that time are as useful and relevant today as when we first wrote them, so for the most part, we have left them unchanged. The cited references are an accurate reflection of the sources that actually influenced us. On the other hand, the section on nursing theory in Chapter 1 contains new material that clarifies the relationship between the domain of nursing practice theory as we have defined it and other types of nursing theory. We have also revised and expanded our discussion of differences between nursing and medicine in their authority over and responsibility for diagnosis and treatment.

The purpose of Chapter 1 is to develop a metatheoretical paradigm—a set of definitions and procedures for the development of practice theory—that will maximize the relevance of such theory to improving the effectiveness of professional practice. We define social practice broadly as the use of social or psychological means or both in attempting to help a client and argue that nursing has great autonomy in determining standards or guidelines for its social practice.

Chapter 2 extends the metatheoretical discussion in Chapter 1 by analyzing the ways to use the various behavioral sciences in developing nursing practice theory, the research methods and strategies most likely to contribute to the rapid development of nursing practice theories, and ways to develop and promote effective collaboration between nurses and behavioral scientists, academic nurses, and practicing clinicians.

CHAPTER 1

DEFINING THE THEORY OF A PRACTICE PROFESSION

Powhatan J. Wooldridge
Robert C. Leonard
James K. Skipper, Jr.

When a social practitioner attempts to help a client, he is guided to varying degrees by existing diagnostic and treatment procedures. These procedures are based in part on theories that state basic principles of effective practice.

The term *practice theory* is likely to suggest a conglomeration of beliefs, philosophical assumptions, and traditions that are used to guide or justify the actions taken by a professional on behalf of a client. Such a theory would contain many nonscientific components, including value assumptions whose truth or falsity could not be tested by research. In this chapter we will take a somewhat different approach to defining and analyzing the practice theory of a profession. In our general definition of practice theory we will include nonscientific theories, but we will focus most of our attention on *scientific practice theory*. By scientific practice theory, we mean theory whose purpose is to predict the salient consequences of professional actions. Theories are scientific if their truth or falsity is determined by the results of empirical research, actions are professional if they involve the use of means over which the profession in question has autonomy, and consequences are salient if they involve goals for which the profession has responsibility.

To identify the boundaries of the scientific practice theory of a profession, we will analyze professional autonomy and responsibility at these two different levels: (1) the authority of individual practitioners of the profession to decide when to use a given kind of treatment or diagnostic means and their accountability for outcomes and (2) the authority of the profession to determine standards for practice procedures and its responsibility for carrying out the research necessary to evaluate their effectiveness. This analysis will itself be scientific and sociological rather than philosophical or ideological. In other words, we will make no statements about what the authority and responsibility of a given profession, such as nursing, *should* be. Instead, we will attempt to analyze the limits of professional authority and responsibility as objective aspects of existing social structure.

In the sections that follow, we will discuss social practice, diagnostic and treatment guidelines, and social practice theories. Each topic is treated first in general terms, applicable to any of the health professions, and then in terms of illustrative applications to the nursing profession. The conceptual framework developed in this chapter provides the basis for the discussion of the relationship between behavioral science theory and social practice theory in Chapter 2.

SOCIAL PRACTICE AND THE HEALTH PROFESSIONAL

Health professionals such as doctors and nurses attempt to help their clients through social and psychosocial means in conjunction with physical means.

When health professionals use social or psychosocial means in trying to help a client, they are engaging in *social practice*. Since social practice involves interaction between a social practitioner and his client, help provided on the basis of friendship, family ties, and the like is not included in our definition of the term. Thus the behavior of a nurse attempting to reassure a patient before an operation is regarded as social practice, provided that the help given can be considered part of her job, whereas identical behavior on the part of a family member is not.

We can think of social practice as comprising two somewhat separate functions—the identification of client needs and the provision of appropriate help. We will refer to these functions as diagnosis and treatment, respectively, using these terms in a broader sense than usual. A nurse's attempts to calm a distraught patient or a social worker's advice are not commonly thought of as treatment; yet in a broad sense they are treatment, that is, action taken by a practitioner in an effort to help a client. Similarly, what a social practitioner learns about a client in the process of friendly conversation is often relevant to the identification of client problems or the selection of effective means of treatment. Such interaction is therefore part of the diagnostic process. Almost all interaction between client and practitioner can be analyzed in terms of diagnosis or treatment. This does not mean that a practitioner's interaction with a client must be entirely a means to an end rather than something enjoyable in itself. It means that one important aspect of any interaction is its contribution toward the goals of social practice. It is the responsibility of the social practitioner to interact in a way that will promote the client's welfare rather than reflect primarily the practitioner's own preferences and desires.

We have defined social practice in terms of a practitioner's attempts to meet client needs by providing appropriate help. Not all client needs are served by any given kind of social practice, and not all means of treatment are appropriate for any given social practitioner to use. For example, if someone has a need to find a wife or to make money, he would not ordinarily seek help from a nurse or a physician. Assistance in meeting such needs would involve a health care professional only in special situations and only to a limited extent. If, for example, a professional football quarterback has a broken finger, a physician may attempt to provide help that will mend the finger in such a way that the player's passing ability and therefore his earning potential are unimpaired. If a person cannot find a spouse because he or she is disfigured, a plastic surgeon might attempt to improve that person's appearance through cosmetic surgery. In these cases, however, the physician's responsibility stops short of actually meeting the patient's need for unimpaired earning potential or for a spouse. It ends with the achievement of a mended finger that has the potential of functioning effectively or with the achievement of an improved appearance that has the potential of attracting a spouse. Reaching the final goal is the client's responsibility even though further help from some other type of social practitioner (such as a football coach or a marriage broker) may be needed. The goals of social practice and the means practitioners are permitted to use to achieve those goals are limited. The limits vary from profession to profession and even for specialists within a profession.

Physicians typically limit their responsibilities and the means they can appropriately use to meet them in a rather precise manner. The trend toward practice specialization has resulted in a situation wherein many physicians have come to define their responsibilities so narrowly that important aspects of patient care—physical as well as behavioral—can be neglected if they lie in an area that is not the clear responsibility of any of the various specialists to whom the patient goes for care. There has also been a trend toward specialization in nursing care. However, nursing has retained a strong commitment to the ideal of a more holistic type of care in which patient needs are diagnosed and help is provided over a broad range of social, emotional, and physical areas. In many settings coordination of the care received by the patient from various practitioners as well as modification or supplementation to make care more acceptable to the patient is primarily a nursing responsibility. However, one must not conclude from the breadth of areas over which nursing has some responsibility for meeting patient needs that all aspects of patient needs are the responsibility of the nurse. In any given situation, analysis of the socially defined limits placed on nursing means and goals is a necessary part of identifying an appropriate focus for the discussion of nursing practice and, by extension, nursing practice theory.

The values of practitioners, their clients, and other personnel with whom they interact determine the responsibility of the practitioner in a given situation. Insofar as values are subject to change over time, the responsibility of a given practitioner and the needs of a patient with a given problem are potentially transitory aspects of social structure and cannot be defined in any permanent sense. *Scientific knowledge can be applied to questions of values only when some particular set of objective values and goals is specified.* This becomes most evident in situations in which there is disagreement about the values to be placed on the consequences of two possible treatments for a client. For example, no scientific theory can by itself tell a physician whether a patient with terminal cancer "needs" a blood transfusion. Some of the probable objective consequences of transfusion may be predicted scientifically—for example, both prolonged life and prolonged suffering—as may the probable effects of withholding it. But scientific theory can be used only to guide practice and only when the values to be placed on the predicted consequences are specified.

Professional autonomy implies a final authority to decide the manner in which care will be given and a corresponding accountability for the outcomes that result. We contend that, in societies that place a high value on science and rationality, professions have a socially defined responsibility to develop theories and do research in the areas in which practitioners are autonomous and accountable for outcomes. In contrast, a profession will have little or no socially defined responsibility for developing theories and doing research in areas in which their practitioners are not autonomous, and accountability in those areas is thus limited to the process itself rather than extended to the outcome for the client.

The concept of professional autonomy does not imply that professional practitioners do not need to coordinate and articulate those aspects of care over which they have authority with care that is provided under the authority of other professionals. Nor does the concept of autonomy imply that a true professional will never carry out tasks and procedures authorized by the members of another profession or dictated by bureaucratic regulations. It is possible to have professional autonomy in some areas, but not in others. It is also possible for "grey" areas of practice to exist in which it is not clear whether a given professional practitioner (1) has the authority to act autonomously and is thus accountable for outcomes as well as process or (2) has only the authority to follow established procedures and is thus accountable for process alone. The existence of many such grey areas is typical of situations in which professional roles and organizational systems are in the process of changing, as is true of many specific nursing roles and of nursing's place in the health care delivery system in general.

Nursing practice and the care of the hospitalized patient

The goal of nursing practice has been defined by nursing theorists as helping the patient meet certain kinds of needs for help that he cannot meet for himself. (See, for example, Henderson, 1956; Orlando, 1961; and Weidenbach, 1964.) The meeting of patient needs in the hospital is sometimes divided by social theorists into two separate diagnostic and treatment processes—patient care and patient cure—with the suggestion that nursing goals are primarily care goals and medical goals are primarily cure goals. Mauksch (1965) ties the distinction between care and cure to Harvey Smith's classic essay (1955), "Two Lines of Authority Are One Too Many." Smith referred to a conflict between the two authorities of profession and bureaucracy, and although he thought of only the physician as a professional, the professional authority of the registered nurse comes no less in conflict with the bureaucratic authority of the administrative hierarchy of the hospital. In addition, the professional authority of the registered nurse can sometimes come into conflict with the professional authority of the physician.

There has been widespread use of the care-cure distinction in theoretical analyses of in-hospital services to patients, and the conceptualization of care resembles (at least on a superficial level) the way that many nursing theorists have conceptualized "meeting patient needs for health." A closer analysis suggests, however, that important transformations in meaning and emphasis occur from one theorist to another and sometimes even within the work of the same theorist. Nursing theorists whose examples are chosen from the hospital setting tend to see the needs for which nurses care as derived from the patient's overall situation rather than from a pathological condition per se. There is often an accompanying emphasis on short-term palliative goals rather than the cure of the patient's condition. For example, Orlando (1961:5) states that "need is situationally defined as a requirement of the patient which, if supplied, relieves or diminishes his immediate distress or improves his immediate sense of adequacy or well-being." This suggests that in the hospital setting nursing care goals focus on the patient's immediate situation rather than on his eventual cure. They incorporate a holistic concern with all the patient's needs, regardless of origin, rather than focusing exclusively on those needs that stem from the patient's pathological condition. In analyzing the hospital setting, sociological theorists have also tended to associate care with psychosocial goals and interventions and cure with biophysical goals and interventions. This distinction is suggested, for example, in Mauksch's opinion (1960) that "modern thinking in psychosomatic and sociosomatic medicine would tend to break down the distinction between care and cure."*

There are several sources of confusion in discussions by social theorists of the care-cure distinction. For example, they sometimes base the distinction on the actual effects of practitioner action and sometimes on the practitioner's motives and goals, regardless of their actual effects. Confusion also results from attempting to classify the practitioner's activities as *either* care or cure. Such distinctions tend to break down, since the same act may contribute to the achievement of more than one kind of goal simultaneously, and the practitioner may have more than one type of goal in mind when performing the act.

The terms *care* and *cure* are used in a number of different ways by medical practitioners and by patients. Some common usages imply that cure relates to the goal of effecting a more or less permanent correction of a pathological

---

*By way of contrast, Leonard (1966) concludes that for there to be any sociopsychosomatic hypotheses, clear distinctions must be drawn between socio-, "*psyche*," and "*soma*." In a full-fledged sociological conception of the situation (for example, Mead, 1934), somatic phenomena become indicators of social process, just as do psychic phenomena; but this does not necessarily imply that no analytical distinction exists.

condition that has or will tend to have undesirable effects on the patient, and care relates to the goal of correcting or preventing an undesirable effect without attempting to modify permanently the source of the trouble. The idea that physicians do not know how to cure diabetics but do know how to care for them is one illustration of this distinction. The term *care* is also used in the generic sense, in which it includes cure. This meaning is illustrated in the idea that the best way to *care* for a patient is to *cure* him.

We will refer to care and cure in this latter sense, rather than using the classic care-cure distinction of Mauksch and of others. We will analyze the practice of nurses and physicians in the hospital setting in terms of each of the major distinctions suggested by the multifaceted conceptualizations of the theorists we have mentioned. These distinctions are as follows:

1. The diagnosed genesis of the patient's need (situationally derived or pathologically derived)
2. The kinds of means employed by the practitioner (psychosocial or biophysical)
3. The goal of the practitioner's action (palliative or curative; short-term or long-term).

The first stage of the care process is usually diagnosis of biological or psychological illness. The nurse's role in diagnosis of illness and in the decision to admit a patient is, at least in theory, subordinate to that of the physician rather than autonomous. Since nurses receive a good deal of training in the biophysical aspects of medicine, they often form opinions about the nature of a patient's pathological condition and about the kind of treatment most likely to be effective. A nurse in charge of receiving patients as they come into the emergency room may have the function of determining the seriousness of the patient's condition, the kind of physician who should see him, and so forth. These decisions are based on a preliminary diagnosis of the patient's pathological condition and they can play an important part in the timing and even the nature of treatment. However, when the physician's diagnosis and/or prescribed treatment for the patient's condition does not correspond with that of the nurse, the nurse's responsibility for attempting to convince the physician to change the diagnosis and the means she can legitimately employ to do so are limited. To some extent, this is true even of nurse-practitioners.

In contrast, the nurse can and often does assume an autonomous role in the diagnosis and treatment of needs that arise from the patient's difficulties in adjusting to the hospital, to being sick, and to his diagnosis. These needs result from the patients' reactions to the situations in which they find themselves, rather than from any pathological condition per se. In other words, such needs are *situationally* derived rather than *pathologically* derived. In general the distinction between a situationally derived need and a pathologically derived need is not based on whether the need stems from a biological or psychological cause. For example, a patient's need for a bedpan can be situationally derived, and a mentally ill patient may have a pathologically derived need for reassurance that the hospital staff are not plotting against his life. If only an individual who actually had a pathological condition would experience the need under the given conditions, then the need is pathologically derived. In any other circumstances the need is situationally derived.

Once the patient's primary pathological condition has been diagnosed, the question of determining and administering appropriate treatment remains. Although physicians usually assume the major responsibility for deciding on curative treatment and determining many of the physical details of treatment, nurses usually assume much of the responsibility for carrying out the procedures ordered by the physician. Unless the primary diagnosis includes a diagnosis of physical abnormality, the handling of the psychosocial and situational aspects of curative treatment is often left largely to the discretion of the nursing staff. Nurses have the major responsibility for diagnosing and meeting the situationally derived needs of most hospitalized patients, including their emotional response to biophysical treatment.

In dealing with situationally derived needs, nurses also have considerable autonomy in employing certain kinds of biophysical means. Most so-called comfort measures fall into this category, as do procedures for physically moving and caring for patients, attending to specific dietary needs within general guidelines, dealing with and/or preventing certain kinds of medication and/or treatment side effects, keeping the patient clean, controlling infection or tissue breakdown, and so on. Physicians tend to have the dominant authority in prescribing medications, regardless of the derivation of the need, and they are usually responsible for making general decisions concerning diet, exercise, the timing of ambulation, and so forth. Nurses, however, have considerable autonomy in determining the details of such care, including some of its biophysical aspects and most of its psychosocial aspects.

The goals of nursing treatment of the hospitalized patient are usually short term and palliative rather than curative. The nurse attempts to meet immediate needs rather than to rectify permanently the circumstances giving rise to the need. For example, a nurse may discuss a patient's fears with him before surgery with the hope of reducing the probability of such complications as postoperative vomiting, urinary retention, or even death during surgery. These needs are situationally derived, since they result from the patient's diagnosis and treatment rather than directly from his pathological condition. Even if a given diagnosis were incorrect and no pathological condition existed, these situational needs would still exist. The goal of the nursing help provided for these needs does not necessarily involve conditioning the patient's psychological reaction to operations in general, with a view to possible future operations. Instead the emphasis is on reducing complications during and after the present operation. Of course, if the patient ever had another operation, such a carry-over effect would probably be welcome, but the primary emphasis is on meeting present needs, rather than on permanently modifying any (quite normal) tendency to react negatively to operations.

Once hospital treatment has been completed, there remains the problem of convalescence and, in some cases, of rehabilitation and readjustment. When situationally derived needs are brought about by a condition or situation that is likely to persist over a long period of time, nursing goals often tend to shift from a palliative emphasis to an emphasis on effecting a more or less permanent increase in the patient's ability to meet needs for himself. This shift of emphasis is typical when a patient must learn to live with a chronic illness, or when treatment for a pathological condition is likely to involve a lengthy convalescence or physical impairment. For example, in caring for the needs of a diabetic patient, physicians are responsible primarily for diagnosing the patient's pathological aspects and prescribing for those needs which derive from it. Physicians directly or indirectly assume responsibility for prescribing medication, determining the correct dosage and procedural details of administration, and specifying the ultimate goals of the basic patient education to be undertaken. However, for these prescriptions to have their intended effects on pathologically derived needs, situationally derived needs for additional information and explanation must be met to ensure the client's acceptance of the procedure as part of his daily obligations. This long-term goal is often a nursing responsibility.

The meeting of situationally derived needs is important for its indirect effects on the meeting of pathologically derived needs as well as for its own sake. In meeting pathologically derived needs a curative emphasis is usually considered preferable to a palliative emphasis. However, the kind of help actually attempted varies with the immediacy of the need and with the probability that the patient will be cured of his pathological condition. Because of the high value placed on cure, a primary consideration in all nurse-patient interaction in the hospital is the probable effect of a nurse's actions on the eventual cure of the patient's diagnosed biological or psychological condition. This high value placed on cure does not necessarily contradict placing a high importance on meeting situationally derived needs. A great deal of evidence indicates that neglect of a patient's situationally derived needs is likely to reduce the effectiveness of curative therapy. Frightened, apprehensive patients make poor surgical risks; lethargic, despondent patients take longer to recover from illness; and angry, resentful patients are likely to impair hospital efficiency and effectiveness in caring for other patients.

In our choice of the hospital setting for a sample analysis, we tried to choose an area in which the role relationships between medicine and nursing are relatively stable and where their relative spheres of authority and responsibility are clear. In this setting, nursing tends to have primary authority over and responsibility for decisions concerning how to meet situationally derived needs for palliative goals through the use of psychosocial means, whereas medicine tends to have primary authority over and responsibility for decisions concerning how to meet pathologically derived needs for cure goals through the use of biophysical means. When the decision involves some elements favoring nursing autonomy but others favoring physician direction, the primary authority and responsibility for decision making vary according to other circumstances. For example, in meeting situationally derived needs through biophysical means, nursing's autonomy varies with the particular means to be employed and the extent to which the goal is curative.

It is sometimes argued that it is unrealistic to speak of nurses having broad areas of prescriptive autonomy in hospital settings. We have even heard some professional nurses talk of "abandoning" the hospital setting as "hopeless" for professional nursing practice, since so much of what the hospital nurse does is in response to medical orders written by the physician, and since the high priority given by the hospital bureaucracy to carrying out medical orders and/ or specific tasks limits the extent to which nurses can actually carry out holistically oriented care procedures, even in those areas where the potential for autonomous nursing practice exists. That such limitations can be hard to overcome is implied by the "reality shock" (Kramer, 1974) suffered by nurses who have been educated to practice holistically and are then confronted with the reality of hospital practice and its numerous task-centered demands. While we recognize that this problem exists, we also believe that in many practice circumstances it is no more time consuming to incorporate psychosocial dimensions as part of practice than it is to practice in an exclusively task-centered fashion. It may even be quicker, if misunderstandings can thereby be avoided, and/or the number of interventions that have to be repeated because of a failure to meet patients' needs can thereby be reduced. Whether or not hospital nurses fully use their potential power and authority to diagnose and prescribe for situationally derived needs, this potential exists, as does its relative freedom from domination by the medical profession. The only major exceptions to nursing's domination of the psychosocial aspects of patient care delivery occur when the means used bear directly on the curative therapy. If, for example, a nurse were to provide information that led the patient to question the effectiveness or necessity of a medical regimen, her authority to provide such patient education might be questioned, particularly if it led to the patient's discontinuing therapy or changing physicians.* In the technical terminology used by social theorists, the 16 possible combinations of the 4 dimensions we used in analyzing the relative power and authority of nursing and medicine constitute a "property space." In our analysis of the patient care process in the hospital setting, the combination of pathologically derived needs, biophysical means, and long-term curative goals tends to be associated with high authority and responsibility of medicine and a correspondingly low professional autonomy of nursing; whereas the combination of situationally derived needs, psychosocial means, and short-term palliative goals tends to be associated with low authority and responsibility of the medical profession and a high professional autonomy of nursing.

If all or nearly all the circumstances we had to consider fell into either of these two combinations, then our analysis and conclusions would be relatively simple. We could invent a name for each of the two extreme combinations (perhaps *care* and *cure*) and reduce the property space to a single, ideal type that would incorporate all of the major analytical dimensions implied by social and nursing theorists in their conceptualizations of the nature of professional nursing practice. Unfortunately, it is apparent that in many cases, health-related services are provided that are best represented by other combinations of the dimensions.

Another way of reducing the property space to less than 16 combinations might be to to drop some of the dimensions that proved less useful than others in distinguishing those areas in which nursing has high professional autonomy. Of the four dimensions, the distinction between long- and short-term goals seems least useful in distinguishing areas of nursing autonomy. While it is true that there is a tendency to emphasize short-term, "acute" goals in the hospital setting, perhaps because of the predominant provision of "episodic" care by a variety of different individuals, this tendency is no less true for medicine than for nursing.

On the other hand, our analysis of the hospital care process did not really deal with nursing care that focuses on primary prevention and health maintenance, and one might also add rehabilitation and the promotion of healthy growth in the absence of pathological conditions as important goals. Although

---

*The degree of nursing's authority in this area is controversial, with nursing claiming a professional responsibility under certain circumstances to inform or educate the patient, even when the information provided may cast doubt on a regimen prescribed by a physician, and medicine claiming a professional responsibility to see that curative goals are not impeded. In the hospital setting, the medical point of view tends to prevail, but nursing's point of view often prevails when nurse-practitioners practice in settings outside the hospital.

the simple palliative versus curative dichotomy was reasonably adequate for our in-hospital example, it would be inadequate for analyzing care goals in primary prevention, health maintenance, rehabilitation, or wellness, particularly if the short- versus long-term dimension were dropped. Accordingly, we would suggest to any analysts wishing to apply our typology to nursing practice in general that they drop the long- versus short-term distinction, but expand the categories used for the goals dimension to include developmental, rehabilitative, and restorative goals. This would result in a property space with 20 combinations.

Other areas of nursing practice

The limits of the nurse's responsibilities for diagnosis and treatment and the extent of the nurse's autonomy vary with the treatment setting, the qualifications of the nurse, the derivation of the need, the means employed, and the goal of the treatment. The role of the nurse in caring for a hospitalized patient with a biopathological medical diagnosis differs in many respects from the role of the nurse in caring for patients in their own homes, in nursing homes, or in mental hospitals. However, the patient needs for which nurses assume primary diagnostic responsibility are usually situational in origin, and the means over which nurses have independent prescriptive authority often have psychosocial aspects that are major determinants of their effectiveness. Many of the supposedly fundamental differences claimed for other areas of nursing practice have, on a more careful analysis, turned out to be only slightly different and not the major exceptions that some of our colleagues initially thought they were. For this reason, we will conclude with a brief analysis of two practice areas that have been suggested as major exceptions to our conclusions.

Nurse-practitioners often exercise considerable prescriptive authority over biophysical means and/or attend directly to pathologically derived needs, often with a curative emphasis. While the legal authority for such activities varies from state to state, there is little doubt that in all states a de facto shift toward greater authority for nurse-practitioners in these areas has begun and promises to continue. It is possible to overemphasize both the amount and rapidity of the changes in nursing autonomy that are occurring as a result of the nurse-practioner movement as well as the *level* at which they are occurring. Professional autonomy applies not only to the diagnostic and prescriptive authority of individual practitioners in applying recognized standards of practice to meet the needs of individual patients; it also implies the authority of the profession itself to determine the standards of practice. In scientifically based professions, this authority is primarily legitimized not through practice but through research. While expanded professional autonomy in practice may eventually lead nurses to do ground-breaking research into new biophysical means to cure patients, the expansion of nursing's prescriptive autonomy in these areas has tended to be limited to those aspects of practice for which available guidelines are well developed and tested. Furthermore, this expansion has often been accompanied by legal and professional pressures to follow existing practice guidelines exactly and to refer possible exceptions to physicians for treatment. In such circumstances, the increased autonomy of nurse-practitioners may be more apparent than real.

A somewhat different (and in our view, stronger) case can be made for the position that psychiatric mental health constitutes an exception in which nurses have diagnostic and prescriptive authority to meet pathologically derived needs, albeit through psychosocial means. Although in legal theory nurse-therapists would practice under the direction of a psychiatrist, in fact they often have considerable autonomy in diagnosing and treating mental illness and behavioral disorders through psychosocial means. Psychiatric nurses have made outstanding contributions in developing and testing new procedures for reducing situationally derived distress in hospital settings through the use of psychosocial means, but so far have been less successful in developing new therapies for the cure of psychiatric illness. This may be simply because it is more difficult to develop curative therapies for patients with pathological psychiatric conditions than it is to reduce situationally derived emotional distress for patients who are relatively free of such conditions. On the other hand, it may also be caused in part by greater restrictions on the freedom of psychiatric nurses to depart from established therapeutic procedures when meeting pathologically derived needs for cure than when meeting situationally derived needs for palliation, development, or restoration. In caring for patients with pathological psychiatric conditions, as in caring for patients with pathological biophysical conditions, the use of biophysical means to cure conditions tends to be dominated by members of the medical profession (that is, by psychiatrists). Even in community mental health settings where the therapeutic role is shared and psychiatric nurses have perhaps their greatest autonomy for curative diagnosis and intervention, psychiatric nurses tend to restrict their practice to psychosocial diagnosis and treatment, with the psychiatrist assuming primary responsibility for biophysical diagnosis and treatment.

We have not intended to imply that we either approve or disapprove of existing differences between the authority and power of medicine and those of nursing. While each of us holds opinions on this subject, they are not relevant to our analysis of the actual differences as they currently exist. We have yet to discover a counterexample in which the values of all three dimensions of our final typology suggest nursing autonomy (situationally derived need; psychosocial means; palliative, developmental, or restorative goal), but the authority* of medicine and/or physicians is clearly dominant. Conversely, we are not aware of any counterexamples of patient-care situations in which all three dimensions of the typology suggest medical autonomy (pathologically derived need; biophysical means; curative goal), but the authority of nursing and/or nurses is clearly dominant. We believe, therefore, that these factors help to differentiate areas of nursing autonomy from areas of medical autonomy in all areas of practice.

GUIDELINES FOR EFFECTIVE PRACTICE

Guidelines for effective practice are technological norms that constitute part of the obligations of the practitioner's role. The technical definition of *norm*, as the term is used here, is a pattern of expected behavior, deviations from which are punished by social sanction. (See, for example, Johnson, 1960:8.) Norms prescribe patterns of behavior that are believed to result in effective practice. Such norms are different from many other norms in that the behavior they prescribe is valued primarily because of a cognitive judgment that it will benefit the client. If in the light of new knowledge a certain procedure is no longer believed to maximize benefits to clients, then some other pattern of behavior will be prescribed in its place. Practice guidelines range from highly complex and abstract formulations that demand a considerable amount of specialized knowledge to understand, to relatively simple admonitions such as "when giving an injection, swab the patient's arm with alcohol to reduce the possibility of infection."

All guidelines for effective practice may be analyzed in terms of three elements: (1) the circumstances under which the guideline is to be applied, or *framework*; (2) the action to be taken, or *means*; and (3) the purpose of the action or *goal* (in sociological terms, the structural context, the prescribed behavior, and the manifest function of the norm). These terms are adapted from Patricia James and William Dickoff's use of "agent," "recipient," "framework," "means," and "goals" (1968a, 1968b) to analyze nursing practice guidelines. They, in turn, are related to terms used by Burke (1945). In the alcohol swab example the framework is any set of circumstances under which the practitioner gives a patient an injection, the means is to swab the patient's arm with alcohol, and the goal is to reduce the likelihood of infection (which meets a situationally derived, short-term patient need by biophysical means).

---

*Authority is not quite the same as power. Authority implies that the use of power is socially defined as legitimate rather than illegitimate. Physicians may sometimes have the power to dictate to nurses even in areas where nurses have a professional right to practice autonomously, but they do not have the *authority* if such behavior is defined as an abuse of power.

As we use the term *framework*, it incorporates any relevant restrictions as to agent and recipient.

The *practice guidelines* of a profession consist of procedures that direct practitioners to perform in a given way the diagnostic and treatment activities for which they are responsible. In sociological terms they are the technological norms or the standards of the profession. It is believed that if practitioners conform to such norms, they will maximize the effectiveness of diagnostic and treatment activities. Such a belief is based on more general *theoretical principles*. For example, the belief that it is beneficial to rub a patient's arm with alcohol before giving him an injection is based on the general principle of antisepsis, which is in turn based on biological and biochemical theories. Similarly, the belief that a pleasant demeanor on the part of a practitioner is beneficial to hospitalized patients is based on the general behavioral principle of "support," which is in turn based on science theory. In recent years practice guidelines and principles of practice have undergone a number of trends:

1. Technological norms of practice have been justified to an increasing extent by their logical relationship to general principles of practice.
2. General principles of practice have become incorporated into systematic theories of practice.
3. The validation of practice guidelines, principles of practice, and theories of practice has come to depend at least in part on scientific criteria that emphasize the examination of empirical phenomena through systematic research.

These trends are most apparent in practices in which physical or biophysical means are used to achieve goals, but the same trends are evident in the field of social practice.

Any guideline for effective practice is based on a cognitive judgment shared by fellow practitioners that if a practitioner performs some act or sequence of acts under a given set of circumstances, the effect of his actions will be beneficial to the client. When the achievement of certain benefits for a client is part of the obligations of a practitioner, and when the procedure specified by one guideline is judged to be more effective in achieving these benefits than any alternative patterns of behavior, the practitioner must follow the preferred guideline whenever the stated conditions apply or he will be subject to societal sanction. The behavior prescribed by a guideline is valued primarily for its benefit to the client. This is indicated by the tendency, when a guideline is not followed, for sanctions to be proportionately severe to the extent of the ill effects suffered by the client and the assurance with which those effects can be traced to the practitioner's failure to follow the guideline. For example, if a nurse is observed to be careless with a sterilization procedure, censure may be relatively mild in the absence of any discernible ill effects on the patient.

If a nurse fails to make sure of the dosage of a drug and the patient dies, apparently as the result of an overdose, the penalties are likely to be much more severe.

In situations in which meeting client needs involves the efforts of practitioners from more than one occupation, some of the practice guidelines followed by practitioners of one occupation may be primarily determined by the practitioners of other occupations. As we have pointed out, the division of labor in terms of what tasks various professionals perform does not always correspond precisely to the division of prescriptive authority. Many guidelines for effective nursing practice originate within the medical profession. This is particularly true of guidelines in which the means are chemical or physical and of guidelines for which the goal involves meeting a pathologically derived need.

Guidelines for nurse-patient interaction

The nurse engaged in direct patient care performs many functions involved in diagnosing and treating biological disease conditions. She may administer drugs, draw blood samples, take the patient's temperature or blood pressure, or perform some other physiologically based procedure. In performing these actions, the nurse is usually gathering information for or carrying out treatments prescribed by the physician. The physiological means used in such procedures are not ultimately determined by the nursing profession, nor is the decision to perform a nonroutine physiological procedure normally made by a nurse. The ultimate authority for setting up procedures to guide aspects of practice involving diagnosis and treatment of physiological illness is held by the medical profession. This does not necessarily mean that physicians directly supervise nurses performing these procedures, but simply that they are the ultimate arbiters of what constitutes effective practice. Such procedures might therefore be called medical guidelines for effective nursing practice.

Even when following medical guidelines, nurses often have wide discretionary powers to prescribe for their own practice and for the practice of others. Nurses, along with nonprofessional personnel whose practice nurses supervise, generally have more face-to-face interaction with hospitalized patients than do physicians in most therapeutic teams. The medical profession prescribes for many of the physiological aspects of this interaction, either directly through the orders of individual physicians or indirectly through medical guidelines for nursing practice. However, to a large extent nurses prescribe for the psychosocial aspects of the interaction.

Insofar as the physician is concerned, the nurse is free to enlist the patient's cooperation in carrying out a medical prescription or simply to impose her will unilaterally. She may decide to explain to her patient precisely what is going on or she may elect to tell him nothing. In short, she may choose from a wide spectrum of subtly different approaches, each of which is likely to make a difference in the way the patient defines his situation. Nursing guidelines for social practice attempt to structure the psychosocial context of this aspect of practice in ways that will benefit the patient. One such guideline might be that when a nurse is ordered to administer an enema to a woman in labor (framework), she should (1) present the idea of having the enema as a fact of the physician's order, (2) explore the patient's response to the idea, and (3) get the patient to consent to have the enema before administering it (means). This will decrease the discomfort produced by the enema, increase the patient's overall satisfaction with the care she is receiving, and increase the physiological effectiveness of the enema (goals). Note that these goals meet situationally derived needs and that they are short-term, or immediate, dealing with the needs themselves rather than with the situation provoking them. In the research report from which this nursing guideline was adapted (Tryon and Leonard, 1965) results indicated significant increases in the achievement of stated goals.

Many nursing guidelines for social practice are vague about framework. The practitioner is usually assumed to be a nurse, though many nursing guidelines could apply equally to nurses' aides or other nonprofessional personnel. Another common assumption is that the interaction between practitioner and client always takes place in a "typical" health care setting; that is, usually one that is typical for the particular kind of nurse who formulates the guidelines (such as a maternity ward, the patient's home, or an emergency room). Such an assumption raises the question of the extent to which a guideline can or should be applied in every setting. For example, time-consuming means may be prescribed with the assumption that their administration will not cause the practitioner to neglect carrying out medical or nursing prescriptions of a higher priority. This may be a realistic assumption for a clinical professor of nursing or for a nursing graduate student, but it is quite unrealistic for a hospital staff practitioner who has an already overcrowded schedule.

Nurses frequently complain that the nursing guidelines they were taught do not apply in the settings they work in after graduation. Rather than that the guidelines themselves are inadequate, this may indicate that nurses do not always understand the theory behind a given guideline sufficiently to be able to adapt the general principles involved to a new framework. For example, in the classic experiment by New, Nite, and Callahan (1959) nurses who had become accustomed to working under the pressure of limited time for carrying out medical prescriptions did not even attempt to carry out time-consuming nursing prescriptions when sufficient time became available. The failure to specify explicitly the framework of a nursing guideline may lead to its rejection as invalid or impractical. Once this happens, the guideline may lose its power to influence behavior even if the framework changes to a situation wherein the guideline is applicable.

Much of what a nurse does to provide psychosocial help for patients' situationally derived needs depends on factors peculiar to the given situation and to the individual nurse. It is occasionally argued that achieving nursing goals through interpersonal relations is an art, the basis for which is inherent in the personality of the nurse. It is further argued that this art can never be studied scientifically nor taught to apprentice practitioners. Although it is true that current scientific explanations of variation in the success of nurses and other social practitioners leave a great deal unexplained, which might be attributed to art, progress is being made in reducing the amount of unexplained variation. Hollender (1959:2) comments on this process in medicine:

> It was Freud and other psychoanalysts who first provided the body of data to fill this gap. In the beginning the focus was on the role of psychological factors in the etiology of illness. More recently it has also encompassed the emotional reactions to disease. With this shift, attention has increasingly been focused on the nature of the interaction between physician and patient. *The so-called art of medicine*, which in the past was based on intuition and experience, can now be more clearly described, formulated and sometimes explained.

While Hollender's comments dealt with physician-patient interaction, they are even more true of nurse-patient interaction.

We do not mean to imply that there is no art of social practice, but rather that there are general guidelines for effective practice within which even the most artful social practitioner confines much of his practice. Furthermore, even artful deviations from common practice are inevitably based on generalizations (conscious or unconscious) about human beings and social order. Much of artistry lies in the skillful application of general principles to specific situations. An artful nurse might be skilled in determining which patient requests should be acted on immediately and which are merely a symptom of an entirely different kind of need. A request for pain medication, for example, might mask a need for a bedpan, as reported by Tarasuk et al. (1965). While general principles can be formulated to help the nurse diagnose and care for patient needs, the effective application of general principles to a specific situation will always depend to some degree on the skill of the individual nurse.

The artistry of individual nurses undoubtedly constitutes a major factor in the successful meeting of patient needs. On the other hand, given that such artistry actually is individual and cannot be generalized and taught, it cannot make a lasting contribution to the average overall success of nurses in meeting patient needs. In other words, such artistry cannot be incorporated into the body of professional knowledge. The subjective, unconscious skill of a given nurse tends to be communicated only in part to her associates, and such an unsystematic contribution to the level of patient care is likely to be "watered down" in subsequent generations. Therefore significant and lasting improvement in patient care will come primarily through improvements in the practice guidelines and theoretical knowledge that structure the activity of nurses. However, the study of unusually successful or artful practitioners can lead to the discovery of the general principles behind their success and thus to the improvement of practice guidelines and general theory.

The medical guidelines that prescribe the nurse's part in the diagnosis and cure of a patient's condition usually describe the required action step by step in great detail; any major deviation can result in severe sanctions against the nurse. In contrast, most nursing guidelines for nursing practice state means in programmatic terms rather than in detail. Sanctions for failing to perform the prescribed action are more likely to be mild. Considering these differences, some behavioral scientists might seriously question whether nursing guidelines constitute a distinct technology. This question is one of degree. Nursing guidelines have an existence independent of medical guidelines to the degree that nurses share common ideas about what is the "right" way to act with patients, to the degree that such activity is justified in terms of helping the patient, and to the degree that nurses' ideas about the kind of nursing activity that will help patients differ somewhat from those of physicians.

At the present time, nursing guidelines probably contribute less than medical guidelines to meeting the needs of the average patient. However, individual nurses may be strongly influenced by nursing guidelines in a way that increases their effectiveness considerably over what it might be otherwise. The socialization of such nurses is the primary goal of both undergraduate and graduate nursing schools, and the evidence suggests that they are often successful. However, nurses with master's degrees account for only a small number of practicing nurses, and the majority do not even have bachelor's degrees. When the average nurse takes action that she believes will help a patient, but that is not prescribed by a medical guideline, nursing guidelines usually direct her behavior only in a very general way. She is left to fill in the details on the basis of her own ideas about human behavior and her artistic inclinations. Furthermore, long-established norms of nursing (for example, the norm against "getting involved" with patients) are sometimes thought to conflict with new, more rational norms for effective practice.

Recognition that a given means is effective does not settle the issue of whether such means may properly be prescribed. For example, whether or not a practitioner should always tell a patient the truth would not be entirely established even if it were possible to show that in a given case a lie would help to cure or care for the patient. There is likely to be a good deal of conflict where there is a policy disagreement between practitioners over the priority of the goals to be achieved or where there is disagreement over the effects of the means to be used. The frequency of both kinds of disagreement is high in emergent professions in general and in nursing in particular. At present, such disagreements weaken the power of nursing guidelines for social practice. In the long run, however, we believe that such guidelines will have an increasing influence on the behavior of nurses and other practitioners as well.

THEORY AND SOCIAL PRACTICE

Theories can be classified according to whether they rely on empirical (scientific) investigation, assertions of value, or both for their validation. The typology generated by considering the various combinations of these two modes of validation is presented in Table 1.*

Scientific theories, including those of the behavioral and social sciences, are stated in such a way that their truth or falsity can, in principle, be determined by investigation of empirical reality—the world about us that we perceive through our senses. In contrast, philosophical theories depend on assertions of value whose truth or falsity cannot be determined by empirical investigation. Prescriptive theories involve the combination of an empirically verifiable statement about a cause-effect relationship between means and goals and an assertion of value that the goals are sufficiently important that the practitioner should employ the means. Prescriptive theories are thus the type of theory most directly related to medical and nursing practice guidelines. Formal theories such as mathematical or other purely logical theories, are those whose truth or falsity depends entirely on the extent to which a theoretical proposition can be derived from a set of axioms and postulates. In addition to these four kinds of theory, there is *metatheory*, or theory about theory, such as this discussion.

Corresponding with each kind of theory are a variety of different kinds of activity, all of which are referred to as theorizing. One kind of theorizing consists of defining terms or concepts in such a way that the terms are linked to form a *typology* (such as that shown in Table 1) or a *conceptual framework* composed of a number of different typologies and interrelated concepts. When metatheoretical guidelines are specified for applying a typology or framework

---

*This typology was originally presented by the senior author with different suggested names for two of the theoretical types (Wooldridge, 1971). The names presented here are more in conformity with current usage.

TABLE 1 ■ Types of theory as defined by their modes of validation

Criteria for the validation of fundamental propositions		
Empirical investigations	**Assertions of value**	**Proposed theoretical type**
Yes	No	Scientific
No	Yes	Philosophical
Yes	Yes	Prescriptive
No	No	Formal

to achieve a given analytical purpose, the result is sometimes referred to as a *paradigm*, or general model, for such analysis (Merton, 1957:50). A more loosely defined term for such a general theoretical model is *theoretical perspective*.

Metatheories, conceptual frameworks, and paradigms are not subject to validation through testing their consistency with logical postulates (as is formal theory), higher values (as is philosophical theory), or empirical observations (as is scientific theory). Their validation is usually in terms of *heuristic potential*—the extent to which those using the metatheory, typology, or conceptual framework manage to develop *substantive theories* (theories that make specific predictions and are thus testable) that are useful for a given purpose. Researchers sometimes do refer to the *testing* of systems theory, adaptation theory, symbolic interaction theory, structural-functional theory, or some other theoretical perspective. What this may mean is that the investigator has conceptualized a substantive theoretical hypothesis from the point of view of the indicated theoretical perspective, has predicted specific empirical findings from the substantive hypothesis, and proposes to gather data to see whether or not the predictions are correct. Whether or not the predicted empirical relationship is found reflects directly on the truth or falsity of the substantive hypothesis, but reflects on the heuristic value of the theoretical perspective only in the most general and indirect manner. The heuristic issue is more involved with whether or not substantive hypotheses developed from the theoretical perspective raise issues whose truth or falsity is relevant to a given purpose, than whether or not the hypotheses are found to be empirically true.

We do not intend to address the issue of which kind of theorizing is most important. All are of value, and since they serve different purposes, they are not really comparable in any strict sense. Instead we intend to focus on a particular metatheoretical purpose—*to define a paradigm for developing practice theory that will maximize the relevance of practice theory to improving the effectiveness of professional practice.*

Practice theory of a profession

General theoretical propositions about how to practice in order to maximize beneficial results for clients can be referred to as *principles of effective practice*. We will define the domain of the *practice theory* of a profession as consisting of principles of effective practice, more general substantive theories designed to articulate principles of effective practice with one another, and all typologies, conceptual frameworks, and paradigms whose purpose is to develop such principles.

To the extent that a set of principles of effective practice is logically integrated, based on empirical evidence, and subject to revision in the light of new evidence, it constitutes a scientific practice theory. Our first metatheoretical principle is that *practice theories should be stated in such a way that the assumed cause-effect relationship between the means and the goal(s) can be empirically tested*. Not all beliefs about the effects of means are part of scientific practice theory. Variables that have no ultimate empirical or sensory referents are excluded, as are beliefs about causal relationships between empirical variables when they are not held provisionally. For example, beliefs about the "state of grace" of an individual or the effects of prayer on a patient's condition would be excluded insofar as grace has no ultimate empirical referents and belief in the effectiveness of prayer is based on faith rather than an objective testing. However, if grace were operationally defined in terms of empirical referents and the effectiveness of prayer were considered to be objectively testable, these exclusions would not apply. For example, the proposal that patients who believe in the effects of prayer will be affected by whether or not they pray and by whether or not they believe others are praying for them could be tested.

The social structuring of prescriptive authority results in an indirect social structuring of practice theories. One function of practice theories is to make generalizations about complex theoretical interrelationships so that practice guidelines can be modified to fit a precise set of circumstances in which the means employed have maximum effectiveness as compared to other means that the practitioner might use. Our second metatheoretical principle is that *practice theories should focus on causal agencies that are manipulable by the practitioner, on effects that are deemed relevant to evaluating the achievement of practice goals, and on those contingent conditions that are applicable to practice situations*. By contingent conditions we mean variables that produce variation in the effect a given cause is likely to have. In practice theories such conditions describe variations between practitioners, clients, and situational contexts in general that tend to produce variation pertinent to evaluations of relative effectiveness. In medical parlance the term *contrain-*

dication is often used to describe a condition under which action that usually affects practice goals positively is likely to affect them negatively.

The principle of asepsis is an example of medical practice theory. As a general principle, it can be formulated in abstract terms. The abstract goal is the prevention of infection; the abstract means is preventing bacteria from coming into contact with the patient under a variety of contingent conditions (open wounds, childbirth, internal examinations, and so forth) in which contact would carry a high probability of causing infection. In a given situation the specific means might be washing one's hands with a special antibacterial soap, pulling on special gloves without touching the outside, wearing a surgical mask, swabbing a patient's arm with alcohol, and so forth. The theory specifies no exact kind of infection nor the criteria for judging that infection exists; in a given situation infection might manifest itself as a swelling and redness around a cut, an increase in body temperature, an increase in white blood cell count, or the observation under a microscope of some wiggly, oddly shaped apparitions.

A general principle for emotional distress prevention through cognitive structuring would be an example of nursing practice theory. Such a principle would use a wide variety of specific means, such as encouraging the patient to talk, asking for his consent to procedures, and telling him as much as possible of what is going on. Manifestations of emotional distress in patients might include a wide variety of empirical indicators, such as postoperative vomiting; urinary retention; increases in blood pressure, pulse rate, or respirations; facial grimaces; as well as verbal statements by the patient. The nursing profession has begun to formulate such theoretical principles, although they are not as precise as principles for preventing infections, the necessary research and theorizing are well under way; and there are indications that psychosocial hygiene may be as important to patient welfare as biophysical hygiene. (See, for example, Chapter 6. See also the series of studies described in Wooldridge, Leonard, and Skipper, 1978.)

We will use the phrase *rationalization of practice* to refer to the process by which the action of practitioners is determined by the objective effectiveness of the action. The addition of a given principle to a practice theory has potential to contribute to rationalization of practice if the principle can be integrated with other statements of causal relationships already part of the practice theory in such a way that fuller, more accurate predictions about practice effectiveness can be made. This potential is realized if the new principle leads to changes in practice guidelines and thus to more effective practice.

Rationalization of practice is closely tied to the professionalization of an occupation.* When a sociologist calls an occupation a profession, he likely means that it has a service orientation, a body of theoretical knowledge, and a high degree of autonomy (Goode, 1960; Hughes, 1963; Sussman, 1966). Professional practice involves interaction between a client and a social practitioner, the goal of which is to meet the client needs for which the practitioner is professionally responsible. The body of theoretical knowledge of a profession includes practice theories about how client needs arise, ways of diagnosing such needs, and ways of giving effective help to the client. Autonomy in this context implies that the professional is free to determine the most effective way to apply his knowledge in the service of his client, subject to the restrictions of professional ethics.

As an occupation becomes a profession, its practitioners assume a collective responsibility for developing their body of theoretical knowledge. We would argue that professional responsibility for increased rationalization of practice through the development of practice theory is bounded primarily by the limits of the practitioner's authority to diagnose and treat independently and of the profession's authority to determine practice guidelines. It is this theoretical focus that defines a *professional practice theory*. Areas of practice in which the ultimate authority and responsibility for diagnosis and treatment are assumed by another profession are not included in this focus. For example, theories predicting the relative effectiveness of different medications administered by nurses would be part of medical theory rather than nursing theory, insofar as they concern means for which the medical profession assumes prescriptive authority. In a similar way, nursing theories can apply to practitioners who are not nurses. Our third metatheoretical principle is that *practice theories developed by a given profession should focus on means for which that profession can assume autonomous prescriptive authority both through direct manipulation in practice and through the structuring of practice guidelines*.

The three metatheoretical principles just enumerated, in combination with the definitions of terms used in this chapter, constitute a paradigm for developing practice theory in a way that will maximize its direct applicability to the improvement of clinical practice and its relevance to professional goals. We have defined practice theory in such a way as to include only those components of prescriptive theory that can be subjected to empirical validation—

---

*We are not implying that only an occupation whose practice is highly rationalized in this way can be labeled a profession. For example, the ministry is a profession whose practice is not highly rationalized. In complex, formally organized societies such as our own, even tradition-oriented professions such as the ministry and law tend to rationalize their practice to some degree. The increasing emphasis on behavioral science theory in these professions is a strong case in point.

the scientific part of prescriptive theory. The value assumptions implicit in this analysis are (1) that the primary purpose of practice theory is to maximize the effectiveness of professional practice under existing social structural conditions rather than to challenge these conditions and (2) that the client's welfare (however defined) is the primary perspective from which effectiveness is to be evaluated. These value assumptions are arbitrary to some degree, but they were not chosen casually. It is necessary to define priorities to have a focus at all and to accept the limitations that any focus implies. The socially conservative and client-oriented aspects of the focus we have chosen emphasize those areas of practice in which the practitioner is most likely to make contributions that will universally be viewed as valuable and legitimate. At the same time, there is ample room for innovation and major breakthroughs in the way that general kinds of means are used with minimum likelihood of negative side effects through territorial disputes with collaborating professionals. Viewed in terms of the short-run interests of the health care delivery system as a whole, this perspective has much to recommend it. Viewed in consideration of long-term trends, this perspective is likely to be rejected to the extent that a health care profession is committed to expanding into areas of practice historically established as within the domain of other health care professions. We do not necessarily mean to imply that nursing has such a commitment. As we will see, there is considerable support for the idea of differentiating nursing regimens and practice guidelines from those of medicine.

Nursing practice theory

When we apply our three metatheoretical principles to nursing, it becomes immediately apparent that theorizing about nurses (why they act the way they do, why they have the opinions they do) is only marginally relevant to nursing practice theory as we have defined it. As we shall see, however, such theorizing may be somewhat more relevant to nursing education theories or to nursing administration theories. It is also apparent that much or even most of what nurses do to promote patient welfare through the use of biophysical means is directed by medical guidelines or rationalized by medical theories. In contrast, most of what nurses do through the use of psychosocial means is either directed by nursing guidelines and rationalized by nursing theories or else is not directed or rationalized at all. There are, of course, numerous exceptions to this generalization. In procedures such as turning and ambulating patients, treating decubitus ulcers, tube feeding, and certain kinds of sterilization and asepsis procedures, nursing exercises a prescriptive authority that is as strong as or stronger than that of medicine. In some cases nurses have done a majority of the applied research directly dealing with a problem, but they have not usually generalized their findings to propose theoretical principles. It is also true that nursing's prescriptive autonomy in the manipulation of psychosocial means might be challenged by social workers and, particularly when the need is pathologically derived, by physicians in general and psychiatrists in particular. However, under most circumstances nurses have considerable prescriptive autonomy for psychosocial means, and they have begun to do applied research and propose theoretical generalizations of their findings (see Sections II and III).

We can derive some confirmation that our characterization of nursing practice theory as tending to focus on the manipulation of psychosocial means to meet situationally derived needs is normatively correct from official governing and regulating bodies. For example, the Commission on Nursing Research of the American Nurses' Association (1975:1) stated that:

> The physical sciences and medicine address biological malfunctions and resulting symptoms. While they can answer the what and how of illness and health, traditionally they have had difficulty in relating this to human behavior. . . . Research in nursing addresses the human and behavioral questions that arise in the treatment of disease and the prevention of illness and maintenance of health.

Similarly, Article 139, Section 6902 of the New York State Education Law (enacted in 1972) stated that:

> The practice of the profession of nursing . . . is defined as diagnosing and treating human responses to actual or potential health problems through such services as casefinding, health teaching, health counseling, and provision of care supportive to or restorative of life and well-being, and executing medical regimens prescribed by a licensed or otherwise legally authorized physician or dentist.

While the nurse-practitioner movement has somewhat expanded the prescriptive authority of nurses, it has not yet led to a major effort by the nursing profession to develop new means of biophysical treatment or new general scientific principles to rationalize the biophysical basis of nursing practice. For these reasons we will lose no generalizability by concentrating primarily on nursing practice theories that concern the effects of psychosocial means on situationally derived needs for palliative, restorative, or developmental care.

The nurse who identifies a nursing technique that she believes effective in meeting patient needs has implicitly formulated a *causal hypothesis*. Such a hypothesis predicts that certain kinds of means will produce certain kinds of effects under a given set of practice conditions. However, when the nurse attempts to specify the theoretical principles on which her technique is based, she is likely to have difficulty conceptualizing the means in a way that will be useful to other practitioners. One problem is that general principles of practice, if they are to be useful, must be formulated in such a way that they will lead to accurate predictions of the effects of means and at the same time be applicable to a wide range of practice conditions. In part, the goals of generality and accuracy are opposed to one another. One way of increasing the precision of a generalization is to limit severely the circumstances under which it is to be applied—which amounts to limiting its generality. The trick is to maximize precision without simultaneously limiting unduly the potential application of the principle. One way that this may be done is by specification of somewhat different principles of treatment for different diagnostic categories.

In nursing there is a need to find out more about how to vary techniques and approaches according to background conditions. Many principles of psychosocial nursing care ignore the impact of cultural, social, and personality variables on the relative effectiveness of alternative approaches. Skillful nurses sometimes take these factors into account when they apply general principles to their practice. However, until such contingencies are systematically incorporated into practice theory, many diagnostic criteria will remain uncommunicated, and much of the potential contribution of nursing theory to practice rationalization will not be realized. Attempts to develop useful diagnostic categories for treating situationally derived needs are often hindered by the medical culture's bias toward biological determinism. This ethnocentric attachment to a biopathological emphasis can result in an overreliance on medical diagnosis in deciding on patient care plans—even when psychosocial means are used to meet situationally derived needs. To the patient who does not share this medical culture or its value system, the medical diagnosis of his condition may not seem the most salient aspect of his situation. Furthermore, the same medical diagnosis is likely to mean different things to different patients. Since the patient's definition of his situation affects both his needs and his response to the nurse's attempts to help him, the nurse can ignore the patient's point of view only at the risk of professional ineffectiveness.

Closely associated with the idea of finding nursing principles that are widely applicable is the idea of conceptualizing principles of effective nursing at high levels of generality. There are both practical and theoretical reasons for formulating the means and goals of nursing in general terms. A general principle can summarize a large number of specific practice guidelines at once as well as relate them to one another. Since general theoretical formulations imply a large number of specific propositions, they have what philosophers of science call a high *informative value* (Zetterberg, 1963:79). Nursing practice theory is composed of principles that are distinguishable from nursing guidelines in that (1) they are more generalized about the means to be employed and (2) their logical integration with other theoretical principles is more explicit.

Our example of a nursing guideline for effective practice concerned the administration of an enema to a woman in labor. It prescribed that the nurse should present to the patient the idea of having an enema as a fact of the physician's order, explore her response to the idea, and obtain her consent before administering the enema. The goals of this procedure were to increase patient comfort and satisfaction as well as the physiological effectiveness of the enema. One of the general theoretical principles on which this prescription was based is "if a patient is approached as a person with the ultimate power of accepting or rejecting the proposed care, then the effectiveness of that care is increased and both patient and staff satisfaction is increased" (Tryon and Leonard, 1965). Note that the means in the guideline are much more specific than the means in the general theoretical principle. While the means in the guideline are easier to carry out in practice, the variables in the theoretical statement are more easy to relate to other general theoretical variables such as "authoritarian versus democratic leadership" and "activity versus passivity." These implicit links to other theories can be useful in suggesting circumstances in which the theoretical principle would be less likely to hold. Would it, for example, apply equally to nurse-patient interaction in a country with strong authoritarian traditions, such as Germany? The general theoretical principle predicts the effects of a wide variety of practitioner actions in a wide variety of situations, while the practice guideline predicts and evaluates the particular consequences of a relatively specific behavior pattern in a relatively specific situation.

Predelivery enemas for mothers in labor are ordered less often now than when Tryon and Leonard did their research, and most physicians write their order so that the enema need not be given if the patient objects. This may lessen the applicability of the original practice guideline, but it in no way diminishes the applicability or importance of the general theoretical principle used to interpret the research results. This theoretical principle applies to all patient care procedures, not just enemas, and the writing of orders for enemas in such a way that the patient actually has the authority to reject the enema entirely should, according to the theory, enhance its effectiveness for those patients who receive it. Even though the new practice situation may make it impossible (or at least unethical) to replicate the research with a control group where the procedure is forced on the patient without discussion and an experimental group in which all patients receive the enema (albeit with discussion), the original research is relevant to the new situation through its logical relation to the general theory, which helps rationalize the new practice guideline. Indeed, it is quite possible that Tryon and Leonard's research findings helped bring about the change.

CONCLUSIONS

Social practitioners occupy a wide variety of occupational roles. Physicians and nurses, lawyers and accountants, ministers and priests, social workers and clinical psychologists, management consultants and systems analysts, teachers and administrators—all engage in social practice to varying degrees. By analyzing any one of these professions from a sociological perspective, we can talk objectively and meaningfully about the theoretical focus of that profession. We start by examining the social process of client-practitioner interaction from the point of view of the practitioner. This leads to a description of the kind of social practice guidelines relevant to the given kind of professional practice. We then shift to an analysis of professional responsibility and authority to determine which of these guidelines are autonomously prescribed by the profession in question. This makes it possible to discuss objectively the theoretical focus of professional knowledge under given conditions of social structure.

Regardless of the nature of the client the practitioner serves, it is possible to define practice goals in terms of meeting client needs for help. First, a distinction between normal (situationally derived) and abnormal (pathologically derived) needs can be made on the basis of an empirical-theoretical description of the typical functional relationship between the client and his environment. Second, we can analyze the means that a practitioner uses in attempting to meet a given need as psychosocial or physiological, depending on the aspects of the practitioner's action deemed to be most relevant to meeting the need in question. Finally, the goals of the practitioner's action can be classified according to whether they involve a curative, restorative, developmental, or palliative emphasis. If client needs are met by changing the environmental structure in which the client functions, then the structure tends to become a client as well, in that the practitioner assumes professional responsibilities for its welfare. For example, the psychiatric nurse who tries to change the family structure within which the child-client functions can become professionally responsible for the welfare of the entire client family.

Guidelines for professional practice are standards of behavior that guide the action a professional takes on behalf of his client. Such a guideline consists of (1) a *framework* that specifies the circumstances under which the guideline is to be applied, including characteristics of the agent and recipient; (2) a description of the *means* to be employed that serves as the basis for process evaluations; and (3) a description of the intended *goals* of the action that serves as the basis for outcome evaluations. These standards can be classified according to the profession in which they originated and which has the socially recognized responsibility for changing them.

Scientific theories of practice predict the relative effectiveness of potentially acceptable means in terms of the goals of diagnosis and treatment. They can be classified according to the professions that have the authority to implement the prescribed means through setting up practice guidelines and through direct practice. The basic questions to ask of a given proposition in determining whether it is part of the scientific practice theory of a given profession are

1. Does the profession have the socially accepted responsibility to determine guidelines for manipulating the variable conceived of as causing the effects described?
2. Are the supposed effects of the manipulation relevant to goals whose achievement is the responsibility of the profession?
3. Are the conditions under which the procedure is advocated likely to occur in practice?
4. Can the proposition be tested empirically?

In a case where the answer to each of these four questions is yes, the proposition is part of the practice theory of that profession. A complete practice theory would consist of a model predicting the effects of all allowable alternatives on all relevant criteria for all sets of circumstances likely to be encountered. To achieve such a complete theory is, of course, a practical impossibility. The development of practice theory is directed toward a series of approximations, each of which improves the extent to which the practitioner will be able to predict the relative effectiveness of alternative treatments.

REFERENCES

American Nurses Association. 1975. Research in nursing: toward a science of health care, pub. no. D-52.

Burke, K.A. 1945. A grammar of motives. New York, Prentice-Hall, Inc. Dickoff and James.

Dickoff, J., James, P., and Wiedenbach, E. 1968a. Theory in a practice discipline. Part I. Practice oriented theory, Nursing Research 17:415-435.

Dickoff, J., James, P., and Wiedenbach, E. 1968b. Theory in a practice discipline. Part II. Practice oriented research, Nursing Research 17:545-554.

Goode, W. 1960. Encroachment, charlatanism and the emerging professions: psychology, sociology, and medicine. American Sociological Review 25:902-914.

Henderson, V. 1956. Research in nursing practice—when? Nursing Research 4:99.

Hollender, M.H. 1959. The psychology of medical practice, Philadelphia, W.B. Saunders Co.

Hughes, E.C. 1963. Professions, Daedalus 92:655-668.

Johnson, H.M. 1960. Sociology: a systematic introduction, New York, Harcourt Brace, Jovanovich, Inc.

Kramer, M. 1974. Reality shock: why nurses leave nursing, St. Louis, The C.V. Mosby Co.

Leonard, R.C. 1966. The impact of social trends on the professionalization of patient care. In

Folta, J.R., and Deck, E.F., Editors. A sociological framework for patient care, New York, John Wiley and Sons, Inc. pp. 71-82.

Mauksch, H.O. 1960. It defies all logic—but a hospital does function, Modern Hospital 94:67-70.

Mauksch, H.O. 1965. The nurse: coordinator of patient care. In Skipper, J.K., Jr. and Leonard, R.C., Editors. Social interaction and patient care, Philadelphia, Lippincott Co., pp. 16-29.

Mead, G.H. 1934. Mind, self and society from the standpoint of a social behaviorist, Chicago, University of Chicago Press.

Merton, R.K. 1957. Social theory and social structure, New York, The Free Press.

New, P., Nite, G., and Callahan, J. 1959. Too many nurses may be worse than too few, Modern Hospital 93:104-108.

New York State Education Law. 1972. Article 139, Section 6902.

Orlando, I.J. 1961. The dynamic nurse-patient relationship, New York, G.P. Putnam's Sons.

Smith, H. 1955. Two lines of authority are one too many, Modern Hospital, March, pp. 59-64.

Sussman, M.B. 1966. Occupational sociology and rehabilitation. In Sussman, M.B., Editor. Sociology and rehabilitation, Washington, D.C. American Sociological Association, pp. 179-222.

Tarasuk, M., Rhymes, J., and Leonard, R. 1965. An experimental test of the importance of communication skills for effective nursing. In Skipper, J.K. Jr., and Leonard, R.C., Editors. Social interaction and patient care, Philadelphia, J.B. Lippincott Co., pp. 110-120.

Tryon, P. and Leonard, R. 1965. Giving the patient an active role. In Skipper, J.K., Jr. and Leonard, R.C., Editors. Social interaction and patient care, Philadelphia, J.B. Lippincott Co., pp. 120-127.

Weidenbach, E. 1964 Clinical nursing—a helping art. New York, Springer Publishing Co., Inc.

Wooldridge, P.J. 1971. Meta-theories of nursing. a commentary on Dr. Walker's article. Nursing Research 20:494-495.

Wooldridge, P.J., Leonard, R.C., and Skipper, J.K., Jr. 1978. Methods of clinical experimentation to improve patient care, St. Louis, The C.V. Mosby Co.

Zetterberg, H.I. 1962. Social theory and social practice, New York, Bedminster Press.

CHAPTER 2

RELATING BEHAVIORAL SCIENCE TO NURSING SCIENCE

Powhatan J. Wooldridge
James K. Skipper, Jr.
Robert C. Leonard

BEHAVIORAL SCIENCE AND SOCIAL PRACTICE

In the first chapter we examined the ways practice theories are generated and developed concepts for analyzing practice theory. We will now examine the various ways in which practice theories serve as links between social practice and behavioral science theory and how the implications of such links can best be tested. We will then apply this perspective to a more detailed analysis of the relationship between the theories of sociology, social psychology, psychology, and nursing guidelines. We will conclude with a sample analysis of some of the ways that behavioral science theory, nursing practice theory, nursing prescriptions for practice, and actual nursing practice are interrelated in the consideration of procedures for reducing patient distress through symbolic interaction.

Behavioral science theory and social practice theory

If we accept or reject theories on the basis of their usefulness for a given purpose, then the nature of the purpose for which the theories are developed will tend to determine the nature of the theories themselves. In distingishing between practice theories and behavioral science theories, therefore, we must begin by considering the differences in purpose between behavioral science theory and practice theory. Behavioral science theory is used to describe and explain the causes of recurring patterns of human behavior. Practice theory is used to predict the effects of socially permissible practitioner activities on the welfare of clients. We refer to practice theories as *social practice theories* whenever the means whose effects are predicted are social or psychosocial.

These definitions seem to imply that social practice theories are special cases of general behavioral science theories, and in a sense they are. However, the emphasis in behavioral science theory is on developing propositions general enough to apply to broad classes of social situations, and the appropriate application of such a broad generality to a particular social practice situation is not always clear. In addition, dependent variables in behavioral science theories are likely to be conceptualized in terms that are ambiguous in their relation to client welfare. Conversely, social practice theories are likely to be conceptualized too narrowly for easy generalization. They are likely to ignore theoretically important behavioral distinctions in the effects of practice when those effects are perceived as irrelevant to the evaluation of client welfare. For these reasons, very little social practice theory can be unambiguously deduced from existing behavioral science theories. Whether or not social practice theories can ultimately be incorporated into behavioral science theories, discussion and analysis of these bodies of theoretical knowledge as separate entities are warranted by the differences that presently exist between them. A number of published works have discussed the general relationship between sociological theory and social practice (Lippitt, 1966; Selznick, 1959; and Zetterberg, 1962). The reader may find it interesting to examine these references for points of similarity and difference with the analysis presented here.

Social practice theories and practice theories in general focus on the effects of appropriate means on pertinent ends and on those contingencies likely to modify the effectiveness of the means. In other words, they are used in evaluating the relative effectiveness of socially acceptable procedures. The means that are appropriate and the ends that are relevant are determined by the occupational role of the practitioner in question. This means that role obligations determine the focus of social practice theory as we define the term. In contrast, a behavioral science theory does not focus on the means appropriate to any given occupation nor on the ends considered relevant by any occupation. Focus is provided only by the kind of behavioral system to which the theory is intended to apply, such as an individual personality system; a system of interpersonal relationships, or small group; a system of interpersonal and intergroup relationships, such as an organization; or a system of interpersonal, intergroup, and interorganizational relationships, such as a society.

Each behavioral science focuses its inquiry on variables that describe aspects of the structure of a given kind of behavioral system, on the relationships between such variables, and on the response of the given system to variation in outside influences. Psychological theory, for example, focuses on variables describing aspects of personality structure and the responses of individuals to stimuli. Sociological theory examines variables describing aspects of group structure and the responses of groups to stimuli. Psychosocial theory focuses on the way that individual responses to stimuli are modified by group membership and the way that group structure is modified by the individuals who belong to the group.

In the sense that we use the term *group*, it encompasses all action systems in which there is a sustained relationship between social positions involving cooperation in achieving common goals. Thus a group might consist of two members acting in their capacity as group members or of an entire society. We have limited our discussion to sociology and psychology to avoid confusing the basic issues. Our description of the focus of sociology would also be appropriate as a description of the basic focus of social anthropology, for example. The major differences in these two fields seem more in methodology and topical emphasis than in the kind of structure analyzed.

Each behavioral science has its own focus in determining which aspects of behavior are selected and evaluated for theoretical relevance. Each social practice theory also has a focus by which behavior is selected and evaluated. While the selective processes of social practice theories are basically different from theories of sociology and psychology, both kinds of theory involve generalizations about human behavior. The focus of a given social practice theory is narrower than the focus of psychology or sociology in the sense that psychological and sociological variables describing aspects of structure other than pertinent kinds of circumstances, means, and goals are excluded. On the other hand, social practice theories often explore causal relationships between variables describing cultural, social, psychological, and physiological systems, while a general behavioral science theory tends to focus more or less exclusively on variables describing its own kind of system.

Differences between the focus of practice theory and the focus of behavioral science theory result in somewhat different criteria for the usefulness of a conceptualization. In sociological theory, conceptualizations of variables are useful to the degree that the variables can be used to describe any group and to the degree that the value assumed by the variable has a uniform relationship to other sociological variables. In practice theories, conceptualizations of variables are useful to the degree that variables describing means are causally related to variables describing goals and to the degree that a variable describing the conditions under which the means are applied alters the causal relationship between means and goals.

A simple though abstract example can be used to illustrate the genesis of differences in conceptualization between behavioral science theory and practice theory. Since all means involve action applied over some measurable interval of time, one general variable describing means is the probable amount of time that it will take to complete a prescribed course of action. Another general variable is whether the prescribed action is completed all at one time or with intervals between stages. A general variable describing the framework of practitioner-client interaction is the probability that a high-priority demand will be made on the practitioner in any given interval of time. Suppose there were theoretical reasons to believe that, for a given kind of client, the use of certain means with interruptions could have serious negative effects. Then the efficacy of prescribing those means to meet the needs of that client would depend on the probability of interfering high-priority demands. This latter variable is obviously the effect of the social structure, but it is not conceptualized in the way that would be most useful to a social theorist. Assumably, the social theorist would analyze the situation in terms of the role of the person initiating the demand, the kind of action demanded, the symbolic meaning of such demands to the practitioner, and so forth. These aspects of the situation would be crucial for the sociologist to see the demand as part of a complex system of action. But they would not be as important in a practice theory of nurse-patient interaction, which would treat the probability of such a demand as a given rather than as an effect of social processes. To conceptualize the contingency in terms of the probability of demands over the probable amount of time necessary to complete the action is to ignore aspects of the social structure that are important to the social theorist, while emphasizing those aspects that are of crucial relevance to the proposed guidelines for practice.

The accuracy with which one can formulate effective guidelines for social practice by simply making general deductions from behavioral science theory is extremely problematical. A guideline formulated in this way should be checked against the practitioner's own past experiences and against other practice theories to see if it appears reasonable. If not, modification of the guideline may be indicated, or the guideline may be subjected to empirical testing to determine whether its invalidity is real as well as apparent. In any case the proposed guideline should be tested by appropriate basic research. If research seems to support the guideline, then other related guidelines for practice can be tentatively reevaluated in light of the general theoretical principles involved. Where reevaluations suggest a modification in the means prescribed for a given kind of practitioner, client, and social framework, then the modified procedure can be tried out in actual practice and the results compared against the results of standard procedures. Only if the new procedure proves more effective is it time to advocate that the practice norm be changed—and even then empirical evaluations of the new guideline should be made periodically. Such precautions are routine when implications for medical practice are deduced from theories of the physical and life sciences. Since social practice principles derived from behavioral science theories are generally not as well developed, precise, or well tested as the theories of the physical and life sciences, it is even more important to test new social practice theories and guidelines before advocating their widespread application to professional practice. This requirement is in no sense an impractical ideal. It is an essential part of achieving real improvement in the effectiveness of practice. The inductive derivation of principles and guidelines from actual practice and the testing of practice guidelines and principles will be discussed later in this chapter.

Behavioral science and nursing theory

Theories of nursing practice state causal relationships between variables that have sociological, psychosocial, psychological, and physiological aspects. These different kinds of variables typically appear in different places in a given nursing practice theory.

Physiological variables are most likely to be pertinent to evaluating the effects of the means employed on a patient or to describing the kind of patient for which a given means is effective. For example, presence of postoperative vomiting, blood pressure, pulse, urinary retention, and/or the ability to walk unassisted are often useful criteria for evaluating the effectiveness of nursing action, both because they are believed to be indicators of success or failure in caring for situational needs and because they can be important factors in the successful diagnosis and cure of the patient's pathological condition. The effects achieved by a given means are likely to vary according to whether one is dealing with a woman in labor, a man who is intoxicated, or someone with a bad heart condition. Physiological variables that characterize a patient make a difference in the effectiveness of nursing prescriptions partly, or even primarily, because of their relevance to the social context in which the interaction takes place. For example, the social and psychological factors that determine the meanings pregnancy and labor have for a woman in labor are often more important than the purely physiological aspects of pregnancy and labor in influencing her reaction to a given nursing act.

Psychological variables are relevant to nursing theories both in evaluations of the effectiveness of treatment and in specifying the type of patient for which a given means has the described effects. Satisfaction, psychological distress, fear, self-esteem, knowledge, and motivation and ability to cooperate in care procedures are typical of the sort of psychological variables relevant to evaluation of practice effectiveness. The effects of nursing treatment are likely to be contingent on acute psychological factors, such as whether a patient is hysterical or calm, and on chronic psychological factors, such as whether he typically feels self-confident or insecure, or has neurotic tendencies, and so forth.

Psychological variables might also be important in characterizing the type of nurse who is likely to be able to use a given approach successfully, but tailoring the approach to match practitioner characteristics has not been emphasized in nursing theory or in social practice theory in general. Instead the emphasis has been on selecting the right kind of trainees and educating them in the use of those means believed to be potentially most effective. While this approach might make sense in the long run, it would be unrealistic to expect that the means potentially most effective would be the most effective for all the nurses involved in actual practice. Personality and social and biosocial characteristics can be very important factors. For example, male nurses often complain that in nursing school they are taught "feminine" techniques of interacting with patients. Use of a feminine technique by a male nurse may lessen his effectiveness in two ways. First, he may feel uncomfortable with the approach and second, the approach may violate the patient's view of appropriate male behavior.

Specialization of nursing practice and the development of different prescriptions for different kinds of nurses has a considerable potential for improving the effectiveness of nursing prescriptions; however, guidelines for professional practice are generally phrased without reference to the psychological characteristics of the practitioner. This is due in part to the professional emphasis on disregarding personal wishes and feelings in deciding what is best for the patient, and to the concept of professional competence in universalistic terms.

Psychosocial variables that describe interaction patterns are important in characterizing the means whose effectiveness is being evaluated. The means may constitute a complex overall strategy designed to structure the actions of the nurse in terms of the responses of the patient. Such strategies are usually divided into stages such as diagnosis, treatment, and evaluation. While a patient's medical care can be split fairly easily into diagnostic and treatment activities, nursing diagnosis and treatment tend to be combined in nursing action. To a degree this is inevitable. Since nursing diagnosis concentrates on situationally derived needs, what a nurse intends as a diagnostic activity can affect the very needs she is attempting to diagnose as well as the ultimate goals of care. It is quite possible, for example, that the communication that takes place between a patient and a nurse attempting to identify the patient's needs may in itself play a major role in reassuring and calming the patient and in helping him to analyze his situation. Thus nursing diagnosis may meet a number of existing needs. Of course, it is also possible that the nurse's attempts at diagnosis may have negative effects on the patient. In other words, it is easier to differentiate between stages of "the nursing process" according to the manifest goals of the nurse than to differentiate in terms of effects.

Sociological variables usually enter into nursing theories as contingent conditions describing framework. The role and status of patient and practitioner, the social structure of the hospital, and the larger, overall social structure are seldom manipulable by the practitioner engaged in direct patient care. A mistake often made in relating behavioral science theories to social practice is to see all the independent variables that are correlated with practice goals as having direct implications for practice theory. *Independent variables have relevance to practice theory only if part of the practitioner's role is to do something about the variables or if the practitioner can increase his effectiveness by varying his approach according to the variables.* For example, there is evidence that in our society, women more often vomit postoperatively than men, but this is not in itself a part of practice theory. Even if we discover the causal process that produces the relationship, we have not necessarily arrived at results that have implications for practice theory. Perhaps, for example, some aspect of the role of women in contemporary society makes them more prone to psychological upsets that tend to cause postoperative vomiting. The causal process relating sociological, psychological, and physiological variables would be of considerable interest to many behavioral scientists, but it would not necessarily have any major implications for the practice of a nurse. The nurse is, after all, not in a position to change women's role in contemporary society. Only if different nursing means for diagnosing or treating psychological stress in women were specified would the relationship have clear implications for nursing theory. To be part of social practice theory, a relationship must imply that if practitioners do thus-and-so under a given set of conditions, they will increase practice effectiveness. From a practice theory frame of reference, the question "So what?" means, "Now that I know, what do I do differently from what I would have done if I didn't know?" This is quite different from the, "So what?" of the social theorist, which means, "Now that I know, what does it tell me about the way a social system (complex organization, small group, person) functions?" Some propositions have implications for both kinds of theory; others are relevant to only one.

So far we have limited our discussion almost entirely to what might be called nursing theories of patient care. For this reason, we have chosen the perspective of the nurse engaged in direct patient care as the basis of our analysis of nursing practice theory. In analyzing the practice theory of the nurse-administrator or the nurse-educator, we would proceed to examine the limits of the nurse-administrator's or nurse-educator's responsibility for goals and means, in much the same way as we analyzed these factors for the bedside nurse. It would soon become obvious, however, that scientific evaluation of the effectiveness of administrative guidelines or educational guidelines in terms of the values of the nursing profession depends on our ability to evaluate the effectiveness of direct care practice. To administer effectively the nurse-administrator must know what kind of behavior on the part of staff members who are engaged in direct patient care will best meet patient needs. To teach effectively the nurse-educator must know the worth of the techniques and procedures taught to the students. If we assume that the ultimate goal is to meet patient needs, then the question, "What will be the effect of a given kind of nursing care on the patient?" is logically asked before the question, "How can we see to it that patients get the kind of nursing care that will be most effective?" We have no intention of denying the importance of learning how to create the most effective kind of organizational structure or being able to train the most effective kind of nurse. But to decide what kind of organizational structure is desirable or what kind of nurse is desirable we must first know what kind of practice is effective.

The impact of nursing's attempts to emphasize psychosocial factors in patient care has been limited by the extent to which their careful reconceptualization into practice terms and empirical testing have been omitted. For example, the symbolic interactionist idea that barriers to communication impede effective practice has sometimes been translated into a general prescription that nurses should talk to patients, and this prescription has begun to affect practice. But stopping to chat does not necessarily improve communication *or* patient care. The potential impact of psychosocial theories of symbolic interaction on nursing theories, prescriptions, practices, and effectiveness provides an important example of the use of a conceptual framework from the behavioral sciences and its translation into nursing theory that may clarify some of the general points we have made previously.

Symbolic interaction and nursing theory

In discussing nursing theories of patient care we have emphasized the importance of diagnosing situationally derived needs and of using psychosocial means to meet these needs. In describing nurse-patient interaction in such diagnosis and treatment processes, we have singled out symbolic forms of communication as being crucial aspects of the interaction. A focus on the symbolic content of interaction has long been a major perspective in social psychology, but it has only recently been specifically incorporated into nursing theories. The distinction between direct and symbolic behavior is based on the culturally defined significance of the behavior rather than simply on whether the behavior is verbal or nonverbal. A single act on the part of the nurse can have both symbolic and direct aspects. For example, giving food to a patient is direct, physical action in the sense that the food will meet certain physical needs of the patient, but the same act may also have for the patient the symbolic meaning that the nurse is concerned about his welfare and is trying to help him. This implies that our previous distinction between biophysical means and psychosocial means depends on the reason the means are believed to have an effect and that *the same act can be psychosocial as well as biophysical.*

The importance of effective communication between patient and staff is generally recognized in nursing. Effective communication is not simply a matter of common sense and good intentions. As Esther Lucille Brown (1963:125) has written:

> To be able to use verbal and non-verbal communication therapeutically is a skill of high order. Without training in its use, staff will continue to find reasons for not permitting patients to talk about their problems.

The student nurse or physician, on first experience with hospital practice, often finds communicating with patients difficult. Under this circumstance the practitioner is likely to decide that the easiest solution to the problem is not to talk at all or to restrict conversation to a set of routine comments and responses. As Brown concludes:

> The concept of "total patient care" is extensively promoted, but it is only in the initial stage of becoming an operational concept. Behavioral scientists would probably question whether it can become more fully operational until communication between staff and patients is greatly increased.

To say that it is necessary for training staff "to use verbal and non-verbal communication therapeutically" implies that the discovery of potentially effective means is not in itself sufficient to improve practice. Many practitioners will need special training to use complicated psychosocial means effectively. However useful this statement may be in leading us to recognize that common sense and a superficial acquaintance with potentially effective guidelines do not always lead to maximum efficiency, it is apt to be misleading if it is taken to imply that common sense communication by the average staff member is inevitably ineffective. This suggests that we need simple guidelines for the practice of average staff members, as well as more complicated guidelines for the practice of communication specialists. To a considerable degree, the development of such guidelines depends on the development of a general theory of nurse-patient interaction.

Thus far we have discussed the importance of symbolic communication as a form of treatment. However, communication also plays an important part in diagnosis. Some patient needs, such as those for medication, food, sleep, and baths, can be inferred with a reasonable degree of accuracy from the nurse's knowledge of the situational context. However, the nurse can often improve the effectiveness of her care by making a nursing diagnosis to confirm the validity of the patient's presumed needs (Tarasuk, Rhymes, and Leonard, 1965). Other needs can be discovered only by communicating effectively with the patient. For example, it may be important for the nurse to find out whether a patient scheduled for surgery thinks he is in danger of dying, whether a pregnant woman is worried about who is taking care of her children, or whether a patient considers taking pills to be partly his responsibility or wholly the nurse's. These and countless other factors are highly important in diagnosing needs and in prescribing means to meet those needs.

Communication, then, is a means to diagnosis, the goal of the first stage of the process by which nursing practice meets the needs of a patient. Since accurate diagnosis of a patient's needs is a prerequisite to effective care, getting the patient to communicate his needs is essential for effective practice. Yet, it is clear from published studies that many patient needs remain uncommunicated. But just what does effective communication consist of? Precisely what activities does it demand of the nurse? The nurse, of course, must talk to the patient, but idle chatter is not in itself likely to lead to the evaluation of pertinent variables. Since it is the nurse who is seeking information from the patient, effective communication obviously involves listening to the patient as well as talking to him; but we need variables to specify further the kind of talking and listening likely to obtain the needed information.

Some behavioral science theories and guidelines concerning interviewing are relevant for diagnosing a patient's needs. Once again, it is necessary to adapt relevant techniques and theoretical propositions to practice before they can be used to improve the efficacy of nursing. The first steps of such an adaptation were proposed in Ida Orlando's *The Dynamic Nurse-Patient Relationship* (1961). Orlando advocated an open-ended interview technique with virtually unlimited probing for use by nurses in diagnosing patient needs, and she illustrated her thesis with numerous examples. She argued that the nurse will increase her effectiveness if she shares her "perceptions, thoughts, and feelings" with the patient. Most behavioral science guidelines for interviewing caution the interviewer against interjecting his own opinions into the interview, since that involves the risk of introducing systematic bias into the data. Orlando's (implicit) theoretical position is

1. The possibility of such bias is overbalanced by the greater abundance of depth information obtained.
2. The patient's desire to have his needs met produces manifest verbal and/or nonverbal identification of a misinterpretation by the nurse.
3. The patient will, under the impact of repeated probing, eventually reveal any original bias so that the nurse can discount it.

Orlando translates this theoretical position into a guideline for effective nursing practice, which can be paraphrased as follows.

1. Observe the patient's verbal and nonverbal activity for possible distress symptoms, such as unusual behavior, nervousness, "inappropriate" affect, and so on.
2. Make a tentative interpretation of these symptoms and then comment to the patient either on the symptom or on your feelings about his behavior.
3. Continue steps 1 and 2 until you and the patient are in apparent agreement on what he needs (if anything) and there are no apparently discrepant symptoms.
4. Take action to meet any diagnosed needs.
5. Validate the effectiveness of your action by asking the patient if his need was met.
6. Repeat steps 1 to 5 if the patient says the procedure did not help or if you observe any discrepant symptoms.

Safety features to guard against bias are included in these guidelines. The nurse is directed to look for symptoms that tend to contradict initial interpretations. Even if the nurse notices no such symptoms, if the action taken to meet the diagnosed needs proves ineffective, then the nurse is encouraged to assume that the fault was primarily in the diagnosis and to start the whole procedure over again.

These guidelines and theories are not simple deductions from general principles borrowed from the behavioral sciences. Orlando's theoretical position was developed from her own experience and from observing numerous nurse-patient interactions. Her guidelines for effective diagnosis and treatment have been tested with a wide variety of distress symptoms used as criteria of effectiveness. Examples include postoperative vomiting, blood pressure and pulse increases, complaints of pain and discomfort, sweating and moaning, and patient dissatisfaction with care. Some of this research is summarized in Leonard et al. (1967). The results suggest that guidelines such as Orlando's can increase effectiveness when the practitioner is a registered nurse selected for sensitivity to patient needs and given additional sensitivity training. (Graduate students at the Yale School of Nursing conducted most of the research specifically designed to test Orlando's general principles and guidelines.) Whether or not instituting these prescriptions would increase the effectiveness of practitioners with less training (as Orlando implies it would) is less well tested. Orlando herself (1972) has, however, attempted to test this generalization of her guidelines; see Chapter 3. The ability of a nurse to recognize discrepant symptoms would probably be less if she had no special sensitivity training, and the very generality of the guidelines suggests that a good deal of empathy and interpersonal skill on the part of the nurse is needed for successful application. A clumsy and mechanical repetition of the steps listed might do more harm than good. Finally, the ability of the practitioner to treat effectively (or persuade others to treat) diagnosed symptoms might be limited for practitioners with less technical skill and authority than a registered nurse.

We doubt, however, that this latter possibility is a major factor in effectively meeting situationally derived needs. Many registered nurses receive little training in the use of psychosocial means, and there is evidence that aides and licensed practical nurses are sometimes more effective in meeting situationally derived needs than are registered nurses. (See Skipper, Wooldridge, and Leonard, 1968.) The need to develop more effective guidelines for patient care is likely to remain the responsibility of the nursing profession even if the practitioners using the guidelines are auxiliary nonprofessional personnel rather than nurses. The development of such guidelines is therefore part of the focus of nursing theory even though the means may be implemented by other nursing personnel.

Once the patient's needs have been diagnosed, the practitioner still has the problem of how to meet those needs. Psychosocial theory emphasizes that an individual's definition of his situation is an important determinant of his behavior. It is easy to see illustration of this principles in patient reactions to the hospital environment and to medically prescribed treatments. How a patient feels about his treatment, for example, is likely to be a major factor in how much he will cooperate with the diagnostic and therapeutic procedures prescribed for him. This has been found to affect even the success of such physiological procedures as predelivery enemas (Tryon and Leonard, 1965).

That psychological factors affect the patient's response to treatment is generally recognized by health practitioners. Many psychological factors are not, however, considered to be readily manipulable by available means. Most nurses have neither the training nor the time to give patients psychotherapy. However, making changes in a patient's basic psychological makeup is not the only way to affect his definition of a given situation. A basic psychosocial principle is that an individual's definition of his situation is affected by his interaction with the "significant others" in his immediate social environment. This implies that what the practitioner does and says when with the patient will have important effects on the patient's definition of his situation and thus on the degree to which his needs are met. It is important to realize that all interaction between a practitioner and a patient has some symbolic meaning to the patient. For example, not discussing a patient's problems may symbolize to him that the practitioner does not care about his welfare or that he is in grave danger and the staff are trying to hide it from him (Orlando [1961:17] reports an interesting example of a patient who made just such an interpretation). That we constantly hear hospitalized patients complain, "nobody ever tells me anything" bears out the significance of this observation.

For the nurse the problem of how to interact effectively still remains. Not only is the overt content of what the nurse does and says important; even choice of language is problematical. Furthermore, the specification of framework and recipient is likely to be an important part of prescribing effective symbolic action. For example, in situations where ordinary rules of privacy must be violated, it may be only through joking that the nurse can interact effectively with the patient (Coser, 1959). Of course, with certain kinds of mental patients, communication is an extremely difficult problem (Sommer and Osmond, 1962).

Some social theories predict the kinds of needs that patients are likely to experience in a given situation. General behavioral science theory provides insight into some of the common problems of hospitalized patients. For example, patients sometimes feel responsible for taking an active part in their own treatment, which conflicts with the passive role into which the hospital casts the patient. Many difficulties between staff and patient and many aspects of patient behavior attributed to his medical condition may be symptomatic of any human in a role-conflict situation, rather than peculiar to hospitalized patients.

Such general sociological theories have direct implications for administrative guidelines, which prescribe for the manipulation of hospital structure, but only indirect implications for nursing guidelines, which take general hospital structure as given. The implications of this statement for nursing guideline formulation would be that (1) important specifications of framework include the degree to which patients are physically and psychologically able to participate in their own treatment and the degree to which the hospital structure prevents patients from becoming involved in their own care and (2) increasing the degree of a given patient's involvement (within the limits set by the hospital structure) is likely to increase professional effectiveness in meeting the patient's situationally derived needs.

This illustrates how behavioral science may be useful in helping identify a problem, but to identify a problem is not automatically to solve it. First, nurses are members of complex organizations that typically give only lip service to the idea that effective communication with patients is an important part of treatment. Much of the social incentive by which a guideline affects actual practice is therefore absent in many of the social situations in which nurses act. Even assuming that the nursing profession, as a matter of policy, attempts to improve the existing situation through formulating guidelines for more effective communication and through high-level negotiations with physicians and administrators, it cannot be expected that effective performance in this area will soon be given the degree of recognition commensurate with its potential for improving patient welfare. Second, there are difficult structural barriers to effective communication between hospital workers and patients. The typical nurse has little specialized training in the use of symbolic means, and communication is likely to be further hampered by differences between the patient's viewpoint and her own. This problem stems from social differences in the role, status, and general background of nurse and patient. Such factors are intrinsic conditions of nurse-patient interaction rather than means that the bedside nurse can manipulate in caring for the patient. Nonetheless, such structural problems could possibly be ameliorated by the use of administrative means by nurse-administrators and educational means by nurse educators. For example, some attempt to match nurse and patient according to general background could be instituted in administrative guidelines if experimental results seemed to indicate that such a procedure would lead to greater practice effectiveness. Also, additional instruction of nurses in different cultural viewpoints and the way that the patient's role in the hospital influences his interpretation of nurses' actions could be incorporated in educational guidelines.

Summary and conclusion

Using our definition of practice theory, we can pose the following questions as matters subject to objective analysis:

1. What is the focus of nursing practice theory under present conditions of social structure?
2. To what degree is the nursing profession actively engaged in rationalizing nursing practice through improving nursing theory?
3. To what degree will the rationalization of nursing practice be advanced by deducing practice theories from general behavioral science theories?

First, we have argued that nursing theory as opposed to medical theory more often focuses on diagnosing and meeting the situationally derived needs of the patient. These needs are often met by the nurse's manipulation through symbolic action of psychosocial aspects of the patient's immediate environment and condition. A secondary focus of nursing theory is on devising guidelines for administrative and educational practices that will result in the practice of that care identified as most effective. The development of guidelines for effective administrative and educational practice is secondary in the sense that it presupposes the identification of effective care procedures, but it is also essential to the improved effectiveness of patient care. These conclusions stem from an analysis of the kinds of decisions for which nurses are autonomously responsible. When a nurse is engaged in carrying out a physician's orders or a medical regimen, her responsibilities are inextricably linked to the physician's. But the focus of nursing practice is separable from that of medical practice in areas of care where (1) the practicing nurse must act on her own responsibility and (2) guidelines for effective practice (and/or the theory behind them) have not been developed by the medical profession. It is primarily in these areas, we have argued, that the nursing profession has a major responsibility for developing practice theories.

While individual members of the medical profession will undoubtedly make contributions in the treatment of situationally derived needs through psychosocial means, the dominant emphases of medical practice continue to be on curing biological pathology and on specialization in terms of diagnostic categories that stress the patient's pathologically derived needs. The physician typically spends much less time with the patient than does the nurse, particularly in the hospital. For these reasons, it seems likely that the professionalization of nursing will involve an increasingly explicit assumption by nurses of primary responsibility for meeting situationally derived needs and an increasing emphasis on the development of nursing guidelines and theories bearing on psychosocial care. This may well occur even as the nurse's administrative and biomedical responsibilities are increased.

A great deal more reconceptualization and research is necessary before the effectiveness of patient care is likely to be increased much by the insights provided by the behavioral sciences. The problem is to identify those principles of social interaction and human behavior that will be useful in formulating theories of nursing practice. It is progress to recognize that common sense and good intentions are no substitute for scientifically tested principles of interpersonal behavior, combined with skillfully supervised clinical practice in applying those principles, but it would be unwarranted optimism to assume that the necessary principles actually have been developed in the social sciences.

Behavioral science theories are not based on research designed to develop principles of nursing practice. They are not specifically addressed to the situations confronted by nurses in daily work with patients. Blind application of any principles based on research done in situations other than nursing is inefficient and possibly fraught with danger. Even if the so-called basic principles are well tested and widely accepted in a particular behavioral science, there may still remain a large gap between the general principle and its application to specific nursing situations. It would be unreasonable to teach abstract general principles and expect the nurse to discover, unaided, their application to practice. This is distinctively the task of nursing research. Such research will also help to test general proposals about human behavior, and new theories in sociology and psychology could quite possibly be developed from studying nurse-patient interaction.

As basic principles of effective patient care are identified, careful study of the roles of patient, nurse, and physician and of role relationships within a medical setting will have considerable potential for developing administrative guidelines that will result in the ultimate improvement of patient care. As Wilson (1963:76) concludes:

> Research into social structure is undoubtedly as important to the future of medical care as is research into cell structure. Patient care is, after all, the crux, the point of application for the virtuosities of medical science.

RESEARCH ON SOCIAL PRACTICE
Formulating a research hypothesis

The first stage in the research process is not unlike the first stage in the patient care process. It consists of diagnosing a need for some kind of knowledge. For the social practitioner interested in developing practice theory, this means that he must identify a researchable question, the answer to which may have potential for improving practice effectiveness. To be researchable the question must contain variables that have empirical consequences and that are ultimately defined in terms of these consequences rather than in terms of value commitments. To be relevant to practice theory, however, the question must have implications for action when considered in the light of professional values. In other words, the *dependent variable* (effect) must be relevant to practice goals and the *independent variable* (cause) must be appropriate for the practitioner to manipulate.

Theory and empirical experience are the two major sources of researchable questions. We have already commented on the need to carefully test implications for social practice derived from general behavioral science theories or even from general practice principles. We have yet to discuss the derivation of testable generalizations from the practitioner's own clinical and research experience. Here the researchable question is derived inductively. The practitioner observes a number of specific occurrences and abstracts from them a general principle. A nurse may observe that if she talks to patients about their scheduled surgery, they become less tense and anxious and seldom vomit postoperatively. From this she may inductively derive the theoretical hypothesis that emotional distress is a cause of postoperative vomiting and that the particular kind of communication process she uses tends to reduce tension and postoperative vomiting (Dumas and Leonard, 1963). This is in contrast to the deductive process involved in deriving a particular implication from a general principle. For example, a nurse may be aware that tension tends to cause vomiting and that a child's reaction to a situation depends to a considerable extent on verbal and nonverbal cues from his parents. From this she may deduce that she can decrease the probability that a child will vomit postoperatively by increasing the confidence of the child's parents (Mahaffey, 1965). Of course, induction and deduction can both play a part in the formulation of the same hypothesis. While both are important in the formulation of hypotheses in any scientific discipline, inductive generalizations from actual practice are particularly important when the relevant body of practice theory is not highly developed. In nursing, inductive generalizations often play a major part in formulating hypotheses for testing.

The everyday practice of the nurse is implicitly based on a wide variety of assumptions about the people with whom she interacts and about the probable effects of her behavior. Much of everyday nursing practice depends on habits that, once established, minimize the necessity for conscious thought. For example, the nurse may assume that a brisk manner and a smile will cheer patients and habitually act in accordance with that assumption. To some degree, habitual behavior is a necessity. It would be impossible to think consciously and deliberately about all the possible effects of everything one does and says. Habitual ways of interacting with patients leave the nurse free to concentrate on aspects of interaction that do require conscious consideration to achieve the desired results. On the other hand, the nurse may rely on habitual responses to patients on occasions when conscious consideration would result in increased effectiveness. For example, a determinedly cheery manner may be upsetting to some patients, particularly if it is perceived by the patient as indicating a lack of concern for his problems. The skillful nurse develops a knack for recognizing when to abandon her habitual responses for more deliberative action. Such a knack is based on general principles of practice, whether the nurse has consciously formulated them or not.

The first step in inductively developing a researchable question is to bring some of the general, unconsciously employed principles of everyday practice to a conscious level, where they can be analyzed and examined. The clinical experience of the nurse can be a very rich source of research hypotheses with direct implications for practice. Usually the hypothesis predicts that some implicit practice guideline on which the nurse acts will produce certain effects. For example, when a patient states that he is in mild pain, the nurse should first discuss the patient's pain with him and then let him participate in the final determination of the action. It is predicted that through this procedure the pain will be more effectively relieved (Moss and Meyer, 1966). Such hypotheses can be thought of as based on a series of trial-and-error experiments performed in the course of nursing practice.

Effective nursing practice requires the nurse to gather facts about the patient and his illness. This is done by observing the patient, communicating with him, and reviewing facts other professionals have been able to collect. Having evaluated general aspects of the patient's condition, the nurse decides on the course of action best suited to meet the patient's needs. After help has been given to the patient, the nurse examines the patient's condition to find out whether any changes have occurred and if they were the ones expected. If the expected changes occur, then the nurse evaluates her efforts as successful. However, if there were no changes, or if there were unpredicted changes, the nurse must try to discover why. Perhaps this calls for a complete review of all the facts about the patient and an evaluation of the original measures, the care procedure itself, its performance and the extent of its success.

All this may sound like nothing more than a combination of common sense and ideal standard operating procedure for good nursing practice, which it is. But it is also implicitly *research practice*. Consider the same example from a research perspective. First, the nurse engages in a descriptive study of the patient and his illness. To do this she employs both observational and interview techniques. Based on a series of general propositions (a theory) about what is the best action to take for a patient with these symptoms, the nurse formulates a hypothesis that a given nursing procedure will cause certain changes in the patient's condition. Measures of the patient's condition are taken before the treatment is started. The treatment is then carried out. Then the nurse tests her hypothesis by measuring the patient's condition again. If the predicted changes are discovered, support has been found for the hypothesis; if not, the hypothesis is not supported and must be reevaluated. The nurse has now completed a very simple before-after experiment. Of course, we do not mean to imply that the nurse typically goes about caring for patients in the self-conscious fashion just described or that the nurse thinks in terms of the exact concepts we have used. But to learn from experience, the nurse must implicitly examine the effects of her practice in some such fashion.

Granted that there are similarities and analogies between research practice and social practice, what are the differences? Certainly we would not want to imply that knowledge of the basic principles of effective nursing must come directly from practice and that systematic research is unnecessary. Practice is directed primarily to the goal of caring for the needs of the moment, rather than to the goal of developing and testing basic principles. Granted that some development and testing of principles does occur in everyday practice, there are innumerable ways in which the practitioner can be misled about the effects he achieves and why he achieves them. For decades physicians bled patients in the belief that they were effectively meeting pathologically derived needs. Their observations seemed to confirm that this technique often helped—after all, the condition of most of their patients eventually changed in the desired fashion. The point missed is that most sick persons eventually get better, at least in terms of objective symptoms, whether or not they go to a physician. It is quite possible that some of the assumptions on which nurses commonly base their practice may be equally misguided. For example, comments such as, "don't worry, everything's going to be all right" may tend to increase patient anxiety rather than decrease it. To argue that this practice is effective, it is insufficient for the practitioner to demonstrate that many patients become less anxious; she must also show that this change was caused at least in part by her own efforts. Furthermore, even assuming that the practitioner's efforts were highly effective, the question of why they were effective must be answered if the practice of other members of the profession is to be improved.

Let us consider the ways in which inferences drawn from clinical experience can be misleading. First, there is the possibility that a patient's condition may normally change for the better under a given set of circumstances, almost regardless of what the practitioner does. We have already given an example of how activities actually detrimental to client welfare can be labeled as effective under such circumstances (the bleeding of patients by physicians and possibly the use of pat phrases of reassurance by nurses). Second, the improvements could result from bias in evaluating the patient's condition before the action, or his condition after, or both. In other words, the nurse may tend to perceive the patient's condition before her action as worse than it actually is or perceive his condition after the provision of help as better than it actually is. A biased evaluation of the ends to which the action was directed is particularly likely in social practice, where the client is often under social pressure to reward the practitioner by expressions of gratitude. Then, too, changes in patient condition could result from the effects of some aspect of the practitioner's action other than the one to which the change was attributed. For example, a nurse might believe that she had calmed a patient's fears by correcting a misunderstanding about hospital procedure, whereas the effect might have resulted from the patient's increased confidence in the desire and ability of the hospital personnel to take care of him. Finally, the improvements could be real, but entirely fortuitous. In other words, there might be no systematic or general tendency for the patient's condition to improve in a given way, but a particular patient might improve for some idiosyncratic reason not associated with the nurse's efforts.

The possibilities just discussed refer to a lack of what the research methodologist calls *internal validity*. If research has high internal validity, then it will lead to valid inferences about the average effects of the means evaluated on the relevant ends for the cases actually studied. In addition, there is the question of generalizing results to bear on other clients, practitioners, and frameworks. For example, a nurse might have very good results with a given approach for adult patients, but the same approach might be entirely ineffective when used with children. If the research were to lead to invalid inferences about the effects of the means evaluated under different circumstances, then a methodologist would talk about a lack of *external validity* (Campbell, 1957).

While external validity is an important consideration in research, it is secondary to internal validity. It is relatively easy to make research cumulative by combining results from a large number of separate studies, each of which is internally valid. If the separate studies do not have a great deal of internal validity, however, we cannot know what the results of each mean. It is extremely difficult to develop a cumulative body of theory from research whose internal validity is questionable, and particularly in the early stages of theoretical development.

Choosing a research strategy

The researcher who wishes to test a hypothesis about the effectiveness of a given kind of action is faced with a number of problems in deciding which kind of research strategy to adopt. Two important general considerations are the importance of external validity to the research goals and whether the research is primarily concerned with the practice guideline itself or with the theoretical principles underlying the practice guideline. Once the research question has been specified, alternative research strategies are evaluated by theorizing about the probability that the results of a given research strategy will produce misleading results. For example, we theorized that a patient's expressions of gratitude were influenced by social pressure as much as by the actual quality of the help received. This was one of the reasons we concluded that the sort of trial-and-error experimentation that is part of everyday social practice has a low degree of internal validity for testing practice hypotheses. Finally, choice of a research strategy depends on ethical and social questions of morality and practicality. How do these considerations apply to the choice of an experimental or survey design, to the means chosen to measure the variables studied, and to the selection of a sample framework?

We have discussed some of the ways a practitioner might draw misleading inferences from his clinical experience. In particular, we discussed the possibility that a patient's condition may usually change for the better under a given set of circumstances, almost regardless of what the practitioner does. Systematic research can attempt to meet this problem by evaluating the extent to which relevant aspects of patient condition would have changed without the use of the means whose effects are to be studied. This is done by studying patients whose care did not include the means in question. These patients are then compared with patients whose care included those means, and differences between the two groups are used to estimate effectiveness. For example, we could attempt to discover whether hospital patients who had been reassured with pat phrases were more anxious or less anxious than patients who had received no reassurance. Furthermore, both groups of patients could be compared with patients who had received the "deliberative" sort of reassurance advocated by Orlando.

The use of comparison groups helps to rule out one kind of alternative explanation, but it introduces new possibilities of error. Suppose that comparison groups are obtained by surveying incidents in which patients express anxiety and classifying the kinds of reassurance provided by the nurse as "no reassurance," "pat-phrase reassurance," or "deliberative reassurance." In actuality, we would probably need at least one additional category for cases that did not seem to fit any of these categories and some cases might involve both deliberative and pat-phrase reassurance. This sort of problem is minimized in experimental designs, which actually manipulate the means whose effects are being studied. Finally, each case is classified according to the patient's level of anxiety after interaction with the nurse. If we performed such a study, any differences in average anxiety level might be because of differences between the groups that existed before the nursing action we were attempting to evaluate. For example, nurses might tend to give deliberative reassurance only to those patients manifesting extreme anxiety, to give pat-phrase reassurance to patients manifesting moderate anxiety, and to make no specific efforts to reassure patients who manifested minimal or no anxiety. Under these conditions, we might find higher rates of anxiety among patients given deliberative reassurance than among patients given no reassurance or pat-phrase reassurance, even if the deliberative reassurance was more effective than either of the other two techniques.

The survey researcher would respond to this problem by comparing patients who seemed to have manifested the same amount of initial anxiety but received different kinds of reassurance from the nurse. This technique is referred to as *ex post facto contingency control*, and it is the main technique used by survey analysts in ruling out spuriousness as an alternative explanation of a proposed cause-effect relationship.* However, it would still be possible that systematic differences affecting anxiety remained between the groups compared. The survey analyst might attempt to control such potential sources of spuriousness by comparing groups similar in terms of such variables as age, race, sex, and social class, as well as in initial level of anxiety. This technique has severe limitations that are most acute in areas where practice theory is relatively undeveloped, such as the psychosocial prophylaxis of anxiety. For

---

*In this context spuriousness refers to an association produced by systematic differences between the groups in background conditions that existed before the means were applied. The logic of control is somewhat different in techniques such as partial correlation. These techniques are subject to many of the limitations of contingency controls, however, and to other possibilities of error as well.

one thing, it is necessary to study large numbers of patients to be able to control for many variables and still have a reasonable number of cases in each specific combination of the control variables. In our previous example, if there were four categories of age, two of race, two of sex, three of social class, and three levels of initial anxiety, then there would be $4 \times 2 \times 2 \times 3 \times 3 = 144$ specific combinations, within each of which the relationship between the approach used by the nurse and the patient's later anxiety would have to be analyzed. Even more important, one can never be certain that all of the possible sources of spuriousness have been controlled. This is particularly true for problems like the example problem, in which no well-developed theory of the causes of patient anxiety exists to guide the analyst in selection of variables to control. For all these reasons, survey research is usually more useful in suggesting causal hypotheses to be tested than in providing an ultimate test of them.

In testing a causal hypothesis it is important to rule out the possibility that the independent variable will be associated with the dependent variable because of one or more antecedent variables that are causes of both. In our example problem we argued that the initial level of patient anxiety might be a cause of the kind of reassurance provided, as well as a cause of the level of anxiety recorded after the nurse-patient interaction. This kind of spuriousness can be ruled out by assigning cases at random to the different kinds of care whose relative effectiveness is to be evaluated (Fisher, 1947). All clients assigned to receive the same means make up a *treatment group*. A treatment group made up of clients from whom a given kind of means was withheld is referred to as a *control group*. In most clinical trials, the control group receives all the care routinely provided but does not receive the additional care components to be evaluated. By random assignment, we mean that the basis of the assignment is not systematically associated with any factors that are potential causes of the effects to be studied. Basing the assignment on a coin toss or choosing from a table of random numbers are examples of procedures that are accepted as random no matter what effects are being studied.

If assignments are determined at random, then any differences between the two groups must be because of differences in the treatment or chance. In comparing the conditions of only a few patients who received one kind of care with the conditions of only a few patients who received another kind of care, it is quite possible that even large differences between the groups could be because of chance factors. For large groups, even small differences are unlikely to be solely because of chance. The precise probability of finding a difference of a given magnitude or greater between treatment groups because of chance alone can be evaluated mathematically. It is only when this probability is very low that the researcher can be confident that being assigned to

one care procedure rather than the other caused some part of the recorded difference between the groups. In general a low probability of a given difference owing to chance alone is directly related to:
1. A large sample of clients
2. A large average effect because of differences in the treatments compared
3. A lack of variation in other causes of the effect studied

There are two keys to successful experimental research on social practice. The first is to assign clients randomly to treatment groups. The second is to control for contingent conditions believed to effect the causal process and for any known important causes of the effects to be studied. This can be done by intervening to prevent aspects of the framework, agent, or client from varying, by choosing a homogeneous sample of cases for study, or both. This makes it difficult to generalize to other conditions but increases the sensitivity of the experiment and the specificity of the conclusions. The latter is particularly important for the development of practice theories, since the practitioner must apply the theory under specific situations. As we have pointed out, lack of external validity is not nearly so serious a problem as lack of internal validity. Whenever internal validity is high, external validity can be developed through replication of the research by other practitioners with other clients and in other settings. Therefore the preferred design for most research on social practice would seem to be systematic experimentation by the practitioner.

Randomly assigning the kind of care provided to patients helps to prevent incorrect evaluation of the effectiveness of care. The question that remains is are such experiments ethically or morally desirable? In one sense, of course, the answer to an ethical question is not a matter of logic or of empirical evidence. It is ultimately a matter of the relative importance assigned to different values. Under one conception of professional ethics the professional is responsible primarily for good intentions and for conformity to accepted practice guidelines, rather than for the actual results of his actions. However, to the extent that a profession accepts responsibility for scientifically rationalizing the practice of its members, good intentions and tradition are not the sole determinants of professional responsibility. In this conception of responsibility the professional ethic includes a responsibility for scientific examination of the effects of the means employed. If such a responsibility is accepted as an ethical value, then it becomes unethical not to test the principles by which one practices. Such tests seem logically to involve the fewest ethical problems when there are differences of opinion about which kind of care is most effective or when facilities are not available to give the means believed to be more effective to all clients. Under such circumstances, a random determination of which client is to receive which kind of care seems as moral a basis as any other. While specific experimental designs may raise ethical issues, in general we believe that the ethical problems of social experimentation are not nearly so great as many practitioners assume.

Questions of practicality are also raised with respect to experiments on patient care. The idea that experiments are impractical often comes from thinking of experiments in terms of scientific laboratories, expensive equipment, nearly complete control over disturbing influences, and highly complex research procedures. Such a stereotype of the scientific experiment simply does not apply to field experiments in social practice. Field experiments use natural settings, work within regular administrative routine, and can often be worked into the everyday practice of an imaginative practitioner. The crucial difference between field experimentation and the everyday, trial-and-error experimentation that is an inevitable concomitant of social practice is that in field experimentation the practitioner randomizes some part of his practice and then systematically keeps track of relevant aspects of his client's welfare. Of course, it is possible to design very complex field experiments. But the basic core of field experimentation is quite simple, and it can provide insights that are unavailable from large-scale surveys. The key requirement in designing field experiments on patient care is, of course, the active and willing participation of social practitioners (physicians, nurse's aides, and so on) who have a socially recognized responsibility for performing the necessary manipulations. The practicality of such research is amply demonstrated by the increasing number of field experiments on patient care actually carried out by health practitioners.

When experimental research is not feasible, the laborious job of indirectly testing causal hypotheses through the collection of masses of nonexperimental data is justified. For example, the establishment of a causal relationship between cigarette smoking and cancer was accomplished largely by nonexperimental research. (Even here, experimental research with animals was used to supplement the data on the association between cigarette smoking and the development of lung cancer in humans.) The tremendous amount of data required and the elaborate precautions taken against spuriousness in the smoking–lung cancer research illustrate the difficulty of establishing a causal relationship through nonexperimental research. In addition, the effects of cigarette smoking on lung cancer are apparently very large—to obtain convincing evidence of smaller effects would be even more difficult. In contrast, it is possible to establish a cause-effect relationship with experiments based on much smaller numbers of cases. In one sense, causal relationships are never completely established, since there is always some possibility of error. We are using the term *established* to mean that the possibility that the interpretation is in error is judged to be very small. In experimental research what we have referred to as spuriousness can be made so improbable that it can be discounted as a reasonable possibility. Unfortunately, the possibilities of a biased measure of the dependent variable or of the effect resulting from a variable that was unintentionally manipulated can obscure the nature of the causal process even in an experiment. Nor does a single small sample experiment present convincing evidence of external validity.

Summary and conclusion

Experimental research is not a panacea; it remains the criterion against which nonexperimental research designs are judged when causal inferences are to be made (Stouffer, 1960). Both practice guidelines and principles, as we have defined them, involve making causal inferences, so randomized clinical trials are the technique of choice for testing such hypotheses. Survey research is particularly useful when its purpose is to describe conditions of practice, rather than test practice theory. Letting 20,000 nurses "tell their story" (Hughes, 1958) can produce research results that are both interesting and informative. Research that finds the percentage of patients in a hospital who have a given complaint about nursing care (Abdellah and Levine, 1964) can have practice implications if such complaints identify a problem that the staff knows how to solve. In addition, such studies can stimulate further research when the exact nature of the problem and the indicated solution are not apparent. Studies that examine the interaction between practitioner and client are particularly likely to have implications for practice, even when the research design is nonexperimental. Our knowledge of the nature of client-practitioner interaction and of the formal and informal structure of medical institutions is almost entirely dependent on such research. In addition, such studies often suggest principles of practice.

While nonexperimental research is capable of producing a wide variety of results of interest to behavioral scientists and social practitioners, it has one major flaw. Because of the possibility that any given observed relationship could be spurious, such research is not the best way to test principles of practice. Experimental research is by no means a panacea, guaranteed to produce inferences of absolutely unquestionable validity. Misapplication of experimental technique can produce misleading research results. Experimental research, properly designed and executed, can produce tests of practice theory with a higher degree of internal validity than can usually be obtained through survey research. Field experiments using random assignment are both practical and administratively feasible when they are performed by a social practitioner who is professionally responsible for the means whose effects are to be studied.

The fact that experimental techniques have not been employed more often in research on social practice suggests that the practicality, feasibility, and validity of experimentation have not been completely understood by many social researchers. Arguments that it is impractical or unethical to manipulate important social variables lose much of their relevance when one of the researchers is a professional social practitioner rather than a behavioral scientist. In developing and testing principles for effective social practice, it would be foolish indeed not to supplement survey research with experimental research whenever possible. We have presented elsewhere a detailed statement on how to design clinical field experiments to be both theoretically relevant and directly applicable to the improvement of practice (Wooldridge et al., 1978).

BEHAVIORAL SCIENTISTS AND SOCIAL PRACTITIONERS

Achieving a productive give-and-take between behavioral science and professional practice is more than a matter of clarifying the relationships between the theories of the two disciplines. It is also more than devising research designs that can contribute both to behavioral science theory and to the improvement of practice. The useful integration of behavioral science and social practice requires the efforts of people—of individual behavioral scientists and social practitioners. These efforts are hampered in many ways by differences in training as well as goals and values between scientists and practitioners. Integration is also complicated by differences in the occupational cultures of scientist and practitioner and by differences in the social environments in which they work and are rewarded or sanctioned against.

Attempts at integration can take at least three forms: (1) social practitioners can be trained to be behavioral scientists; (2) behavioral scientists can be trained to be social practitioners; or (3) ways to achieve effective collaboration between behavioral scientists and social practitioners can be devised.

Nursing education frequently includes a behavioral science perspective, and efforts have been made to develop collaborative efforts between nurse-practitioners and behavioral scientists. In this section we will comment briefly on efforts to use a behavioral science perspective in nursing education. We will then consider the problems of research collaboration between behavioral scientists and social practitioners. We will conclude with a brief analysis of the potential function of the university-affiliated professional school as a buffer organization in which much of the work of coordinating behavioral science and social practice can be accomplished.

Behavioral science and the nursing curriculum

Instruction and courses in applied social science have become quite common in nursing schools. Most nursing schools require at least one course in basic psychology and sociology for undergraduate students. Applied instruction emphasizing behavioral research and theory directly connected with patient care is often considered to be more helpful to the nurse than basic sociology and psychology courses. This view ignores several salient aspects of the current status of the behavioral sciences and the nursing profession. The potential for application of behavioral science to the health field is much greater than what has already been achieved, but it is within this limited area of application that we restrict the nursing student if we limit the nurse's behavioral science education to applied topics. This is not to say that the nursing student's interest cannot be stimulated by the illustration of general behavioral science principles with specific patient care situations. A thorough familiarity with the best and most relevant studies of applied behavioral science helps the student to see the relevance of general principles to specific nursing situations. In our opinion, a solid preparation in the social sciences in the sense of a liberal education can be even more important than the teaching of already developed applications. However, in current educational programs there is often an inclination to take the findings of basic behavioral research and immediately try to apply them to nursing situations without further testing.

The incorporation of "new knowledge" in the education of nurses can result in serious conflict between the newly trained practitioners and the health organizations in which they practice. Most hospital nurses work in a highly authoritarian environment. This environment is governed by time-honored rules and a hierarchy with physicians and hospital administrators at the top levels. Sometimes the nurse does not have the authority to put into practice what she has learned in school. Instructing nurses in improved means is a necessary condition for the improvement of nursing care, but not in itself sufficient. Such instruction can have the desired effect only if the nurses are permitted and encouraged to use their newfound knowledge in daily practice. How to achieve the necessary changes in hospital organization is an appropriate topic for social research and an important area in which the behavioral sciences can be applied to problems of health and the health professions. New theories of clinical practice may be relatively useless to the professions until the necessary changes in the organizational context of practice have been identified by appropriate research and the necessary organizational changes have been effected. Sometimes college-graduate nurses refuse to work in hospitals because they do not find the opportunity to put into practice what they have learned. For a discussion of this point and of the pressures on the practicing nurse from the profession and health organizations, see Davis, 1966.

In integrating behavioral science into the nursing curriculum, it is important to avoid unrealistic expectations of what behavioral science has to offer, and to discourage uncritical application of behavioral science theory and method to the nursing context. Attempts to apply behavioral science theory to nursing practice should be seen as routinely requiring clinical testing of concepts and principles. For the most part, in their current stage of development the social sciences can offer an orientation, a frame of reference suggesting variables to be taken into account, and some research methods for testing the relevance of these variables in any particular situation. This must be nursing research at the same time that it is social research.

Behavioral research is a necessary part of professional social practice. Emphasis must be placed on experimentation, inquisitiveness, speculation, and critical thinking, rather than conformity and deference to time-honored ways of doing things. Student nurses must learn some technical skills and safety measures that are of necessity governed by strict procedures (principles of asepsis, selection of injection sites and so on, which are dictated by microbiological, anatomical and physiological principles). On the other hand, mastery learning is not possible in learning how to provide effective psychosocial care. A clear understanding of the principles underlying social practice guidelines is a prerequisite to effective social practice. This is true of almost all aspects of nursing where psychosocial means are employed. (See the discussion by Mereness, 1967.)

A nurse must have scientific attitude to design and carry out effective research and to develop an ability to critically judge material from the behavioral sciences for potential applicability to nursing. The scientist thinks in terms of questioning, reevaluation, suspended judgment, and cumulative and never-ending progress, rather than final solutions to problems. The development of such an attitude must become an integral part of the professional role if practice is to become truly rationalized. The nurse who will benefit most from courses in the behavioral sciences develops a critical and analytical way of thinking. This is as true for the nurse-practitioner as it is for the nurse-researcher. Moreover, this type of nurse is most likely to contribute to the integration of behavioral science and nursing.

Collaboration between scientists and practitioners

From the perspective of the academic disciplines, the most important goal of behavioral science is the development of knowledge for its own sake. It is pure research on which the academic disciplines place highest value and for which they pay the greatest rewards to the researcher. The major consideration is whether there will be an increase in the knowledge of the science.

Immediate benefits for society at large are given low priority. In the practice professions, however, the priority of values is reversed.

The professional is inclined to value action over contemplation and to prefer practical research to theoretical research. This is especially true of the professional who is employed by a complex organization whose primary objective is not pure research but some improvement in the production and distribution of goods and services. As Schneider (1957:97) has pointed out, the overall objective of an organization must be the production of profit. Profit, however, may be conceptualized broadly. Thus profit for a hospital may be effective care for patients, for a university, the education of students. The health professional as a member of a hospital organization is interested primarily in the rendering of services that will help care for, and possibly aid in the cure of, ill individuals.

This difference in orientation can lead to difficulties in collaboration between scientists and health practitioners. As Cottrell and Sheldon (1963) comment in their analysis of problems encountered by the Russell Sage Foundation in placing behavioral scientists in practice settings, the health practitioner

> is trained to see his problems in terms of the individual organism or segments of it; the social scientist conceptualizes his problems in terms of interaction among organisms. If the medical man thinks of the environment, it is primarily the physical environment that he considers important. Attempts of the social scientist to analyze the process of social interaction, the development of roles and their systematic relations in institutional patterns and the relating of these facts to illness and health, are likely to strike the medical man as lacking in reality and relevance.

Because of this difference in research orientation, the behavioral scientist who attempts to do research in the health field may be caught between the expectations of his behavioral science colleagues and those of the health professionals with whom he must work. On one hand, his research will be judged by the contributions it makes to his own academic discipline, while on the other hand, his research will be expected to produce useful results for the improvement of the health of society. The behavioral scientist can receive acclaim from health professionals and yet have his work ignored by the members of his own discipline (Reader and Goss, 1959).

If the behavioral scientist tries to limit his work to pure research, the members of the health professions with whom he works are not likely to see this exclusive orientation toward academic values as legitimate. Since the behavioral scientist must work with or around health professionals to collect his data, he is especially vulnerable to such criticism. Of course, it is our contention that mutually beneficial collaboration is possible. We especially stress integration of behavioral science into professional practice through research.*

The professional practitioner in an academic department may experience many similar conflicts. The practice of locking oneself behind closed doors and communicating only with a typewriter for hours and even days at a time can seem unnatural to those in the health professions. On the other hand, the health practitioner does not usually face one problem that the social scientist does when he joins forces with a practice profession. While senior colleagues in an academic discipline often advise younger members that involvement in applied research is not likely to lead to professional advancement, the health professional finds that affiliation with an academic discipline can lead to professional advancement, in spite of the resentment it sometimes engenders among professional colleagues.

The conflict between the ideals of academic disciplines and practice professions is often cast as an issue of basic versus applied knowledge and research. Whereas applied research may have negative connotations to some behavioral scientists, the value of basic research is sometimes denigrated by health professionals. Although this is a familiar dichotomy in behavioral science, we do not subscribe to the position that knowledge or research with immediate practical implications is necessarily on a lower level than any other kind (Wald and Leonard, 1964). Nor is practice theory necessarily less abstract—it is simply different in focus.

Health practitioners cannot expect behavioral scientists to tell them what their practice goals should be; this is a policy decision to be made by the practitioners themselves and is already sufficiently complicated by opinions from other health practice fields. Neither can nurses expect to be given principles of practice that can be recommended without further testing or to be told what means are ethically acceptable in reaching their goals. Professional practitioners cannot expect the behavioral scientist to have detailed enough knowledge of the research setting to avoid blunders. Practitioners cannot expect behavioral scientists to provide them with methodological tools that will automatically answer practice questions.

On the other hand, behavioral scientists cannot expect cooperation in re-

---

*For related discussions by sociologists, see Marvin Sussman, 1964; Hans Zetterberg, 1962; Alvin Gouldner and S.M. Miller, 1965; and Amitai Etzioni, 1965. For an example of such an integration by a behavioral scientist who is also a nurse, see Chapter 5; for an example of collaboration between a nurse–behavioral scientist and a nonnurse–behavioral scientist, see Chapter 6; for examples of collaboration between nurse-scientists and behavioral scientists, see Wooldridge et al., 1978.

search that can make no contributions to practice theory or in research that depends on violations of professional ethics. They cannot expect to be told what sort of research is necessary to solve a given problem, but they can and should expect help from the professional practitioner in identifying the problem. They cannot expect that the average practitioner will know enough about research and academic values to understand always the necessity for methodological rigor. Expecting the health professional to carry out research procedures without an understanding of their purpose is not realistic, nor would it result in good research. It is easy to violate the purpose of a procedure by following it mechanically in situations to which it should not apply. On the other hand, it is possible to ignore a research procedural detail because it seems unimportant when it is in fact essential to guarding against biased results. Truly productive collaboration demands mutual understanding as well as mutual trust.

Finally, the behavioral scientist must be cognizant of, and learn to have patience with, the fact that the incorporation of new social knowledge into any practice profession is likely to be difficult, to be met with resistance, and to be fraught with seemingly endless delays. As Cottrell and Sheldon comment (1963:127):

> The structure of medical institutions is frequently more rigid and authoritarian than the somewhat more informal and much less authoritarian pattern of academic life in which the social scientist is trained.

Sharp (1964) defines three areas of differences between behavioral scientists and nurse researchers: subcultural differences, status differences, and role differences. We conceive of many of the difficulties in collaboration between scientists and practitioners as matters of role conflict, division of labor, and the divergent conflicting values of two cultures. Perhaps the academic scientist must value knowledge for its own sake, while the professional practitioner must replace doubt with action when the demand arises and not when "all the facts are in." In one sense this frees the behavioral scientist to examine a variety of social and psychological phenomena that are outside the perspective of the professional practitioner. On the other hand, it is not unreasonable for the practitioner to insist that the results of research be ultimately applicable in practice. We must agree with Sharp (1964) that nurse researchers and behavioral scientists who wish to collaborate should

> constantly use their interpersonal skills at a maximum level, especially early in the collaboration in order to establish the kind of personal association which can overcome the inevitable frustrations of looking at a given research problem from differing points of view.

The professional school as a buffer organization

Armchair speculation as well as laboratory and other kinds of research with no known practical applications are completely legitimate exercises in the ivory towers of colleges and universities. The aim of research in the strictly academic disciplines is to test theory, and the aim of theory is to guide research (Merton, 1957:103). Practical uses of a theory of the pure sciences are not a matter of concern for most scientists. Theory in nursing also has the function of guiding research, but it has another aim too—to guide professional practice. The practical end point of nursing research imposes an added burden on the researcher, since it places certain restrictions on his fancy; yet this additional aim of research can be a source of added satisfaction as well. What is perhaps less obvious to academicians is that a focus on practical ends is the entry price to be paid for admission into the research opportunities offered by the professional practitioner's access to ongoing social reality.

When the challenge of designing research relevant to both practice and basic behavioral science is understood and accepted, the results can be excellent. Unfortunately, many well-meaning scientists and practitioners fail to understand the issues involved or appreciate the benefits to be gained. While the practitioner may not have the skills and motivation to engage in basic research on social practice, the scientist is likely to be deficient in the requisite clinical knowledge and to lack the professional competence or legal status to obtain it. These are common reasons why research of this kind is not done more often and why the results may prove disappointing when it is attempted.

What is needed to facilitate research into professional practice is a buffer organization, a point of transition from the ivory tower to the day-to-day demands of professional practice. Such an organization would strike a balance between the academic community's long-term commitment to knowledge and the larger society's commitment to short-term, tactical demands for action. The university-affiliated professional school seems ideally situated to perform this function. In the professional school practitioner-researchers know a great deal about how to get the results society demands of their profession, but they do not restrict themselves to direct action. Instead, they affect practice through published works and the education of practitioners. The major part of their role is developing knowledge and transmitting it, rather than applying it. If within these professional schools the values of commitment to professional service and to knowledge can be simultaneously cultivated, there can be a meeting ground for the basic scientist and the skilled practitioner.

The richness of the professional practitioner's clinical experience makes it an excellent source of theoretical hypotheses to test, and the possibilities extend beyond field experimentation to participant observation research and survey research as well. The professional practitioner's thorough immersion in the realities of clinical practice can help the behavioral scientist identify empirical associations deserving of rigorous research, and the practitioner can also supply him with information on the administrative feasibility and practicality of a research design. For this collaboration to be really successful, the behavioral scientist must learn to respect the practitioner as an equal and value his judgment. Collaborative research with practitioners can provide the opportunity to do superior behavioral research through experimental testing of causal theories, while at the same time providing contributions directly applicable to professional practice. Clearly such collaboration offers unique and valuable opportunities for the behavioral scientist as well as for the professional practitioner.

Field experiments tend to be neglected by social scientists because they are not in a position to personally execute them. In contrast, practitioners must experiment to perform their role. In a social practice situation it is not only possible, but necessary, to manipulate social phenomena in a real-life situation. Such manipulation is an explicit obligation of the practitioner's role. Since the outcome for the client is always somewhat uncertain, this manipulation is in a sense experimental. The long-term improvement of practice can come only through making experimentation serve the advancement of knowledge as well as the improvement in welfare of the individual client.

The place of the professional school within the university setting has usually been marginal. The professional school has often been seen as a technical or vocational training program that does not meet the academic standards of the university. The professional school's ideals of service to humanity may be seen as conflicting with the university's ideals of knowledge for the sake of knowledge. The unique buffer function of the professional school is often unrecognized by the school itself, the university administration, or for that matter most social scientists. We have commented on the emphasis on rote teaching methods often found in professional schools and how this can limit the student's critical or reasoning powers. Perhaps from the university's point of view this type of professional instruction is foreign to the ideals of liberal education. However, if the professional schools can accomplish their goals of service to society at the same time that they fulfill their commitment to increasing knowledge, they will have a unique function in the university community. They will provide a link between the ivory tower and the real world. We suggest that recognition by both the basic sciences and the practicing disciplines of the contributions each can make to the other is the way to create a truly *professional* school.

Summary and conclusion

The behavioral scientist is trained to suspend judgment, question existing knowledge, and search for new knowledge. His main concern is not with the application of knowledge, but with its development. The professional practitioner, on the other hand, is trained to accept and use existing knowledge and to value the benefits it may bring his client. His main concern is the use of knowledge, not its development. This difference in basic orientation may make it difficult for anyone to excel simultaneously as a practitioner and a behavioral scientist. However, this does not negate the possibility that individuals can understand the difference in orientation or develop skills in both spheres.

In point of fact, the pure practitioner who naïvely accepts everything he is told and rushes out to apply it does not exist in reality any more than does the pure scientist who accepts nothing and lives in a continual paralysis of suspended judgment. All individuals normally fluctuate between one role and the other, first tentatively accepting principles as a basis for attempts at problem solving and then (consciously or unconsciously) examining principles in light of the results. The basic difference between the scientist and the practitioner is in the relative emphasis they give to each role. It is not necessarily true that skill in testing and developing general principles implies a lack of skill in applying existing principles to a situation. Nor does skill in the application of principles necessarily imply a lack of skill in theory building.

We have discussed some of the social barriers to effective integration of behavioral science and social practice. To understand that these obstacles exist, or even to understand the reasons why, is not to overcome them. On the other hand, the practitioner who attempts to relate social theory and social practice will benefit from an understanding of the social obstacles he faces. There can be no sure method of overcoming them, but one must make the attempt. In our opinion, there has been a tendency to use social obstacles as an excuse for not attempting necessary research and theorization. Too little effort and ingenuity has been spent on considering ways in which social obstacles can be circumvented. The acceptance of adverse stereotypes of scientists by practitioners and of practitioners by scientists is often an excuse for avoiding collaborative projects, even when such an effort is clearly indicated. Similarly, the too-ready dismissal of randomization experiments on social practice as impractical or unethical may be an excuse for employing research techniques that are less appropriate. Finding a way to carry out a piece of important research can require both the methodological expertise of the behavioral scientist and the clinical knowledge and professional prerequisites of the social practitioner. Such research can be extremely difficult for either to design and carry out alone, but it is often relatively simple to accomplish as a collaborative effort.

While the social barriers to effective collaboration between behavioral scientists and professional practitioners are not insurmountable, they do present difficulties. The contemplative ideals of the ivory tower can conflict with the action-oriented ideals of the service organization. Such subcultural differences, if unrecognized or misunderstood, can lead to unrealistic expectations and feelings of frustration and indignation on both sides. Social problems are compounded when the collaboration takes place either in an organization almost entirely devoted to the immediate achievement of practice goals or one that provides few opportunities for engaging in actual social practice. The university-affiliated professional school avoids either of these extremes, and for this reason it provides an organizational context with a high potential for mutually productive collaboration between social scientists and social practitioners. When this potential is fully recognized, we believe that many more collaborative projects will be attempted to the benefit of both behavioral science and social practice.

THE RATIONALIZATION OF SOCIAL PRACTICE

The similarities and differences between the theoretical structure of an applied social discipline and that of a behavioral science have often been a source of confusion for practitioner and scientist alike. In many circumstances such confusion causes relatively little disruption of social relationships and is not obviously detrimental to practice effectiveness or to the theoretical development of the behavioral sciences. The role of the behavioral scientist encourages behavior that is reasonably functional for the development of basic theory, and the role of social practitioner encourages behavior that is reasonably functional for effective practice. The major problem arises when behavioral scientists and social practitioners attempt to collaborate on a research project or when the same person attempts to act as both a social practitioner and a behavioral scientist. Under these circumstances, inability to relate cognitively the role of practitioner to the role of scientist, or to relate behavioral science theory to social practice theory, can be a major obstacle to the development of theory and to the long-run improvement of practice.

The major analytical distinction between behavioral science theory and social practice theory is not particularly hard to make and is difficult to apply only insofar as it is rather abstract. A body of theory is defined by its unifying focus, which expresses the intended use of the theoretical formulations in question. Theories in the behavioral sciences explain how social structures are interrelated to form a system and how structural change in one part of the system has objective consequences for the system as a whole. Practice theories are phrased in terms of a functional frame of reference in which socially acceptable alternate structures (practice guidelines) are examined in terms of their objective consequences for the specific goals of the practitioner. This focus emphasizes means that can be manipulated by the practitioners and consequences that can be evaluated in terms of the practitioner's goals.

Causal relationships explaining the effects of the practitioner's activities on the client have important theoretical implications for the behavioral sciences. Practice theories often implicitly include sociopsychosomatic causal chains. Such practice theories can provide a basis for constructing linkages between the theories of the various basic sciences. Such interrelationships are of interest to sociologists and psychologists, as well as to a variety of health practitioners.

A major problem in integrating behavioral science theories with practice theories, and vice-versa, is that somewhat different concepts tend to be used in each kind of theory. Concepts are devised to make abstract distinctions that are important for the kinds of theories in which they are used. Practice theories tend to use concepts that stress abstract distinctions between stages in the helping process and different kinds of success in attaining practice goals. Such terms as *meeting patient needs, acting on assumptions, deliberative nursing, patient welfare,* and so on may seem hopelessly vague to the behavioral scientist, since they make distinctions of a low order of relevance to behavioral science theory. Of course, the opposite problem is also present. Behavioral science concepts often do not make distinctions of key importance to practice theory. (We prefer to take no position on the largely semantic issue of which distinctions are more "basic." Such issues provoke more heat than light and seem to have little substantive content.) There is no easy solution to this problem. The interrelationship of behavioral science theory and social practice theory is further complicated by the fact that both types of theory are in relatively early stages of development. Many of the concepts used by behavioral scientists and social practitioners are unclear in meaning or of doubtful utility. Attempts to interrelate behavioral science concepts and social practice concepts are likely to meet with difficulty. On the other hand, such attempts are well worth the effort involved, since they can stimulate badly needed theoretical clarification and provide useful insights.

In the early stages of theory building there is often a tendency to generalize principles far beyond the conditions and operational contexts in which they have been studied. Such overgeneralization can be a useful counter to the common tendency to look at issues too narrowly, but principles not thoroughly grounded on scientific testing are purely speculative. Scientifically based principles for psychosocial care are fairly new in nursing, and debates over what kind of action is best are likely to be based more on polemical assertions and counterassertions than on carefully evaluated evidence. To the extent that such debates serve as stimuli to needed research, they are functional for the development of practice theory. However, we strongly suspect that in nursing practice, as in almost any kind of human relations situation, the most effective approach will be found to vary markedly with the circumstances in which it is to be applied.

Surveys and other nonexperimental research can be useful in suggesting causal hypotheses pertinent to practice and in describing practice problems for which solutions need to be found; laboratory research can test the solutions under limited conditions. But implications for practice derived from nonexperimental clinical or laboratory research should be tested by carefully designed clinical experiments. It is difficult to pay more than lip service to the idea of developing social practitioners with the desire and ability to question, test, and continually reevaluate, when the application of such an orientation to everyday practice is left unclear. One means of developing a critical ability in the social practitioner is to include experimental research on the effects of the practitioner's own practice as part of the formal educational process. Since the practitioner is evaluating the results of his own practice, this type of experience can increase the practitioner's clinical skill at the same time that it increases theoretical knowledge and research capabilities. In the long run the development of social practitioners (such as nurses) with research abilities and a scientific orientation will contribute to behavioral science theory as well as practice theory. The results are likely to be particularly rapid if such practitioner-theoretician-researchers make explicit efforts to relate practice theory to behavioral science theory. Even if no such efforts are made, however, the development of social practice theory can serve as an intermediate step between behavioral science theory and actual practice.

The debate over whether the professional should be free to practice according to his individual inclinations or whether his practice should be restricted by collectively determined professional standards is common in the social practice professions. Emergent professions tend to become highly concerned with setting up prescriptive guidelines justified by their presumed effectiveness in meeting client needs. In scientifically oriented societies such prescriptive standards are developed and justified through cognitive theories of practice, which are subject to empirical testing in one form or another. This leads to the phenomenon we have called the *rationalization of practice*, in which the behavior of professional practitioners is increasingly guided by prescriptions and theories which are subjected to empirical testing and retesting.

The rationalization of practice may or may not lead to immediate increases in the effectiveness of practice. Whether or not practice effectiveness is increased over the short run will depend on the validity of the theories used to guide practice and on whether each theoretical application is carefully tested prior to widespread adoption as a guideline. The results of behavioral science applications to social practice have often been disappointing. The reasons are that the behavioral science theories applied have often been vague or invalid and that many social practitioners have advocated general application of the guidelines derived from behavioral science theory before adequately testing them. In part, prescriptions have not been adequately tested because randomization experiments on the effects of social and psychosocial means have not been considered valid by social practitioners or recognized as feasible by behavioral scientists. In addition, the education of behavioral scientists has sometimes tended to denigrate the value of applied research, and the education of social practitioners has sometimes fostered attitudes that are inimical to research in general. On the other hand, recent developments in the education of health science practitioners in general and nurses in particular hold a great deal of promise for an improved understanding of the relationship of behavioral science to social practice. If this potential is recognized through better focused theory building and research, then we believe that major breakthroughs in the effectiveness of health care delivery may be achieved in the near future. Such an eventuality would be important not only for the benefits derived by millions of patients; it would also be important for its implications for behavioral science theory.

REFERENCES

Abdellah, F.G., and Levine, E. 1957. Patients and personnel speak. Washington, D.C., USPHS pub. no. 527.

Brown, E.L. 1963. Meeting patients' psychosocial needs in the general hospital, Annals of the American Academy of Political and Social Science 346:117-125.

Campbell, D.T., and Stanley, J.C. 1966. Experimental and quasi-experimental designs for research, Chicago, Rand McNally.

Cottrell, L., Jr., and Sheldon, E. 1963. Problems of collaboration between social scientists and the practicing professions, The Annals of the American Academy of Political and Social Science 346:127-128.

Coser, R.L. 1959. Some social functions of laughter, Human Relations 12:171-182.

Davis, F. editor. 1966. The nursing profession: five sociological essays, New York, John Wiley & Sons, Inc.

Dumas, R.G., and Leonard, R.C. 1963. The affect of nursing on the incidence of postoperative vomiting: a clinical experiment, Nursing Research 12:12-15.

Etzioni, A. 1969. The semi-professions and their organizations: teachers, nurses, social workers, New York, The Free Press.

Fisher, R.A. 1947. The design of experiments, Edinburgh, Oliver and Boyd.

Gouldner, A.W., and Miller, S.M. 1965. Applied sociology, New York, The Free Press.

Hughes, E.C., Hughes, H.M., and Deutscher, I. 1958. Twenty thousand nurses tell their story, Philadelphia, J.B. Lippincott Co.

Leonard, R.C., Skipper, J.K., Jr., and Wooldridge, P.J. 1967. Small sample field experiments for evaluating patient care, Health Services Research 2:46-50.

Lippitt, R. 1966. The process of utilization of social research to improve social practice. In Shostak, A.B., editor. Sociology in action, Homewood, Ill., Dorsey Press, pp. 276-281.

Mahaffey, P.R., Jr. 1965. The affect of hospitalization on children admitted for tonsillectomy and adenoidectomy, Nursing Research 14:12-19.

Mereness, D. 1967. Freedom and responsibility for nursing students, American Journal of Nursing 67:69-71.

Merton, R.K. 1957. Social theory and social structure, New York, The Free Press.

Moss, F.T., and Meyer, B. 1966. The effects of nursing interaction upon pain relief in patients. Nursing Research 15:303-306.

Orlando, I.J. 1961. The dynamic nurse-patient relationship, New York, G.P. Putnam's Sons.

Orlando, I.J. 1972. The discipline and teaching of nursing process, New York, G.P. Putnam's Sons.

Reader, G. and Goss, M. 1959. The sociology of medicine. In Merton, R.K. et al., editors. Sociology today, New York, Basic Books, Inc., Publishers, pp. 240-241.

Schneider, E. 1957. Industrial sociology, New York, McGraw-Hill, Inc.

Selznick, P. 1959. The sociology of law. In Merton, R.K. et al. editors: Sociology today. New York, Basic Books, Inc., Publishers, pp. 115-127.

Sharp, L.J. 1964. The behavioral scientist in nursing research, Nursing Research 13:327-330.

Skipper, J.K., Jr. 1965. Communication and the hospitalized patient. In Skipper, J.K., Jr. and Leonard, R. editors. Social interaction and patient care, Philadelphia, J.B. Lippincott Co., pp. 120-127.

Skipper, J.K., Jr., Diers, D.K., and Leonard, R. 1967. Research collaboration between professional practitioner and behavioral scientist. In Abrahamson, M. editor. The professional in the organization, Chicago, Rand McNally and Co., pp. 136-143.

Skipper, J.K., Jr. and Leonard, R. 1968. Children, stress, and hospitalization; an experimental study, Journal of Health and Social Behavior 9:275-287.

Skipper, J.K., Jr., Wooldridge, P.W., and Leonard, R. 1968. Race, status and interaction between patients and hospital personnel, Sociology Quarterly, Fall, pp. 35-46.

Sommer, R., and Osmond, H. 1962. The schizophrenic no-society, Psychiatry 25:244-255.

Stouffer, S.A. 1960. Some observations on study design, American Journal of Sociology 55:355-361.

Sussman, M. 1964. The social problems of the sociologist, Social Problems 11:215-225.

Tarasuk, M., Rhymes, J., and Leonard, R. 1965. An experimental test of the importance of communication skills for effective nursing. In Skipper, J.K., Jr., and Leonard, R.C., editors. Social interaction and patient care, Philadelphia, J.B. Lippincott Co., pp. 110-120.

Tryon, P., and Leonard, R. 1965. Giving the patient an active role. In Skipper, J.K., Jr., and Leonard, R.C., editors. Social interaction and patient care, Philadelphia, J.B. Lippincott Co., pp. 120-127.

Wald, F., and Leonard, R. 1964. Toward development of nursing practice theory, Nursing Research 13:309-313.

Wilson, R.N. 1963. The social structure of a general hospital. The Annals of the American Academy of Political and Social Science 346:67-76.

Wooldridge, P.J., Leonard, R.C., and Skipper, J.K., Jr. 1978. Methods of clinical experimentation to improve patient care, St. Louis, The C.V. Mosby Co.

Zetterberg, H.L. 1962. Social theory and social practice, New York, Bedminster Press.

SECTION TWO

Nursing theorists and practice theory

THE NOTION that nursing does have or should have *a* theory in the sense of a single conceptual framework or orientation for all nurses to follow is not one that we would advocate. Most nursing theories (or, more correctly, most nursing theorists) present a combination of metatheory, philosophical theory, prescriptive theory, scientific theory, and formal theory. Different theorists present different mixes of these theoretical elements and place a different degree of emphasis on framework, means, and ends in proposing conceptual frameworks.

In this section, five major nursing theorists have been selected for intensive analysis. The first three show the developmental continuity of some of the earliest theorists; the last two represent more recent theorists of quite different types. In each case the work of the theorist is examined in terms of the mix of various kinds of theory and the ways in which the theorist's work fits into the practice theory orientation defined in Section 1. The relationship of the theorist's work to that of major behavioral science theorists is also examined, as is the extent to which the theory has been tested directly or indirectly.

The primary purpose of this section is to illustrate the use of our approach in analyzing nursing theorists and not actually to analyze all the leading theorists. After reading this section the reader is invited to attempt a comparable analysis of a favorite nursing theorist as an exercise.

CHAPTER 3

THE CURRENT STATUS OF PRACTICE THEORIES IN NURSING

Madeline H. Schmitt

The first chapters of this book provided a metatheoretical framework for defining social practice (especially nursing) theories and understanding their relation to behavioral science theories. This framework was illustrated by examples of theory and research taken mostly from the late 1960s, when the original version was first proposed (Wooldridge, Leonard, and Skipper, 1968). At that time the major nursing theorists were theorists of the nursing role process; there was only a single journal devoted to nursing research (*Nursing Research*, begun in 1952). The *Journal of Health and Human Behavior* (now the *Journal of Health and Social Behavior*) had been founded as a reflection of the growing importance of health-related research to behavioral and social scientists, and Simmons and Henderson had only recently published the first compendium of nursing research, *Nursing Research: A Survey and Assessment* (1964). Since that time, there has been a tremendous growth in the literature of nursing theory and in the amount of research devoted to nursing practice problems. The addition of several new nursing research journals, such as *Research in Nursing and Health* and *Western Journal of Nursing Research*, and compendiums summarizing nursing research activities, such as Krueger, Nelson, and Wolanin (1978), reflects the expanding volume of theory and research activities in nursing. Such growth has been and remains critical to the development of the profession. The Joint Commission on Nursing and Nursing Education report issued in 1970 pointed to the absence of nursing theory and research into practice as a major deficit in the development of nursing.

In the 1960s and throughout the 1970s there were increasing numbers of nurses educated through the doctoral level (Pitel and Vian, 1975). These nurses and others have contributed to the expansion of the literature in nursing theory development and in research oriented toward problems of nursing practice. Yet as Batey (1977) noted, adequate conceptual-theoretical frameworks for research remain at a serious deficiency, and Henderson (1977:164) noted that nurses in general still have a great deal of difficulty undertaking studies that might "revolutionize practice."

Simultaneously with these changes in nursing there has been a continuous growth of interest in research and theory building regarding health behavior by several behavioral science disciplines. Medical sociology, which first established itself as a substantive area of sociology in the 1950s (Olesen, 1975), experienced steady growth through the 1960s and 1970s, though there are concerns in medical sociology about its atheoretical nature (Johnson, 1975). In 1973 *Psychological Abstracts* established a special Medical Psychology subsection reflecting psychology's increasing interest in individual health and illness issues (Asken, 1975). Other recent discussions attempt definitions of this field (Asken, 1979; Masur, 1979). Medical anthropology, not known as such prior to the 1960s (Foster, 1975), has also been growing steadily as a field since the 1950s, though there had been an "ethnomedical" tradition in anthropology well before this time.

To confuse the situation even further, many of the nurses receiving doctoral preparation up through the 1970s have studied in these same disciplines, that is, sociology, anthropology and psychology (Pitel and Vian, 1975). Knowledge of this is essential in comprehending the nature of the nursing theory that has been generated and the kind of research that has been conducted by these nurses.

What is the nature of the growing body of nursing theory? What is its present relevance to the practice of nursing? The purpose of this chapter is to describe the development of some nursing theories and to evaluate the extent to which they have focused on practice theory and practice-oriented research.

Theoretical frameworks and data-gathering techniques for problems of nursing practice have traditionally been derived from two domains: biological sciences and psychosocial sciences. Henderson (1977) talks about the biologically oriented research that some American nurses were exposed to as part of their training in the early 1900s. It emphasized investigation into the procedures of nursing practice, but few nurses actually continued with a biologically oriented research career. Recent doctoral preparation of nurses for research has not typically been in the biological sciences (Pitel and Vian, 1975). Thus the nursing theories that have been developed have been derived largely from the social sciences. There are, however, recent notable exceptions to the psychosocial emphases of most nursing research and theory development. The work of Verhonick et al. (1972) on prevention and treatment of decubitus ulcers* and the work of Walike et al. (1975) and others on tube feeding† are biophysical nursing research examples that could be subjected to a meta-theoretical critique similar to the one given in this chapter for psychosocial nursing research and theory.

FRAMEWORK FOR THE ANALYSIS OF NURSING THEORY

The social practice dimension of nursing involves the use of social or psychosocial means in attempting to meet certain patient needs that the patient cannot meet by himself and to encourage movement toward self-help. Among the needs that are the special responsibility of nurses are those arising from

---

*See *Research in Nursing and Health* 2 (1979) vi-vii for a complete bibliographic listing.
†For early examples, see De Somery and Walike (1977) and Heitkemper, Hanson, and Hansen (1977).

the state of being sick and the patient's response to sickness or those arising from the situation of being at risk of future illness or at a reduced level of wellness. As we defined nursing theory in Chapter 1, not all needs resulting from sickness provide a legitimate focus for nursing theory and research. Only those needs that are potentially resolvable through means over which nursing has control and that are consistent with goals that are the responsibility of the nursing profession can fall within the domain of nursing practice theory. Scientific nursing theory encompasses only those aspects of theories that can potentially be verified by empirical research. Philosophical nursing theories, which articulate the overall values and goals of the profession, are important and determine the domains in which scientific nursing theories ought to be developed but are not subject to empirical validation. Philosophical theories may, as Henderson (1977:164) puts it, "revolutionize practice" by defining professional goals, but they will not revolutionize the effectiveness of practice in meeting the established goals of the profession.

Stevens (1979) in her analysis of nursing theories notes that to date most nursing theories are of the "ought" variety, in which philosophical theory predominates or is mixed in with the scientific theory. This book makes a strong argument for the expansion of the "how can the effectiveness of what already exists be improved?" variety of scientific theory, which contributes directly to the rationalization of practice. This sort of analysis of nursing theories is an essential component in responding to appeals to use research findings in practice (Krueger, Nelson, and Wolanin, 1978) since it is scientific nursing theory that provides a perspective for generalizing and integrating research findings. If Stevens (1979) is correct that most nursing theories to date have been of the philosophical variety, and if much of nursing theory has been formulated from the perspective of general social science rather than the perspective of practice theory, then it is not so hard to explain why nursing has experienced difficulty in applying research findings to improve the effectiveness of everyday clinical practice.

In the discussion of nursing theories in this chapter, the following paradigm will be used as a guideline for theory analysis.

1. Identify the *general purpose of the theory*, as stated by the author. Is it to improve practice by improving patient welfare? Does it identify a specific problem of practice as its focus?

2. Identify the *patient need or problem addressed.* Is the need or problem addressed situational? Does it involve the patient's response to sickness or the prevention of sickness?

3. Identify the *goal of nursing action* in meeting the need. Is it oriented primarily to palliation, development, restoration, or adaptation? Are these goals for which the nursing profession is generally held to be responsible and accountable?

4. Identify the *means proposed to meet the need*. To what extent is this means within control of the nursing profession? Is the means proposed currently regarded by the nursing profession as legitimately manipulable? Are there normative limitations on the kind of practitioner who can legitimately use the means? The issue of legitimacy is distinct from the issue of reliability and feasibility.

5. Identify the *areas of practice that might be affected* (scope) if the theory received support empirically. Is the scope narrow or broad, specialty focused or general? Does the means require special preparation of practitioners?

6. Identify *attempts to operationalize and test the theory*. What would be required to operationalize and test the theory? Has it been done? Has the theory received any support? If so, is there any evidence that it has significantly influenced practice?

In the discussion that follows, this paradigm is applied to the work of several major nursing theorists who were early contributors and whose ideas have generated sustained research efforts.

EARLY THEORISTS OF THE NURSING ROLE PROCESS

With the historical exception of Florence Nightingale's work (Schlotfeldt, 1977), the construction of systematic theories of nursing practice by nurses is an activity less than 30 years old. The publication of Peplau's *Interpersonal Relationships in Nursing* (1951) can be identified as a landmark that has been followed by a long series of attempts to write theories of nursing practice.

In retrospect, the emphasis of the early period of theory building seems to have been on defining the nurse's role and the scope of activities (means) theorized to contribute to desired changes in patient health behavior. Literature on the subject during this time came both from behavioral scientists and nursing theorists. A key influence from which this literature evolved was the work of Talcott Parsons, perhaps the most prominent grand theorist in sociology. In *The Social System* (1951) Parsons discusses the instrumental role of the physician in relation to the patient, comparing it to the instrumental role of the father in the family system. By extrapolation the nurse becomes the expressive mother. The role definitions of the two central health care figures help define the patient role as well. If the physician is the father substitute and the nurse is the mother substitute, then the patient has many characteristics of the dependent child. The most he can do is cooperate with professions who act on him to keep him comfortable and get him well. The nurse "cares," the physician "cures." Behavioral scientists of this early period were intent on describing the profession of nursing from this perspective (Corwin and Taves, 1963; Saunders, 1954; Schulman, 1958; Skipper, 1965). Nursing theorists of the period seemed more intent on moving away from uncritical acceptance of a substitute mother role and toward conceptualizations of the way expressive characteristics associated with the nursing role (means employed by nursing) might operate to benefit patients (Schmitt, 1968). One might call this a period of rationalizing the expressive role. Because I believe these early efforts have been a root source of major progress in design of nursing interventions as well as a continued source of some of the most serious failures, representative theorists of the period will be analyzed in some detail here.

Peplau's theory

The publication by Peplau (1951) of *Interpersonal Relationships in Nursing* was the first attempt to develop a general theory for nursing practice. Many social and psychological theorists were influential in Peplau's conceptualization of the role of nursing and the means employed by nurses to assist patients. They include George Herbert Mead, Harry Stack Sullivan, Erich Fromm, Carl Rogers, Edward Sapir, Karl Maslow, Karen Horney, and E.R. Hilgard. From Mead, Peplau derived her emphasis on social determination of behavior and its accessibility to change, her concern with basic processes of communication, and her focus on the possibility for change and growth existing at the level of self-conscious communication, role playing, and role taking. Many of these themes were also present in Sullivan's work because of Sullivan's early association with Mead. Sullivan was probably Peplau's most powerful intellectual influence. She used Sullivan's model of prototaxic, parataxic, and syntaxic communication types, the idea of anxiety as a socially communicated experience, and the idea of dynamisms as ineffective patterns rooted in the interpersonal situation. Her list of basic human needs also followed Sullivan's theory. From Fromm, she derived her emphasis on different kinds of love, mature democratic behavior, and the nurse as democratic leader. From Sapir, she took an emphasis on symbols and feedback processes; from Hilgard, the idea of learning in a therapeutic context; from Maslow, the ideas of growth and self-actualization. From Sullivan and Rogers she took the ideas of the participant-observer role and the nondirective interview as a therapeutic technique. What integrated these diverse social science ideas and rooted them in nursing was the definition of illness as a basic threat to one's life and the importance of one's learned processes for dealing with threat in determining which coping behaviors to use. Peplau believed the potential for teaching patients more effective coping strategies based on the threat implied by illness to be the motivating force for new learning and growth on the patient's part and the basis for nursing intervention.

Overview

According to Peplau, the threat deriving from illness consisted of the patient's perceiving a barrier to the attainment of his goals (the satisfaction of his needs). The patient might be expected to respond to the interference by:
1. Retaining the goal and the means previously chosen for its accomplishment
2. Retaining the goal but changing the means for achieving it
3. Substituting a new goal
4. Feeling blocked from any goal seeking, resulting in a state of severe anxiety

The blocking reflected the reappearance of developmental conflicts, and regressive and maladaptive behavior might be observed as a defense against anxiety caused by blocking. Effective nursing is defined by Peplau as activity that moves a patient away from feeling blocked and anxious (item 4) into one of the adaptive states described in items 1 to 3. She sees the nurse as being the professional with whom the patient had the greatest amount of direct contact. It followed that nurses had a unique opportunity to help the patient overcome the threat of illness and blocks to goal achievement by encouraging new and more effective patterns for coping with daily living problems. The encouragement of more effective coping is to be achieved by the use of an interpersonal relationship in which the nurse would provide information, support, and technical expertise and would act as an object to be identified with. The main section of Peplau's book consists of an elaboration of the stages of nursing as a "significant, therapeutic, interpersonal process" (1951:16). This process has four phases that, though overlapping, are hypothesized to occur in a specific sequence. These are phase of orientation, phase of identification, phase of exploitation, and phase of resolution.

The *phase of orientation* has its theoretical basis in the work of Mead and Sullivan. The emphasis is on discovering the meaning of the illness to the patient based on his past experience and his current total life situation (Kurt Lewin's field theory [1935] is also relevant here; illness is one experience in the total life field at a given point in time) and helping him to more fully comprehend and integrate the illness experience into the total life field. Part of the process is focused on the patient receiving orientation to the hospital and to the professional medical "meaning systems." Orientation is accomplished through nurse behavior organized into four roles—resource person, counselor, surrogate, and technical expert. The emphasis in technique is on nondirectiveness, so that the patient is not inhibited from full elaboration of the situation from his perspective.

The *phase of identification* has its theoretical basis in Freud and Sullivan. Patient and nurse are both subject to respond to each other more or less unconsciously and to greater or lesser degrees as if each were some significant other from an interpersonal past. The association for the patient could easily be toward the mother image because of the expressive and physical caring components of the nurse's role. In the phase of identification patients' associations from the past are identified and assessed for their value in facilitating growth in the current illness situation. Based on the patient's past experiences of receiving mothering he is likely to respond in one of three ways to this new (implied or actual) dependence:

1. Counterdependence—behaviorally seen as the patient who refuses to have anything done for him
2. Overdependence—behaviorally seen as the patient who wants everything done for him
3. Limited dependence—acceptance of the immediate need for some dependence without fear and self-threat

In the identification phase learning is accomplished through working with past identifications to have an impact on changed and changing behavior. The nurse is usually more consciously aware of this process than the patient.

The *phase of exploitation* is the phase of actual relearning. Behavior fluctuates between hanging on to old patterns and committing to new ones. This phase occurs in varying depths. The extent to which this phase is developed depends on variables such as:

1. Illness problems
2. Degree of the patient's inadequate personality functioning
3. The ability and desire of the nurse and patient

The *phase of resolution* is a period of solidifying gains in learning and giving up secondary gains of old patterns. The patient assumes responsibility for continued growth and breaks his dependent tie with the nurse. Fromm's democratic bias is evident here in Peplau's emphasis on the "desirable" traits of independence, aloneness, and responsibility. The nurse helps the patient reintegrate learning into the situation to which he will return. This is difficult if the patient is still operating within the context of old meanings.

Chapters 4 through 11 in Peplau's book provide the elaborated theoretical base that underlies these phases. She examines four developmental tasks that can be seen in relation to the central issues of the four phases. These are

1. Counting on others and the phase of orientation
2. Learning to delay satisfaction and the phase of identification
3. Learning to identify oneself and the phase of exploitation
4. Developing skills in participation and the phase of resolution

The tasks are outlined sequentially and follow Sullivan's discussions of tasks of infancy through adolescence. They also follow the process of moving anxiety from prototaxic through parataxic to syntaxic modes of communication.

Finally, Peplau outlines the problem-solving process associated with her definition of the nursing process. The process outlined is descriptive in that it provides a system by which all relevant data are collected; it is analytical in that it is based on theoretical ideas identified previously and predicts a sequence and development; it is evaluative in that it provides means whereby one can see what has been accomplished and make appropriate plans for the future.

Observation comprises the assessment component. Peplau discusses several dimensions important to observation as assessment. These include type and sequence of observation, where one moves from random to more systematic and increasingly self-conscious observation. She talks of hypotheses as imposing organization or system on the observation. She talks about unitization of observation so that segments of interaction can be compared with each other, and she talks about the range of roles one can assume in the observation situation—from spectator to interviewer to data collector to participant. For Peplau, who focuses on the interpersonal aspects of patient observation, the system or framework against which interaction is compared is her phases and the participant-observer role. An important part of interaction in this context is evaluation of the shared meaning of an illness event to the participants, which often can be seen as the interpersonal goal toward which the interaction moves. According to Peplau (1951:263):

> The aim of observation in nursing, when it is viewed as an interpersonal process, is the identification, clarification, and verification of impressions about the interactive drama, of the pushes and pulls in the relationship between nurse and patient, as they occur.

Communication is the intervention component, and *consensual validation* provides the means of evaluating whether and to what degree shared meanings have evolved. The tool devised for summarizing this approach to the nursing role and process is the *process recording*, which is a record of the verbal exchanges and nonverbal expressions of nurse and patient in sequence. It also contains a column for the nurse's analysis of the meaning of the exchange.

Following the guidelines just listed, what is the significance of this very early theory of Peplau's for the development of practice theory?

Analysis and evaluation

General purpose of the theory ■ The general purpose of the theory as stated by the author is to clarify the role of the nurse in helping the patient deal with the threat of illness in such a way that his overall growth in life and his ability to achieve chosen goals will be enhanced. The focus is on the use of nursing means to promote patient welfare rather than on the broader knowledge-development goal of social science so the theory has a practice orientation. The extent to which this theory had arisen from the problems of patients in clinical situations Peplau had experienced is not provided (although illustrative practice examples are presented), but there is considerable discussion of the relationship of her theory to those of prominent social and psychological theorists. This implicitly suggests that Peplau's practice theory was more deductively derived from the social science frameworks to which she had been exposed than inductively derived in a grounded fashion from clinical practice.

Patient needs or problems addressed ■ The needs Peplau lists are derived from basic human needs taken from a Sullivanian framework. Peplau argues that these basic needs have situationally derived counterparts that arise from illness. The patient's need to respond effectively to illness is clearly situationally derived. The patient's developmental need to learn how to respond to future illnesses is less clearly situational (unless a cure is impossible). The patient's need to learn how to handle life stresses in general is even less clearly situational.

The goal of nursing action ■ The nurse's goal is to contribute to the patient's overall growth and development by fostering characteristics of independence, aloneness, and responsibility as well as ability to cope with the immediate illness and its implications. These goals are oriented more to restoration, development, and adaptation than to palliation. The nurse's goals of assisting the patient to achieve his life goals and of fostering patient growth in life may be somewhat broader than the goals for which nurses are generally held to be professionally responsible and accountable. In acute physical illnesses, for example, nursing responsibility seldom goes beyond the object lesson of physical illness in meeting adaptation goals.

The extent to which such broad goals are directly the responsibility of the field of psychiatric nursing as compared with psychiatry, neurology, and so on is a source of confusion in the development of this field (Sills, 1977:205). Peplau was conservative in defining the goals of her theory as arising from the situation of illness and the means for responding to them as nursing means. Some psychiatric nurses define the goals of their specialty as similar to those of psychiatry itself—that is, the treatment of a pathological condition. They often advocate means that have traditionally been regarded as psychiatric (medical) means—for example, medication clinics, psychoanalytical techniques, and so forth. Although nurses may employ psychiatric means for the treatment of pathological conditions, from the perspective of this metatheory such goals and means do not contribute to the development of nursing practice theory, nor should they be the bases on which nurses build their practice-oriented research.

Means proposed to meet the need ■ The means proposed by Peplau for achieving the general developmental goals is a four-stage complex interpersonal relationship between the nurse and the patient. Because interpersonal relationships involve both patient and nurse, an important part of the framework is the patient's willingness to engage in the relationship, since this is an aspect obviously not fully within the nurse's control. To fully implement an interpersonal relationship involves significant expertise on the part of the nurse in symbolic communication (for example, in the phase of identification). The framework minimally involves availability of the patient for the duration of this unfolding relationship, and Peplau gives little attention to situational limits placed on the feasibility of employing such means, such as the length of hospitalization. In contrast, the means essential to the immediate situationally derived goal of mastering the illness situation are more within the nurse's power to manipulate. The nurse's handling of anxiety generated by the patient's response to the illness threat is crucial to helping the patient achieve mastery of the illness situation. This involves a high degree of communication skill.

Areas of practice that might be affected ■ Peplau's perspective is that of psychiatric nursing, and the goals she identifies for nursing interaction with patients are influenced by and should be evaluated from that perspective. Psychiatric nursing has broad goals relating to the growth and development of individuals and the development of specific individual characteristics, so the development of skills in nurses to employ such interpersonal means with psychiatric patients is a legitimate aim of the specialty. The means would be seen as most legitimate if employed by a psychiatric nurse or, perhaps, a primary nurse or a nurse practitioner who is the primary care source for the patient. The means might also be legitimate for a public health nurse. They would probably be viewed as somewhat less legitimate for use by a nurse with little psychiatric training or one who was involved in the patient's care in a fragmentary or peripheral way. To my knowledge there has been little exploration of this theory's potential usefulness in areas other than psychiatric nursing, though Peplau intended the theory to apply broadly. Such potential usefulness should not be rejected out of hand. Exploration would necessarily lead to questions of:
1. The legitimacy of the prescribed goals in other areas of nursing
2. Limitations on the means, including the ability of nonpsychiatric nurses to implement the means
3. Situational limitations of the treatment setting, including the willingness of nonpsychiatric patients to engage in such interpersonal activities.

The last factor would of course be very much a function of the extent to which patients identified needs that approximated those outlined by Peplau. Even if such needs were identified, alternative means to Peplau's might also be explored.

Attempts to operationalize and test the theory ■ The theory of nurse-patient interaction proposed by Peplau is complex, and many aspects of it would need to be operationalized for full empirical testing, for example:

1. Standards for diagnosis of the patient's anxiety level (as it arises from illness) and the meaning of the illness to the patient (as associated with blocked goal achievement)
2. Manipulation and measurement of the extent to which each of the four phases of the relationship is achieved
3. Measurement of the patient's increased ability to cope with illness and of increased effectiveness of the patient in goal achievement
4. A research design adequate to test empirically the cause-effect relationship hypothesized to exist between the means (item 2 in this list) and the goals (item 3 in this list)

Peplau's own contribution is the development of a framework for systematic observation in the form of a process recording to document various aspects of the development of the interpersonal relationship (means). Indirectly, portions of Peplau's theory have been tested through its influence on and relation to other more limited theories of nursing practice that have been more extensively operationalized and tested; for example, Orlando's.

Orlando's theory

Orlando's theory of nursing was proposed in the late 1950s. Its first and perhaps clearest statement is in *The Dynamic Nurse-Patient Relationship*, published in 1961; although Orlando's later book (1972) expands on her earlier statement, it does not change the basic characteristics of her theory.

Overview

According to Orlando, "Learning how to understand what is happening between herself and the patient is the central core of the nurse's practice and comprises the basic framework for the help she gives to patients" (1961:4). This involves discovering the meaning of the illness to the patient based on his past experience and current life situation as it relates to professional meanings. In contrast to Peplau, who is concerned with a developmental process whose aim is patient growth, Orlando is concerned primarily with sustaining the patient in his immediate need. In fact, Orlando's proposed nursing process can be perceived as an intensive examination or elaboration of Peplau's orientation phase.

Patient behavior is assumed to indicate an unmet need ("a plea for help") whose specific nature may not initially be communicated accurately. The patient needs in an illness situation to which nurses must respond are of three types:

1. Needs generated by physical limitations
2. Needs generated by setting
3. Inability to communicate

The behavior may be nonverbal (motor activity, physiological activity, noises) or verbal (complaints, questions, requests, refusals, demands, comments, statements). The patient's automatic needs consist of common needs assumed to apply to all patients, which are met by organizational routine, and needs as diagnosed and prescribed for by another professional practitioner (such as a physician), which are met by following orders.

Nurse reaction is problematic. The tendency to apply generalized (automatic) expectations of patient role behavior to the situation is great. The nurse must continue a "deliberative" process until persuaded that she knows what the patient's behavior means (what his needs are) and what nursing activities will meet those needs. The only assumption the nurse must operate on, consistent with Mead's theoretical orientation, is that every person's experience is unique, that nothing can be assumed; therefore, she must communicate to the patient her perceptions, her thoughts in response to her perceptions, and her *feelings* in response to her perceptions and thoughts. To do this, nondirective techniques are used in the form of reflective and restatement communications and verbally stated perceptions, thoughts, and feelings. Once she clarifies the patient's immediate need through this process, the need itself may even be met by another nurse or by a nurse's aide.

Nurse activities (instructing, suggesting, directing, explaining, informing, requesting, questioning, making decisions about the patient, handling the body of the patient, administering medications or treatments, changing environment) are then of two modes. They can be automatic activities based on general assumptions or previous diagnosis, or the nurse can go through a prior, simultaneous, or follow-up period of deliberativeness that adjusts the automatic assumptions of need and meaning to the unique situation of the individual patient. Regardless of which route is taken the results should be evaluated. In general, evaluation of deliberative compared to automatic nursing behaviors should reveal "better" behavior—that is, greater consistency between verbal and nonverbal behavior (1961:65-66) or improvement in verbal and nonverbal behavior (1972:22, 54-55), including verbal and nonverbal indications that a helpful outcome has been achieved either in palliation of needs or in the discovery of solutions to problems (1972:61). Assumptions that the patient's needs have been met that are based on objective criteria should be subjectively validated by a deliberative exchange with the patient.

In summary, Orlando puts heavy emphasis on adequate assessment of the

immediate nurse-patient situation by encouraging exploration of the meaning of the situation to the patient and discouraging premature hypothesizing
about what the patient behavior means. In addition, she emphasizes use of a
similar technique for evaluating the impact of any nursing activity.

Analysis and evaluation

The *general purpose* of her theory, according to Orlando, is to make clear
the process by which nurses identify and respond to individuals' needs for
help in the immediate situation of distress or contribute to an immediate sense
of adequacy or well-being. This process, called deliberative nursing (1961) or
the nursing process discipline (1972), is what distinguishes nursing as a
profession. It is offered as a solution to the perceived problem of ineffective
nursing, that is, those nursing actions that do not achieve desired effects. By
definition the focus of the theory is on the use of nursing means to promote
patient welfare, rather than increased knowledge; thus it has a practice orientation.

Unlike Peplau, Orlando does not cite previous theorists in her work, so the
behavioral science derivation of her theory is a bit harder to assess. The assumptions of her framework seem to be related strongly to the theoretical
orientations of George Herbert Mead. This is particularly true of her emphasis
on the importance of personal meanings of illness. There also appears to be a
theoretical connection to the work of Peplau. Despite these theoretical connections, it is clear that Orlando's strongest evidence for her theory is more
in her presentation of convincing clinical cases than in some logical assem-
blage of theoretical pieces. The theory is primarily "grounded" in the observation of ongoing practice (Glaser and Strauss, 1967) as opposed to being
deductive. Orlando's approach reflects her belief that social science theories
that predict and interpret behavior only from general characteristics of patient and setting too often lead to misdiagnoses when they are used automatically. She argues that only specific assessment of each individual cared for
will produce the sort of data needed to meet that patient's needs.

In Orlando's theory the *patient needs addressed* by the nurse are situationally derived by definition and, in content, relate to needs of the patient to
cope with physical limitations, the patient's need to cope with adverse reactions to the setting, and communicational difficulties of the patient in relating
the first two types of needs.

The *goal of nursing action* is the immediate improvement of the patient,
"an increased sense of well-being or a change for the better in his condition
. . . which contributes simultaneously to the patient's physical and mental
well-being" (1961:91). This goal is primarily one of palliation, related as it is

to meeting those immediate needs of the patient that arise out of the illness situation. Orlando does indicate that an additional effect of the deliberative approach may be an improvement in the individual's ability to take care of himself, but this is not developed as a major goal within Orlando's framework. There is a sense of stasis about a process that provides no way of carrying one beyond the immediate situation and the achievement of short-term goals. The process would have to be modified to be applied to the achievement of long-term goals that necessitate frustration of more immediate goals. For Peplau, the motivation for accepting this immediate frustration in deference to long-term goals would exist in the ongoing quality of the relationship established between nurse and patient, the aim of which would be development of the patient's specific interpersonal skills. The deliberative process would also have to be greatly modified (or dispensed with entirely) in certain emergency situations wherein the patient's automatic need and the required automatic activity are apparent (cardiac arrest, to give an extreme example).

The *means proposed to meet the needs* is a specific form of communication process initiated and carried through by the nurse with the patient as recipient. The means Orlando focuses on seem most directly related to reducing communication difficulties between the patient and the nurse. The nurse's evaluation of outcomes also focuses almost exclusively on communication aspects of the patient's verbal and nonverbal behavior. Specific means to meet the other needs identified in Orlando's framework, for example, the patient's physical limitations and adverse reactions to setting, are not dealt with. Put another way, Orlando's theory focuses on a process by which patient needs may be more accurately identified but does not focus on the content of the nursing activities that will most effectively meet those needs.

In her emphasis on the immediate situation and on nurse actions in the immediate situation she provides a way of delivering nursing care that is not dependent on "extra" time (in fact she argues that her process is a time saver) taken away from established nursing activities and is not necessarily dependent on an ongoing relationship between patient and nurse.

Implementation of the process described by Orlando requires training. In fact, it is this training, according to Orlando, that transforms the nurse's identity to a professional one (1972:32-43). Because of her argument that this process is at the heart of professional nursing, the *areas of practice* intended to be affected by this theory are many. Every nurse who aspires to be professional, then, should have training in the deliberative process. Because the process focuses primarily on communication difficulties and judges improvement largely through patient communication without much specification of content, the deliberative process is not unique to professional nursing. It is easy to imagine how social workers, lawyers, physicians, and other professionals might also improve their effectiveness by using a deliberative process to assist clients in articulating their needs and exploring possible ways to meet those needs. For this reason we do not consider Orlando's theory as specifying a principle of effective practice unique to nursing. Orlando's assertion (1972:20) that the deliberative process is distinct to nursing is not supported by her research; since she examined only nursing practice, she had no data on whether or not similar principles are used by other professionals.

Some basic problems stemming from Orlando's concentration on process to the exclusion of content become clearer in her *attempt to operationalize and test the theory* (1972). As with Peplau, the means designed to gather data on this process is a process recording. The format is quite similar, in expanded form, to sections of Peplau's original process recording format. Additionally, Orlando employed audiotapes. In her study the goal was to develop a tool for objectively measuring the process discipline and then to assess the effectiveness of the process with a group of nurses trained to use the process discipline (deliberative nursing). The content analysis scheme developed to measure the degree to which the discipline was implemented and to measure the outcome of the process was fraught with reliability problems and produced data only weakly supportive of the theoretical hypotheses.

Efficient, valid, and reliable measurement of social interaction processes is difficult. Nursing interaction as a major independent variable has only occasionally been well documented descriptively in research studies and even less often measured quantitatively. In one sense, then, Orlando's attempt to rationalize components of her theory through quantitative measurement is an important step toward making her theory testable. She measures outcome only by verbal report, however, while a successful outcome depends not only on the degree of clarity with which a need is communicated and understood but also whether there are reliable nursing means for meeting the specific need. The nurse's use of an approach that meets Orlando's theoretical criteria may be necessary to effective nurse-patient interaction, but it is not sufficient in itself to achieve desired goals.

The problems with Orlando's particular test of her theory do not necessarily imply a lack of usefulness of the theory in guiding practice or research. In the 1960s there were a number of experimental studies that employed her definition of deliberative nursing to operationalize and test the effects of nurse-patient interaction (for example, Anderson, Mertz, and Leonard, 1965; Dumas and Leonard, 1963; Elms and Leonard, 1966). These studies examined outcomes other than verbal statements as measures of the extent of effectiveness. The addition of content-specific dependent variables was helpful in clarifying the significance of Orlando's theory with respect to outcome. Unfortunately, these studies did not systematically describe nursing intervention except in terms of Orlando's general theory with some illustrative case examples; the nursing activities designed to meet the identified needs were not systematically documented. In addition, factorial designs would have to be used to separate analytically the contribution of deliberative communication per se from the effects of variation in nursing activities designed to meet the stated needs. Whereas these early studies employed simple two group designs, later studies have begun to overcome these difficulties but have departed somewhat from the original concept of deliberativeness as Orlando described it.*

Ujhely's theory

A third major contribution to the development of nursing role process theories is Ujhely's *Determinants of the Nurse Patient Relationship* (1968). This book was published somewhat later than the works of Peplau and Orlando, but was conceived during the late 1950s and early 1960s and is intellectually indebted to its forerunners.

Overview

The social science foundations for the development of Ujhely's theory are somewhat different than those for Peplau's. Major emphases involve theoretical ideas from Wilhelm Reich, Carl Jung, Rollo May, Paul Tillich, and Carl Rogers, more for their psychophilosophical contributions than for basic psychological or therapeutic techniques. She was influenced also by a variety of social psychologists and sociologists in her emphasis on situational restrictions to nurse-patient interaction.

She explains that in the nurse-patient situation her view of human nature is possibly "more useful" than some others. In this view, which draws heavily from psychophilosophical contributors, individuals are seen as a synthesis of good (man is basically rational and requires education), evil (man is bad/irrational and requires control), and social (man is a tabula rasa and can be shaped by his environment) influences. These three influences manifest themselves in a layered way in an individual's personality structure, with the social layer being most accessible and the "good" core accessible only by dealing with the social and "evil" layers. The perception of the social layer is influenced by Reich's ideas of *character armor* and the good core by Jung's ideas of the *collective unconscious*.

Ujhely's view of human nature directly influences her elaboration of the

*See, for example, Diers et al. (1974), in which a content analysis scheme is used to document systematically the manipulation of nursing process; and Powers and Wooldridge (in press), in which both content analysis and a factorial design are used. A detailed discussion of methodological and theoretical issues as they apply to attempts to test Orlando's theory is contained in Wooldridge et al. (1978).

nurse-patient relationship. Her emphasis is on sustaining the patient in the experience of his illness (similar to Orlando) and, by and large, helping an individual cope with role changes at the social level of personality. This means helping him to use what controls he has developed to contain the occasional "bursting through" of evil and good influences to the surface. This is done by helping the patient identify and elaborate *content themes*—what the illness means to him, often as expressed in role change terms. Unlike Orlando and like Peplau, this elaboration of meaning in the form of content themes is done over time within the context of a relationship whose limits have been explicitly defined by the nurse and agreed to by the patient. The relationship has three phases.

1. *Orientation phase.* This is the beginning period in which the limits of the relationship are defined, content themes are identified by nurse and patient (the nurse may also tentatively identify mood and interaction themes for herself at this time), and beginning work with the content theme is done. This orientation phase differs from Peplau's in that it specifies the types of meaning (content) that will receive priority but shares the commitment to beginning a relationship, through the nurse's leadership, that will provide the patient with a means of active coping with his illness. This dimension differs from Orlando's more exclusive emphasis on the patient and his immediate experience, with the nurse engaging in interaction that is limited by that immediate experience.

2. *Working phase.* This phase fully engages the patient in elaboration of the content theme, focusing his conscious awareness of the meaning of his illness at this level. In addition, depending on many factors such as available time, nurse's comfort, the patient's readiness, and so forth, the nurse may begin to help the patient focus conscious awareness on *mood themes*— to elaborate how he feels about the illness. Movement of the relationship to this level makes it likely that the second ("evil") layer of personality will invade the relationship, and the nurse must be prepared to help the patient accept increased awareness of negative feelings about himself and others as expressed in the context of the illness.

Full development of the working phase involves moving beyond elaboration of content and mood themes to an increase in the patient's elaboration and awareness of *interaction themes*. Interaction themes deal with how the patient relates to the nurse as a person. This fully elaborated working phase, including interaction themes, is comparable to Peplau's identification phase. Its aim is personality change as opposed to sustaining or maintenance functions. Ujhely does not see the illness experience (as Peplau does) as one that necessarily focuses on personality growth. By making the identification phase a more optional and individually paced part of the therapeutic relationship, she creates an opportunity to increase gradually the intensity, emotional involvement, and commitment to change in the relationship. This assumes a gradual increase in the skill of the nurse in helping the particular patient and a gradual increase in the patient's ability to use the resources the nurse has to offer and to develop resources of his own.

3. *Termination phase.* This phase is similar to Peplau's resolution phase. What has been learned by the patient and the nurse in the relationship is reviewed. The patient's thoughts and feelings about termination are explored.

A major contribution of Ujhely's is the identification and elaboration of situational restrictions to the development of the nurse-patient relationship. The possible situational restrictions are of three types: what the nurse brings to the interaction, what the patient brings to the interaction, and the context in which the interaction takes place. With regard to the first, she points out that nurses may vary according to basic values and attitudes about human nature, their physical and emotional condition, their educational and experiential background, and their preference for some of the variety of roles a nurse may potentially fulfill.

Greater emphasis on what the patient brings to the interaction provides broader perception of the flexibility and limits within which the nurse and patient work. Two basic dimensions govern what the patient brings: his ability to experience and his illness. Ability to experience has three components: (1) perception, (2) interpretation, and (3) response to interpreted perception (this is close to Orlando's ordering of experience in terms of perceptions, thoughts, and feelings). Illness has two subparts: the illness state and the patient's experience related to that state.

The limits of the patient's ability to experience require modifications in the nurse's approach. The illness state and the patient's experience of it provide the focus of the interaction and exploration of meanings, with the goal being acceptance of the illness state. Nurses help patients work toward acceptance by responding to the illness state itself and by helping the patient experience the state through the processes described in the various phases of the nurse-patient relationship.

In her emphasis on the indirect effects of responding to the patient's illness state on his acceptance of it (as well as affecting his experience of it directly), Ujhely integrates an emphasis on physical needs and technical skills as important aspects of the nurse's role (1968:208):

> Although in itself a truism, this statement, as formulated here . . . [reciprocal relationship between the patient's condition and its meaning to him and his capacity to experience] . . . has . . . tremendous implications for nurses. As members of one of the healing professions, nurses share in the overall

obligation to do everything in their power to foster a positive outcome of the patient's state; and as members of the nursing profession, they have the specific responsibility, I think, of sustaining the person in his *experience....* Therefore, whether they are aware of it or not, nurses have a potentially crucial role to play with respect to both axes of the patient's predicament—his experience and his condition. By lending knowledgeable physical and emotional support to the patient, and by skillfully carrying out delegated medical tasks and nursing procedures, nurses can exert a favorable influence upon the way in which the patient perceives, interprets and responds to his condition as well as upon the condition itself; and since these two factors influence each other, her positive influence upon one of them may well lead to improvement in the other.

Furthermore, by trying to gain an idea of what his condition means to the patient and, if possible, helping him to correct any misconceptions he may have concerning it, the nurse may be able to disrupt much of the negative interaction that may occur between his state and his experience of it.

The third situational restriction discussed by Ujhely is the context or setting in which the interpersonal relationship between the nurse and the patient takes place. Whether the interaction occurs in the context of a hospital, long-term care setting, or home suggests differences in the patient's condition, in the patient's experience of his condition, and in their possible effects on the nurse's own attitudes and opportunities for the development of a relationship. The actual themes that emerge as central to the interaction will also vary as a function of setting.

Ujhely does not spell out any specific assessment and evaluation process to accompany her elaboration of the intervention component of the nursing process. The nature of the required assessment is implied by the goal, which is sustaining the patient in his experience. Assessment must include measurement of the patient's ability to experience, the nature of his condition, and his current experience of his condition, taking into account both nurse and setting restrictions. Evaluation would involve reassessment of these three elements after a period of intervention.

Analysis and evaluation

The nursing problem identified by Ujhely was that teaching mental health concepts as such and emphasizing their relevance to the various specialities within nursing are not sufficient to develop skills for the social practice of nursing (the use of psychosocial means). She felt additional guidelines for the application of these concepts should be offered. Thus the *purpose of the theory* is to describe a more specific means of nursing the patient and to take into account several classes of variables she felt to have a significant influence on the implementation of means.

She drew on a wide variety of theories—philosophical, religious, sociological, and psychological—in describing these several classes of variables. Since the focus is on variables that affect the nurse's ability to nurse, and thereby assist the patient, it is clear that the theory is practice oriented.

The *patient need or problem addressed* is that of coping with the experience that brought the patient into contact with the nurse in the first place. Ujhely defines the domain of need rather broadly. Needs might include overcoming illness, making the best of personality, finding a place in a new community, being a good parent, or living within the confines of a handicap (1968:92). She points out that many situations in which persons seek nursing assistance are not situations of illness per se. Ujhely's broad definition of patient needs appropriately addressed by nursing intervention emphasizes assistance with personal growth as well as assistance with illness. This bears a resemblance to Peplau's definition of patient needs. Though one might argue that growth needs are not truly situationally derived, the surfacing of such needs and the opportunity to contribute to their favorable resolution may be situationally derived. Ujhely argues that nurses are often found in situations where such needs are likely to be expressed.

The *goal of nursing actions*, according to Ujhely, is to make tolerable situations that would have been intolerable without nursing intervention. She also indicates that it is a nursing responsibility to help the patient make use of his experience in his own personal growth. Questions can be raised about the responsibility of nursing as a whole for this goal, although it is clearly a nursing responsibility in psychiatric nursing, Ujhely's own specialty.

The *means proposed to meet the needs of the patient* and to achieve the goals of the nurse involve a three-stage interpersonal relationship, which has some major similarities to Peplau's proposed sequence. The major theoretical difference arises from Ujhely's recognition that there are many factors—some within the nurse's control, but most not—that affect the feasibility of the relationship and that may alter its character. These include patient, nurse, and setting factors. By definition, not all nurses are prepared to implement such a relationship and not all patients are likely to agree to or benefit from it as fully elaborated. Ujhely does not go beyond the broadest outlines of the conditions under which her three stage interpersonal relationship might be effectively applied.

The *areas of practice potentially affected* by this theory remain ambiguous. Since the nature of the relationship may be strongly influenced by variables related to areas of practice, significant modifications in the theorized relationship may occur. To the extent that modifications are made one may need to ask whether it would still be Ujhely's theory of relationship that is employed.

Attempts to operationalize and test this theory as it stands would be problematic. There is much ambiguity about the content of the variables to be used in testing the establishment of the relationship and its potential impact on the patient's welfare.

Summary

We have presented three theories as representative of an early period of theorizing about nursing. They share a similarity in focusing on the nursing role process and nurse-patient interaction though they differ somewhat in their description of the independent variable. Peplau and Ujhely emphasize the developmental aspects of interaction and Orlando emphasizes the individual encounter. All three point to the patient's perceptions of illness as crucial data for determining nursing interventions. This focus on the importance of the patient's perceptions implies that the patient is a much more active participant in the care process than was implied by Parson's model of health provider–patient relationship that was pervasive in social science thinking of this period. Ujhely, in addition, focused attention on the importance of the patient's state (as related to his diagnosis), the care setting, and the nurse's own capacity for relationship as classes of variables affecting the nature of the developing nurse-patient relationship.

The relative emphasis of the theories discussed is on variables that effect the immediate and long-term relationship between nurse and patient with the implication that factors of relationship have importance for outcomes. Remaining imbedded and unarticulated in these theories (the extended quote from Ujhely suggests these) are other kinds of nursing activities that have potential importance for outcomes. These include the skillful implementation of nursing procedures, which have their own potential direct effects on patient outcomes as well as indirect effects on the patient's psychological experience, and informational activities by which, to use Ujhely's phrase, nurses, "correct misconceptions [about the patient's] state [and] disrupt much of the negative interaction that may occur between his state and his experience of it" (1968:209).

The scientific investigation of therapeutic aspects of relationship—in Ujhley's words, "sustaining the person in his experience"—involves a clear articulation of the concept of support as well as the dynamics of support and measurement of its characteristics. These are only now being developed by the multiple social sciences whose knowledge is relevant to these aspects of nursing practice. Many other variables potentially produce random as well as systematic effects on the nature of relationships built in nursing practice. These might best be understood as *nurse effects* paralleling the *experimenter effects* written about so extensively by Rosenthal (1976). Nurses' attempts to study some of these effects have lacked theoretical connection to any overall frame of reference, so the completed studies have remained isolated, noncumulative contributions to the discipline. Several categories of studies, then, have emerged from these early theoretical considerations. They include the following:

1. Studies that emphasize the importance of the expressive role of the nurse—where a supportive, reassuring figure engages in listening behaviors as patients share their fears, conceptions of what is happening, and meaning of the illness in their daily lives. Representative of this approach are some of the studies reported in Skipper and Leonard (1965). Studies in this area have been subject to the limitations we have cited.

2. Interaction studies, which were attempts to create quantitative methodologies for studying nurse-patient interaction, adding to the early qualitative technique of process recording. See, for example, Conant (1965), Diers and Leonard (1966), and Diers (1971). Theoretical limitations as well as methodological problems have plagued such studies.

3. Studies focusing on the role of patients' perceptions of health care events in the design of nursing interventions that emphasize the informational aspects of nurse-patient exchange. See, for example, part of the discussion of Johnson's work in Chapter 6.

4. Studies emphasizing the importance of the patient's active participation in events in the health care setting. See, for example, Skipper and Leonard (1965), Leonard et al. (1975), Wooldridge et al. (1978), and part of the discussion of Johnson's work in Chapter 6.

OTHER THEORETICAL APPROACHES TO THE DOMAINS OF NURSING PRACTICE THEORY

The early nursing theorists we have described were strongly influenced by psychiatric-psychological theories of intrapersonal and interpersonal behavior that focused on the individual and individual one-to-one relationships. Other nurses were strongly influenced by or were educated through the doctoral level in disciplines allied to nursing other than psychology or psychiatry. Theoretical emphases current in those disciplines were adopted and adapted to nursing theories. Examples of those theories are discussed in the remaining sections of this chapter.

Rogers' theory

A much different approach to the domain of nursing practice theory is presented in Rogers' *An Introduction to the Theoretical Basis of Nursing*

(1970). Rogers' nursing theory is concerned with man's health but in its broadest sense as well as in the narrower sense of individual survival and growth. In the broader concern Rogers focuses on the human life process, how to maintain it, and how to encourage its evolution.

Overview

Rogers' theory of nursing practice is best understood within the context of the references she cites in the areas of evolutionary theory, Lewinian field theory (and other holistic formulations of humans in the world), electrodynamic theory, and communication theory. From an evolutionary viewpoint, Rogers is acutely aware of human beings as an evolving species. The time perspective for her theoretical formulations includes individuals' development over their lifetime and the human race's general development over centuries (the life process in general). Human development is described as continuous, creative, evolutionary, and uncertain. Rogers views the individual and the human race in this evolutionary process as a whole. She argues against approaches that separate humans into mind-body parts. She perceives humans in their wholeness, acting in the midst of a field of dynamic forces. Thus her theory is concerned with the identification of categories of variables (forces) that affect human beings as a whole; the categories of variables proposed as the focus of nursing theory and research are closely tied to space and time dimensions as important environmental forces in human life. In addition, her concern with electrodynamic forces places some of her theory within a physics frame of reference. Finally, the potential of humans to understand and alter such forces in the human life process is a function of their superior neurological development, which brings a conscious self-awareness and ability to communicate increasing knowledge of the environmental forces affecting evolutionary development. Rogers suggests that nursing theory and research are (or should be) a science concerned with human beings as a whole and environmental forces that affect humankind as a whole. To this end, she articulates five general assumptions about human characteristics that are rooted in the theoretical domains just described. For example, her second assumption is "Man and environment are continuously exchanging matter and energy with one another" (1970:54). In addition, she identifies four general principles of nursing science, inherent in her theoretical views, that interpret changes in the life process of man. For example, her principle of reciprocity suggests that all understanding of humans' health-illness state is achieved only by reference to the complex forces operating between them and their environment.

According to Rogers, nursing theory, research, and practice are intimately related. She views nursing practice, in both its individual and evolutionary responsibilities to the human race, as the nurturance of the life process through achievement of maximal states of health. The key to effective nursing practice is viewed as nursing research expanded to build a body of knowledge relevant to nursing interventions. This body of knowledge is concerned with interaction between man as a whole and environmental forces that impinge on and interact with that wholeness. Rogers suggests several key categories of variables as examples of possible significant human-environment interaction. Her proposed focuses for nursing research include

1. Perceptions of time and space—memory, vision, hearing
2. Diurnal cycles and other rhythmic patterns
3. Effects of motion
4. Population effects (concerns with personal space)
5. Communication processes
6. Electrodynamic forces; for example, radiation phenomena

She feels that these variables, which lie at the interface between humans and their environment, influence the individual's life process as well as the human race's evolutionary process. Thus nursing interventions based on a knowledge of these effects can have an impact on the lives and health of human beings. Rogers gives two examples to illustrate the translation of this theory into meaningful practice terms. She notes that jogging as an activity to promote health grew out of research on the relationship between physical exercise and improved physiological functioning of various kinds. She transforms this idea into a more general idea that motion, or human movement in space, might be a key variable in the effect of physical exercise on the developmental life process (1970:105). This is a novel way of thinking about possible relationships, consistent with her theoretical constructions, that opens a wide range of research possibilities for studying the effects of motion on overall development (see, for example, Porter, 1972). On the basis of findings of such research, manipulation of motion to enhance development might become part of nursing practice guidelines. Another specific application of her ideas to nursing practice is that nursing actions can either disrupt individual rhythmic patterns (such as sleep-wake patterns governing human perceptual interaction with the environment) or be supportive to them, thereby either inhibiting or supporting human tendencies toward self-maintenance and survival. Nursing research needs to explore and describe such patterns of self-maintenance before it designs nursing interventions to enhance self-maintenance capabilities.

Analysis and evaluation

Rogers' *general purpose* is to propose a conceptual model of humans as a "reference for envisioning relationships between events" (1970:111), which could be the basis for development of research hypotheses with potential for applications to nursing practice. Though she cites many potential research areas there is no focus on a specific problem of practice but rather a primary emphasis on obtaining new knowledge. The domains she suggests as areas for research are derived primarily deductively from several domains of general theory that she views as relevant to the development of nursing's understanding of the life process.

The general *need* identified by Rogers is sustaining the individual and the human race in the life process. The *goals* are focused on maintaining and promoting human health and providing evaluative, therapeutic, and rehabilitative services to people (1970:82). This reflects an understanding of the relationship between those services, the maintenance or restoration of health, and the life process itself.

It is clear from the examples given by Rogers that at least some of the needs that might be identified using her theory would be situationally derived. For example, the suggestion that traditional hospital routines may interrupt individual rhythmic patterns important for the self-regulation of health and maintenance of the life process describes a situational need arising from the presence of the pathological process requiring hospitalization. Surely, techniques for the education of individuals in ways they might act to maintain their own rhythms for healthful purposes might well fall within the domain of nursing practice theory. On the other hand, a difficulty with Rogers' theory is her suggestion that nursing is responsible for the development of a scientific knowledge base about basic rhythms of the life process, which seems to imply that nursing theory broadly encompasses knowledge about the life process and human adaptation, whether or not it is directly relevant to the design of nursing interventions to restore or maintain health. Another example of this difficulty is Rogers' suggestion that it is a basic responsibility of nurses to do research on electrodynamic energy fields to see if they are associated with the life process. The relevance of such endeavors to the possible development of practice theory is not clearly articulated, though some consider the work on therapeutic touch as falling within this domain.

The major reason for the difficulties in defining nursing's theoretical and research responsibility broadly has to do with the means available to nursing. Even if basic descriptive data on the relationships between variables and health status were available in areas of study proposed by Rogers—for example, the effects of motion, electrodynamic forces, diurnal cycles, and so forth—the means to create and maintain such relationships in life are well beyond nursing's domain of professional practice. On the other hand, the knowledge of such relationships might have powerful implications for the development of practice theories, principles, and guidelines in the support of patients when illness and the treatments for it threaten to alter the patient's capability for maintaining proper relationship to those aspects of his interaction with the environment. The old hospital joke about patients who are never able to sleep because the nurses are always waking them up for treatments gains serious significance when looked at in the context of the possible relationship between sleep-wake patterns and self-regulation, or self-maintenance, of health.

The potential *scope* of Rogers' theory seems broad, since she addresses large numbers of phenomena broadly applicable to many areas of nursing practice. Implementation of changes in nursing practice suggested by research developed along the lines proposed by Rogers might range from general guidelines broadly applicable to nursing care procedures to sophisticated, specialty-focused interventions requiring considerable skill.

Since Rogers' theory is developed at a highly abstract level, it is impossible to *operationalize and test the theory* directly. She has suggested broad domains in which research might be undertaken and in which the utility of her theory might be measured by how productive the exploration of each domain becomes. Considerable research developed from the domains suggested by Rogers' theory has been undertaken.

The concepts, hypotheses, and research programs of Barnard and Neal (1977) in the area of maternal-child nursing are derived in part from the theoretical work of Rogers. The framework discussed by Barnard in the context of the Nursing Child Assessment Project (NCAP) is related very generally to Rogers' emphasis on human-environment interaction and development, emphasizing the study of variables of infant-environment interaction and their influence on infant developmental patterns over time. The framework developed by Neal focuses more specifically on a set of concepts, including motion, sensation, cognition, and affiliation, and their general relationship. This is more narrowly derived from Rogers' work and more clearly directive of domains of research activity. These researchers are guided in the development of substantial research not only by the nursing theory of Rogers and others but also by substantial research and theory building from other scientific disciplines. The descriptive research on normal sleep-wake patterns in infants and the prescriptive theory building associated with the study of the effects of disruptions on sleep patterns (such as prematurity and health provider disruptions) could not have been undertaken without the ready availability of basic theory, research, and technology on sleep-wake states. Similarly, the concern with that aspect of environment-infant interaction that focuses on parent-infant interaction draws heavily on research and theory on maternal attachment-separation processes, infant temperament studies, and so forth.

Space considerations preclude a complete discussion of the research programs of Barnard and Neal but they can be described as a mixture of basic research and theory development—for example, they describe the differences in sleep-wake patterns between premature infants and full-term infants—and applied prescriptive theory building—for example, they describe disruptions of sleep-wake patterns by health care providers and their consequences on infant behavior and development. Variables such as health care provider disruptions are particularly within nursing's domain of legitimacy and are potentially manipulable.

Quite a different matter is the work of such theorists as Kreiger (Kreiger, Peper, and Ancoli, 1979; Macrae, 1979; Quinn, 1979), which can also be described as work derived from Rogers' framework. These theorists draw particularly from those aspects of human-environment interaction that focus on energy concepts. In employing theoretical paradigms such as Rogers', movement to the level of development of effective practice principles must incorporate both substantive theoretical hypotheses and research that meets the usual scientific requirements for design. Kreiger presents her work as within the domain of science, claiming a physiological explanation for the efficacy of therapeutic touch as a nursing practice modality: " . . . transfer of energy from healer . . . [to] the patient . . . appears to be done physiologically by a kind of electron transfer resonance . . . " (1979:660). Yet, neither a body of substantive theory nor studies meeting minimum requirements for proper research design are a part of her reported work. She does not employ more orthodox nursing practices in comparative studies to assess the extent to which they produce desired outcomes as compared to therapeutic touch. Yet, Kreiger claims that therapeutic touch, "is *proving* to be a useful adjunct to orthodox nursing practices."* She and the nurses she trains use it to relieve pain and even, in one reported instance, to shrink fibroid tumors.

One has the sense in reading Kreiger's and other's accounts of their use of therapeutic touch that the focus is on something other than scientific exploration of potential principles of effective practice. It is important to note that Kreiger's ideas could be scientifically investigated, though she has not chosen to do so. Comments such as, "I have found therapeutic touch holds its own in the midst of sophisticated technology and offers a new dimension to modern nursing," (Macrae, 1979:664); "Nursing is, after all, 'a special case of loving,'" (Quinn, 1979:663); and, "we are no longer separate from [the client] . . . we are part of the same open energy system," (Quinn, 1979:663) suggest that this work may have more to do with a felt absence of aspects of the humanistic side of nursing than with a scientific effort to define effective principles of practice. This is both laudable and probably necessary by way of philosophical assertion, but it should not be confused with what it is not, namely, scientific investigation into principles of effective practice.

Overall, Rogers' framework provides a very strong alternative for those

*Italics added by the present author.

nurses who feel that much more determines the dimension of "sustaining the patient" than the interpersonal relationship between the nurse and the patient. In Rogers' theory the total environment, including the nurse, is in interaction with the patient and has significance for him. Variables such as the light and sound properties of the room, the number of patients in a unit, the individual's perceptual abilities or disabilities (here there is an overlap of concerns between Rogers and Ujhely), the frequency and nature of treatment routines—variables under direct and continuous control of nurses—become part of nursing's practice theory domain.

Leininger's theory

A final theoretical statement to be considered, one that has sparked research efforts of a different type, is that of Leininger. Most of her papers can be found in *Transcultural Nursing: Concepts, Theories and Practices* (1978). A comparison of Leininger's theory to others already discussed helps clarify her contribution. Peplau focuses on creating a model of an ideal nurse-patient relationship wherein nurse actions facilitate patient coping and growth. She pays little attention to the limitations of nursing practice situations in achieving this ideal relationship in practice. Orlando, on the other hand, focuses on a common limitation to effective nurse-patient relationships in the inability of the nurse who does not use a "deliberative process" to understand the meaning of the illness to the patient, which leads to inability to motivate his participation in the care process by making nursing interventions compatible with patient meaning systems. Ujhely expands the focus on limitations by focusing attention on major classes of variables that may limit nurse effectiveness in the patient-nurse relationship, while keeping the ideal relationship a focus of her writing. Rogers' focus is on open systems, on communication between man and environment, and is evolutionary in scope. Leininger's focus is on *cultural* meaning systems. With this focus she comes close to Orlando's concern for assessing the meaning of illness to patients as it affects interaction and delivery of nursing care. However, Leininger emphasizes cultural meanings that are broader than Orlando's intrapsychic and interpersonal emphasis on personal, idiosyncratic meanings. Leininger does not readily develop a model of an ideal nurse-patient relationship as Peplau and Ujhely do, largely because such an ideal would be culturally determined and in Leininger's theoretical framework ideals might vary considerably from culture to culture.

Overview

In an early paper on the relevance of culture to nursing (1967), Leininger refers specifically to the problems of helping patients with differing cultural backgrounds. She illustrates these problems through the example of a student who, in interacting with a Mexican-American mother in a manner consistent with her American cultural background, creates fear and alienation when her behavior is interpreted negatively by the mother because of her Mexican background. The effect of the nurse's behavior is exactly opposite to that intended because the nurse did not understand her patient's cultural viewpoint on health and illness issues.

In a 1968 paper, Leininger speculates in a more generalized fashion about the total impact of cultural differences between patients and nursing staff and discusses the potential advantages and disadvantages of nurse-patient assignments being based on similar cultural backgrounds. She suggests that such assignments create ready identification between the patient and the nurse and lead to decreased patient anxiety, thereby facilitating the development of the nurse-patient relationship in initial and working phases. Although she does not discuss it, the impracticality of implementing such a change widely must have been obvious to her, considering the overall differences in nurses' backgrounds and the patients they serve. While professional awareness of this discrepancy was probably an important impetus for expanding concern about the access of minority students to programs in nursing education, the alternative consideration, that of increasing nurses' knowledge of variation in culturally based beliefs and attitudes towards health, illness, and its treatment, led to the recognition of a problem of equal magnitude. Anthropologists, from whom one might expect to obtain data on cultural variations in such beliefs, had rarely focused systematically on this aspect of culture.

In a paper written in 1969, Leininger refocuses her attention from the immediate nurse-patient situation to the need for gathering basic data on systematic cultural variation in the health/illness beliefs and behavior of humans to develop an accurate baseline from which the nurse can know and help a patient of a given cultural heritage. She identifies a descriptive method, *ethnoscience*, as an approach in ethnography helpful to nurse-scientists in gathering such data. Ethnoscience is described as the use of a traditional ethnographic anthropological perspective, but applied with more rigor in light of advances in ethnographic and linguistic methods, and with use of scientific principles in collecting and analyzing data. She illustrates the use of the ethnoscience method in describing the organization and responsibilities of health and illness practitioners in the Gadsup society of New Guinea she studied as an anthropologist. She gives examples of how Western medical and nursing practitioners might "fit" into this culturally specific health and illness organization in order to provide health care in a manner acceptable to this particular group of people.

The overriding problem Leininger articulates is the lack of available basic knowledge on health/illness issues in other cultures. A major emphasis in her later papers is that of conceptualizing *transcultural health care* as a special, interdisciplinary area of study focusing on a "body of knowledge and practices regarding health-illness care patterns from a comparative perspective of at least two or more designated cultures in order to determine the major care features and the health services of cultures" (1976:3). She sees the development of such knowledge as a priority and a key to successful collaboration in health goals between Western health professionals and native peoples.

Leininger (1976) offers a transcultural health model for the comparative study of health care systems, of which her study of Gadsup society is one example. The model involves four classes of variables to guide data gathering and theory development in transcultural health care. The classes of variables moving from the most general to the most specific are (1) the social structural features of the society, (2) cultural and health care values, (3) health care systems and typologies, and (4) roles and functions of the health professionals. These data about a particular group provide the basic information required by a Western health provider who attempts to integrate Western health care with native health/illness belief systems and native medical structures.

From the provider's viewpoint, Leininger articulates two additional problems that arise out of attempts to deliver culturally relevant health and nursing care services (1971, 1973). The varying abilities and motivations on the part of Western health care providers to adapt to culturally different systems of care result in several "types" of behavior patterns exhibited by Western providers. Many of these behavior patterns result in rejection of the Western practitioner. A second problem she points to is the difficulties in assessing the nature and strength of traditional health and illness beliefs as they become mixed with Western ideas and as various ethnic groups begin to approach both traditional and Western healers in care-seeking attempts. This is particularly relevant to groups that remain as ethnic subcultures of American society. Both of these problem areas specific to transcultural health care are in need of useful theoretical conceptualization and research and, ultimately, have direct implications for the delivery of health and nursing care.

Finally, Leininger articulates nursing's unique interest in transcultural health care studies as "the systematic study of comparative caring beliefs, values, and modes of behavior of different cultures . . . as caring is held to be the basis for nursing as a discipline and profession" (1978:10). Effective professional transcultural nursing interventions cannot be designed and delivered without knowledge of and articulation with such culture-specific data. The theoretical work of transcultural nursing involves three phases (1978:39).

The first, the interdisciplinary phase, involves the gathering of data from several cultures of general relevance to transcultural health care in the four areas described previously. From these general data, nurses derive and develop a specific classification of care constructs across several cultures, whereas physicians would focus on culturally specific and culturally universal cure constructs. A beginning list of such constructs derived from the writing of anthropologists and transcultural nursing studies is provided by Leininger (1978:39). They include comfort measures, support measures, compassion, empathy, helping behaviors, touching, and so forth. The extent and specific nature of these caring activities vary from culture to culture, and the comparative study of these can lead to hypotheses explaining the variation. This sort of work would be viewed by Leininger as nursing's contribution to the development of basic scientific knowledge. The applied aspects of transcultural nursing include formulation and testing of professional nursing interventions based on the classificatory scheme and analysis of data.

Analysis and evaluation

There are two *general purposes* for which Leininger has articulated her theory of transcultural nursing: comparative study and analysis and use of the knowledge in providing culturally relevant nursing care practices. Her earliest writing makes it clear that she was acutely aware of problems of nursing care delivery to diverse cultural groups, with professional nursing practices often generating unintended negative consequences because of the lack of sensitivity to the patient's cultural background. However, as with Rogers' framework, the modification and ultimate improvement of nursing practice depends on the availability of (in Leininger's case, cultural) data that have never been collected and analyzed. Therefore an initial purpose of her theory is to provide a framework for the collection of such data. She is more explicit and specific than Rogers in identifying the shared responsibilities of several disciplines, including nursing, for the collection of the most general cultural data having relevance to the health/illness domain; the more specific responsibility of nursing for the classification of caring behaviors, and the most specific responsibility of nursing to modify and improve the nature of nursing care delivery through making it culturally based. Since most of the activity of Leininger and her associates to date has been devoted to the gathering of basic cultural data and the creation of a caring taxonomy, little specific practice theory has evolved from her work yet. This will become evident as we analyze her theory. However, it is also clear from Leininger's writing that she anticipates such a period of development of practice theory in the future (1978:49).

The *patient need or problem* is not defined in terms of specifics of health and illness, as it was in other theories we have discussed. This remains an underdeveloped part of Leininger's theory, perhaps because it is specific to knowledge of cultures that is yet to be obtained. Rather, the need is defined in relation to her goals for accrual of knowledge: "people have a right to have their cultural values, beliefs, and practices understood, respected, and considered." (1978:85) More specifically, patients have a need for nursing assistance that is sensitive to and integrated with their own cultural beliefs, values, and behaviors.

The *goals of nursing actions* are to assist people with these daily living and health needs, foster behaviors that promote and sustain health, or contribute to recovery from illness. These goals are differentiated from medicine's curative emphasis.

It is clear from Leininger's writing that a particular cultural group will have its own goals for health and ways of achieving these. Nursing has general goals for health and, according to Leininger's framework, should incorporate a specific culture's own goals in working with any given culture.

The *means proposed to meet this need* is the modification of current nursing practices that are ethnocentrically based in American scientific medical values to be more compatible with the beliefs, values and behaviors of a given patient's culture; is theoretically within the control of the nursing profession; and is manipulated through the modification of standards of the profession, the educational programs offered, the attitudes developed, and the nursing care procedures taught. The *scope* of Leininger's theory is broad in the sense that all areas of nursing practice are potentially in need of modification for the purpose of making practice culturally relevant. For any given culture, the implementation of culturally relevant care would potentially require nurses specifically qualified through background or study to understand and communicate with the particular cultural group. Leininger does make it clear that the subtleties of cultural meaning cannot be assessed or responded to through only a superficial acquaintance with the culture.

As with previously discussed frameworks this framework is of value largely because it sensitizes us to a whole set of variables relevant to nursing care. Its ultimate utility will be measured by the extent to which knowledge of cultural variables identified as important by the framework do indeed lead to modifications of nursing practice that improve effectiveness.

There is an implicit problem that provides a serious limitation to this framework, which cannot be fully articulated without studies in specific cultures. Leininger's current emphasis is on the need to gather data pertaining to health-illness interpretations in a variety of cultures. From a nursing practice viewpoint these cultural interpretations are given and cannot be modified directly by nurses. Rather, nurses fit their care to the culture. However, it may well be that some caring practices in diverse cultures, believed by members of the culture to contribute to health, contribute directly to disability of spread of disease. As long as health and illness are interpreted strictly as cultural definitions, no nursing actions would be indicated. Ethically, a serious dilemma is presented. No scientific modification and testing of professional nursing practices can resolve this sort of dilemma. It would seem that as the purpose of Leininger's work moves from descriptive data gathering to designing nursing interventions, some issues such as this will have to be grappled with in their complexity.

Many nurse researchers have been influenced by Leininger to engage in transcultural nursing research. Leininger's *Transcultural Nursing* (1978) provides many examples of this work. As noted previously, much of this research is directed toward obtaining knowledge of the health/illness dimensions of specific cultures and only the most general implications for research into nursing practice in culturally diverse populations have been proposed.

SUMMARY

The theories we have discussed do not by any means exhaust the array of nursing theories that have been developed to date. Other theories may well have profited from this sort of discussion, and I urge readers, using the frame of reference proposed here, to subject their "favorite" theorists to such analysis. I suspect it will become apparent that other so-called nursing theories, as well as those discussed here, have been developed at a very general level. Though they focus on practice, they do not do so specifically enough to suggest clear hypotheses for testing that might facilitate the development of practice guidelines. They are general paradigms (models) that identify categories of variables for the practitioner-theorist to consider, and ways in which these categories of variables might be interrelated. In this sense they are metatheories (theories about theories) rather than substantive (content specific) theories that can be directly tested. I believe it is a mistake for such metatheories to be judged by objectives they were never intended to serve, namely, the generation of specific hypotheses for testing. Nurses writing such metatheories have often, because of their dual identity as nurses and behavioral scientists of one type or another, been able to present articulately potential links between variables in the basic sciences on which nursing depends and from which nursing research and nursing knowledge can evolve. Simultaneously, they have brought to the basic science of which they are a part suggestions for further exploration of the nature of the science itself. Nurses who continue to prepare themselves in a basic science and remain in touch with nursing will continue to have opportunities as well as skills to contribute to the growth of both basic science and applied nursing science knowledge. However, it remains for nursing as a whole to identify the concepts and variables of these metatheories that have the most importance for the development of nursing practice theory on the basis of clinical significance and potential for control by the nursing profession. The ultimate test of the usefulness of such "grand theories" of nursing practice lies in their ability to call attention to categories of variables and/or theoretical considerations that might otherwise be overlooked in developing only middle-range theories.

REFERENCES

Anderson, B., Mertz, H., and Leonard, R. 1965. Two experimental tests of a patient-centered admission process, Nursing Research 14:150-157.

Asken, M.J. 1975. Medical psychology: psychology's neglected child, Professional Psychology 6:155-160.

Asken, J.J. 1979. Medical psychology: toward definition, clarification, and organization, Professional Psychology 10:66-73.

Barnard, K.E., and Neal, M.V. 1977. Maternal-child nursing research, Nursing Research 26:193-200.

Batey, M.V. 1971. Conceptualizing the research process, Nursing Research 20:296-301.

Conant, L. 1965. The use of Bales' interaction process analysis in studying nurse-patient interaction, Nursing Research 14:304-309.

Corwin, R.G., and Taves, M.J. 1963. Nursing and other health professions. In Freeman, H.E., Levine, S. and Reeder, L.G., editors. Handbook of medical sociology, Englewood Cliffs, N.J., Prentice-Hall, Inc., pp. 187-212.

DeSomery, C.H. and Walike, B.C. 1977. Effects of parenteral nutrition on voluntary food intake and gastric motility in monkeys. In Batey, M.V., editor. Communicating nursing research, Nursing research priorities: choice or chance. Boulder, Colo. Western Interstate Commission for Higher Education 8:176-187.

Diers, D. 1971. Studies in nurse-patient interaction. Final progess report, USPHS Grant NU 00179, New Haven, Conn. Division of Nursing, Bureau of Health Manpower.

Diers, D. and Leonard, R.C. 1966. Interaction analysis in nursing research, Nursing Research 15:225-228.

Diers, D. et al. 1972. The effect of nursing interaction on patients in pain, Nursing Research 21:419-428.

Dumas, G., and Leonard, R.C. 1963. The effect of nursing on the incidence of postoperative vomiting: a clinical experiment, Nursing Research 12:12-15.

Elms, R.R., and Leonard, R.C. 1966. Effects of nursing approaches during admission, Nursing Research 15:39-48.

Foster, G. 1975. Medical anthropology: some contrasts with medical sociology, Social Science and Medicine 9:427-432

Glaser, B.G., and Strauss, A.L. 1967. The discovery of grounded theory, Chicago, Aldine Publishing Co.

Heitkemper, M., Hanson, R., and Hansen, B.E. 1977. Effects of rate and volume of tube feeding in normal human subjects. In Batey, M.V. editor. Communicating nursing research; optimizing environments for health, nursing's unique perspective. Boulder, Colo. Western Interstate Commission for High Education, 10:91-95.

Henderson, V. 1977. We've "come a long way" but what of the direction, Nursing Research 26:163-164.

Johnson, M.L. 1975. Medical sociology and sociological theory, Social Science and Medicine 9:227-232.

Krieger, D., Peper E., and Ancoli, S. 1979. Therapeutic touch—searching for evidence of physiological change, American Journal of Nursing 79:660-662.

Krueger, J.C., Nelson, A.H., and Wolanin, M.O.: 1978. Nursing research: development, collaboration, and utilization, Germantown, Md., Aspen Systems Corp.

Leininger, M. 1967. The culture concept and its relevance to nursing, Journal of Nursing Education 6:27-37.

Leininger, M. 1969. Ethnoscience: a promising research approach to improve nursing practice, Image 3:22-28.

Leininger, M. 1972. Using cultural styles in the helping process and in relation to the subculture of nursing, Nursing papers at the Illinois Psychiatric Institute, May 13-14, Chicago, 1971, Illinois Psychiatric Institute, pp. 43-61.

Leininger, M. 1973. Becoming aware of types of health practitioners and cultural imposition. In American Nurses Association 48th Convention Papers, Kansas City, American Nurses Association, pp. 9-15.

Leininger, M. 1976. Towards conceptualization of transcultural health care systems: concepts and a model. In Leininger, M. editor. Transcultural health care issues and conditions, Philadelphia, F.A. Davis Co., pp. 3-22.

Leininger, M.: 1978. Transcultural nursing: concepts, theories and practices, New York, John Wiley & Sons, Inc.

Leonard, R.C. 1975. The application of behavioral science to patient care as illustrated by the etiology and control of stress in clinical settings. In Verhonick, P.J. editor. Nursing research I, Boston, Little Brown & Co.

Lewin, K. 1935. A dynamic theory of personality, New York, McGraw-Hill. (D.K. Adams and K.E. Zenner, translators.)

Macrae, J. 1979. Therapeutic touch in practice. American Journal of Nursing 79:664-665.

Masur, F.T. 1979. An update on medical psychology and behavioral medicine. Professional Psychology 10259-264.

Olesen, V.L. 1975. Convergences and divergences: anthropology and sociology in health care, Social Science and Medicine 9:421-425.

Orlando, I.J. 1961. The dynamic nurse-patient relationship, New York, G.P. Putnam's Sons.

Orlando, I.J. 1972. The discipline and teaching and teaching of nursing process, New York, G.P. Putnam's Sons.

Parsons, T. 1950. The social system, New York, The Free Press.

Peplau, H. 1951. Interpersonal relations in nursing, New York, G.P. Putnam's Sons.

Pitel, M. and Vian, J. 1975. Analysis of nurse doctorates: data collected for the international directory of nurses with doctoral degrees, Nursing Research 24:340-351.

Porter, L. 1972. The impact of physical-physiological activity on infants growth and development, Nursing Research 21:210-219.

Powers, M.J. and Woolridge, P.J. 1982. Factors influencing knowledge, attitudes and compliance of hypertensive patients, Research in Nursing and Health, 5:171-182.

Quinn, J.F. 1979. One nurse's evolution as a healer, American Journal of Nursing 79:662-664.

Rosenthal, R. 1976. Experimenter effects in behavioral research, New York, Halsted Press.

Rogers, M.E. 1970. An introduction to the theoretical basis of nursing, Philadelphia, F.A. Davis Co.

Saunders, L. 1954. The changing role of nurses, American Journal of Nursing 54:1094-1098.

Schlotfeldt, I.M. 1977. Nursing research: reflection of values, Nursing Research 26:4-9.

Schmitt, M.H. 1968. Role conflict in nursing, American Journal of Nursing 68:2348-2350.

Schulman, S. 1958. Basic functional roles in nursing: mother surrogate and healer, In Jaco, E.G. editor. Patients, physicians, and illness. New York, The Free Press, pp. 528-537.

Sills, M. 1977. Research in the field of psychiatric nursing 1952-1977, Nursing Research 26:201-207.

Simmons, L.W. and Henderson, V. 1964. Nursing research: a survey and assessment, New York, Appleton-Century-Crofts.

Skipper, J.K., Jr. 1965. The role of the hospital nurse: is it instrumental or expressive? In Skipper, J.K., Jr. and Leonard, R.C., editors. Social interaction and patient care, Philadelphia, J.B. Lippincott Co., pp. 40-48.

Skipper, J.K., Jr., and Leonard, R.C. 1965. Social interaction and patient care, Philadelphia, J.B. Lippincott Co.

Stevens, B. 1979. Nursing theory: analysis, application and evaluation, Boston, Little, Brown and Co.

Ujhely, G.B. 1968. Determinants of the nurse-patient relationship, New York, Springer Publishing Co., Inc.

Verhonick, P.J., Lewis, D.W., and Goller, H.O. 1972. Thermography in the study of decubitus ulcers: preliminary report, Nursing Research 21:233-237.

Walike, B.C., et al. 1975. Patient problems related to tube feeding. In Batey, M.V., editor. Communicating nursing research: critical issues in access to data, Boulder, Colo. Western Interstate Commission for Higher Education, 7:89-112.

Wooldridge, P.J., Skipper, J.K., Jr., and Leonard, R.C. 1968. Behavioral science, social practice, and the nursing profession, Cleveland, Press of Case Western Reserve University.

Wooldridge, P.J., Leonard, R.C. and Skipper, J.K., Jr. 1978. Methods of clinical experimentation to improve patient care, St. Louis, The C.V. Mosby Co.

SECTION THREE

Nursing researchers and practice theory

THIS SECTION contains three chapters written by nursing researchers who we asked to discuss the way that theory affects research and research affects theory in terms of the development of their research, emphasizing:

1. The way that theoretical formulations influenced the study design and/or the interpretation of quantitative and qualitative results
2. The way that the research results led to the confirmation or modification of various aspects of the theory
3. The way that theory was combined with initial research results to generate further research and theory development

Each author was further directed, "write your chapter your own way, so that it reflects the ways that *you* use theory in your research and develop theory from your research."

The three chapters in this section show in some ways a sharp distinction between the abstract ideals in the first two sections and the reality of actual research and theory building. They were chosen to

117

represent differences in developmental stages of research and theory building as well as differences in methodology and theoretical orientations. For the most part, these chapters are presented as the authors wrote them, but we have edited some sections to clarify the relationship between the point the author is making and the ideas in first section of this book. Although each of the authors had read *Behavioral Science, Social Practice, and The Nursing Profession* (Wooldridge, Skipper, and Leonard, 1968), only the chapter by Benoliel makes much use of the analytical terms presented in Section One, and none of the authors explicitly uses the concepts and terms of the nursing theorists in Section Two. You are encouraged to examine these presentations in terms of the general principles presented in the first section of the book and to reach your own conclusions as to (1) where each use of theory fits in the paradigm and (2) the strengths and weaknesses of the research and theoretical interpretations in clarifying implications for clinical practice. Once you have attempted your own analyses, you can compare them with the analyses of Wooldridge and Schmitt in Section Four.

CHAPTER 4

DEVELOPING THEORY FROM PRACTICE
alternative models in nursing care

Ida M. Martinson
Paul V. Martinson

DEVELOPING A DESCRIPTIVE BASE
Initial assumptions

The study discussed in this chapter grew out of a conversation with a neighbor, Dr. John Kersey, a pediatric oncologist. One evening he mentioned a 10-year-old boy, Eric, who had leukemia with central nervous system complications. Eric had reached the end of cure-oriented treatment. During this conversation, I remembered my experience 2 years before, when my family cared for my dying father-in-law at home. As a nurse I had helped make this process possible, and the whole family appreciated those last days. I suggested to Dr. Kersey that perhaps nursing support would enable Eric's parents to keep him at home. The following day he told Eric's parents of my interest in helping them care for Eric. They called that night, and the next morning I made my first visit, 17 days before Eric died at home.

Before this time I had been giving considerable thought to the nature and practice of nursing research. What was nursing research? Nursing research had to do with health care, but what type of research was appropriate? It was important to demonstrate within the health care system that nursing research could make a difference. One of the ways this might be done was to explore alternative methods of delivering care and to evaluate the feasibility and desirability of such care. Allowing children with terminal illness to die at home through the provision of nursing care might provide a good focus for nursing research. The combination of this incident with my interest in nursing research began a process of research and practice that has spanned several years.

A major benefit of the process has been the opportunity to rethink the whole question of nursing research. Initially I thought nursing research was the systematic investigation of anything having to do with patient care. This idea has proven inadequate for a number of reasons, most important of which is the discovery that the total patient situation must be accounted for and that individual and discrete studies must be done within this total perspective. This led me to an expanded definition of nursing research: nursing research is a systematic investigation of patient care that takes into account the total patient situation as a complex set of interactions between physical, psychological, emotional, social, and cultural factors. Among other things, such research involves the patient as primary care receiver, and the family (or immediate social unit) as the larger unit of care, both being cared for because of illness. The research of a nurse is distinct from the research of a physiologist, who studies physical factors in relative isolation from the psychosocial environment. It is distinct from that of the psychologist, since physical factors are directly assessed along with psychological ones. It differs from that of the anthropologist, since the nurse as a researcher is an *active* agent involved in a situation that changes during the very process of research. Not only does the situation continually undergo change, but the nurse, who is no mere observer, is an *active* agent who continually interacts with the situation during the very process of study. The nurse-researcher is different from the medical researcher because nursing care takes all of the named factors into account in addition to medical needs. As the American Nurses Association definition (1975) states, nursing research is research "having to do with the interface between the behavioral and physical sciences."

Clarifying the question

As I began my initial research experience, I was troubled by many questions. The most important of these were: Would parents who are laypersons be able to provide all of the care required by a sick child in the final stage of cancer? Would the child's home provide a suitable facility for such care? What would be the effect on siblings? Would the nursing profession be willing and able to help families provide the care at home? Would the physician be willing to make the decision to end cure-oriented therapy, thereby acknowledging the irreversible and terminal nature of the disease? What would be the reaction of neighbors; would they indicate disapproval of the home rather than the hospital as the place of death? These and other questions could be summarized in one basic question: "Is home care feasible for a child dying of cancer and if it is feasible, is it desirable?" The next 7 years were essentially devoted to developing the descriptive base that would answer this basic question. Could it be done? Could a child dying of cancer be cared for at home?

Findings

Between 1972 and 1976 the study continued with a case method approach. In 1976 funding was received from the Department of Health, Education, and Welfare, National Cancer Institute for a 3-year nursing research study (Grant #CA 19490). During the first 2 years of the project, 58 families with a child who died of cancer participated. Of these children, 46 died at home, 11 reentered and died in a hospital, and 1 died in an ambulance en route to a hospital. Data in the project are from three principal sources: medical records, service documentation, and interviews.

The child's medical record provided the essential data included in the history of the child's disease. Not all data proved to be of equal value. That which we found most helpful concerned the time of diagnosis, the course of the disease, and the nursing and medical management. The types of cancers involved were acute lymphoblastic leukemia, acute nonlymphoblastic leukemia, congenital leukemia, Ewing's sarcoma, neuroblastoma, ependymoma, astrocytoma, medulloblastoma, Burkitt's lymphoma, lymphoblastic lymphoma, rhabdomyosarcoma, malignant histiocytosis, and undifferentiated lymphoma. As the project continued, various checklists were developed to ease the problem of data collection, and at the time of the 2-year postdeath interview the parents completed the symptom checklist (SCL-90-R; see Martinson, 1978).

The second important data source was the service documentation. This documentation was extensive and thorough. Not only did it help answer questions initially identified, but it raised new questions and also helped to answer them. Throughout the project, nurses involved with the family kept detailed accounts. Every home visit and telephone call was recorded, the time and an indication as to who had been the initiator was noted, and the content of the contact was stated.

Not only was the third source of data, the interview records, the most extensive; it also served as the core for project analysis. The procedure was quite thorough. The parents were interviewed in their own homes at four times. The regularly scheduled interviews were at 1 month, 6 months, 12 months, and 24 months after the death of the child. Notes were taken by trained interviewers during the greater part of the first 2 years. During the third year of the project, most interviews were tape recorded. This was done by a trained interviewer who had also lost a child to cancer and had a personal sense of the most appropriate questions to ask. The recordings were then transcribed for analysis. In the case of the few families that preferred not to be taped, the interviewer recorded the interview by shorthand and then prepared a typewritten script for analysis. Others were interviewed in addition to parents. These included 84 nurses who had served as either primary, coprimary, or backup nurses; 27 physicians, with 3 physicians interviewed twice; 12 members of the clergy; 29 siblings, either in groups or individually; and 22 grandparents.

One family of the 58 did not wish to be interviewed after the death of their child. Another family was interviewed 3 times, but declined the 24-month interview. A third family refused the 6-month interview, but one of the parents called later wishing to take part in the remaining 12- and 24-month interviews. On one occasion, when the interviewer failed to keep an appointment, the family chose not to reschedule that interview. In that case the remaining 24-month interview was later completed. To date, 234 parent interviews have been completed. This high rate of continued involvement was of great benefit to the study. Perhaps this is in part because of the appreciation for the service provided by the project. However, most families indicated that the interviews gave them an opportunity to help others in the future as well as to talk to someone who understood what they had been through. This last reason held especially in the case of the interviewer who herself was a parent who had lost a child.

It is from this base of data that we were eventually able to answer many of the questions that had initially concerned us. The question concerning the feasibility of the home as a health care facility proved to be the easiest to answer. Some of our initial concerns in this area related to matters of convenience (such as access to the bathroom and stairs), equipment (IV setups and oxygen) and tasks requiring specialized equipment and skills (such as administration of oxygen). As it turned out, all these potential problems proved to be relatively easy to avoid or overcome.

Let us take, for instance, the example of equipment and its management. It was discovered that in the majority of cases of children who died at home (24 to 46), no hospital-type equipment was needed. A variety of equipment was needed for the other 22. Six children required oxygen, which family members were able to handle without mishap. Four children required suctioning, and a suction machine was obtained and the parents were trained in its use. Four of the children required intravenous fluids, and securing the necessary equipment was no major problem. All intravenous feedings were initiated by a health professional, but parents or other family members supervised the infusion. Only two children required indwelling urinary catheters, which were inserted by nurses. The parents cared for the catheter subsequently. The condom urinary catheter worked well for three boys. Only one child had a gavage feeding tube, which was inserted in the hospital; feedings continued at home. In no case did a child return to the hospital because of a lack of equipment available for use at home.

We similarly discovered that a majority of cases did not require even more ordinary hospital furnishings. Wheelchairs were used by 14 of the children, and a hospital bed by 7. Several children did not even require supplies such as Chux, swabs, and similar items.

Other factors of initial concern, such as the convenience of the bathroom to the ill child, were not mentioned as difficulties by any of the families in the study. In fact, most of the children wanted to be in the living room or family room, in the center of family activity. While the home environment did not offer the ready availability of specialized equipment (though all necessary equipment was procurable), the home provided an atmosphere, quite in contrast to the institutional setting, in which the parents could feel in control.

Another initial concern was the adaptability of nurses to the different sort of role they would be asked to play. A major determinant in our model of nursing for home care was the role of the parents. In contrast to institutional nursing care, home care would involve the parents as the primary care givers. To be sure, this care giving would not be possible without the active participation and guidance of the nurse, but the nurse's role would tend to be more supervisory than direct. The history of the project demonstrates clearly that nurses have the resources and ability to adapt to this alternative health care delivery system and its many differing kinds of demands.

After a successful experience with the first family, the physician questioned whether the care provided could be replicated. His suspicion was that factors that went beyond strict nursing factors accounted for its success. Perhaps certain matters of personal background and skill on the part of the nurse were involved. The next case involved a family 250 miles away. In this case a nurse in that area provided services. The third family requested to be involved with home care. The physician involved in that case made the referral to Dr. Kersey, the physician with whom I had been working. We worked together with this family, and the child did die at home. It was now quite apparent to me that home nursing care could provide for the medical needs of dying children, and subsequent experience continued to confirm this.

For each of the families, we needed to locate a nurse who would be available and close enough to make a home visit whenever the family requested. One half of the children lived outside the Minneapolis-St. Paul area, including rural areas and neighboring states. While more time was spent locating a nurse in these areas, a nurse was always found. In fact, a total of 58 different nurses served as a primary or coprimary nurse, and for almost all of the nurses this was a new experience. One half of the nurses had baccalaureate degrees. All but four were registered nurses. Most of the nurses had not previously been in a situation in which they were on call 24 hours a day, 7 days a week; however, after the experience the nurses made no real criticism of that requirement.

One of the important conclusions we derived from our study was that parents could become the primary care givers with the nurse as the key health professional who counseled and guided them with respect to caring for their child. At the same time both the nurse and the parents maintained a close relationship with the physician, who served as consultant at a still more general level. Other members of the health team were not routinely involved but sometimes served as consultants to the nurse, the family, and the physician as needed. Other than the clergy, these other members of the health care team did not become involved except by referral from the primary nurse involved.

Another initial concern was whether the physician would find it possible to stop cure-oriented therapy when the child was cared for at home. In many cases, physicians did make such a decision. Several were quite clear in their acceptance of responsibility for deciding whether or not to continue cure-oriented therapy. Others continued to treat beyond the point where cure-oriented therapy seemed medically indicated, feeling that they were thereby "helping the family retain hope."

While the question of when to stop cure-oriented therapy did not pose much of a problem for the care givers in the home, the physicians had varying attitudes as to the advisability of home care. Some physicians were willing to attempt it whereas others were adamantly opposed. In one situation the physician was not supportive of the program but the family had requested to be involved. The home care nurse remained in close contact with the physician, and the family gave their child excellent care. After this experience the physician was much more open to home care as an option. Other physicians believed they were already providing home care, since one or two of their patients had died at home; however, they did not make the program generally available to all their patients.

It was rather surprising to find that though neighbors were generally supportive there were several incidents in which misunderstanding or insensitivity was apparent. Although the attitude and support of neighbors is by no means as critical as the other factors we have mentioned, it is nonetheless important for the parents to have a sense of acceptance within their wider community. The data bearing on this issue were not systematically quantified, but one example may illustrate the kind of misunderstanding that sometimes arose.

A mother telephoned me and started the conversation by saying, "I think you need to hear this." Inwardly apprehensive, I listened as she related an incident. While she was on her way to the grocery store, a neighbor stopped her and remarked, "Oh, isn't it too bad you didn't get your child to the hospital before he died?" As I listened, the mother paused and I wondered what to say. Then she began to laugh and said, "She doesn't know where it is at, does she?" When interviewed later, this mother told us that she would probably have thought the same herself until it happened to her own child. In her experience, she learned how much it meant to her child to be at home until the end.

Probably the most difficult question to answer was whether the siblings of the dying child might be negatively affected by having the child die in the home. Preliminary analysis of the data indicates that before the child's death, most siblings were frightened at the prospect of the child's dying. However, of the 29 siblings interviewed afterward, all expressed the sentiment that the dying wasn't "scary." Following the death of her eldest daughter, one mother wrote:

> One of the heavy burdens for me was the feeling of such major responsibility for meeting the emotional needs of the other children. Having Brenda at home helped immensely, because they were able to verbalize with her as well as with me. Having her at home seemed to reassure them a lot and seemed to make death a much less frightening thing and heaven more real to them (Martinson, 1979).

Certainly, the death of a sibling is difficult for the remaining children; however, the available evidence consistently indicates that the siblings and their parents believed that having the child die at home had actually lessened the sibling's fears from what they might have been otherwise.

The following case study is included to provide an illustration of a family's reactions to having their child die at home. Data for the case study were abstracted from the 1-month and 6-month interviews with the parents and interviews of the family minister, hospital nurse, and home care nurse, as well as from the home care nurse's case notes, project staff notes, and physician comments and medical records.

The patient was a 14-year-old girl with neuroblastoma. Her disease had been diagnosed 5 years before her death, and she had had seven hospitalizations for surgery, chemotherapy, or radiation. At the time of her referral to the home care project, she was in a Minneapolis-St. Paul area hospital, although the family lived in a small town over 100 miles away. The father was a skilled blue-collar worker with high school and vocational school degrees, and the mother was a homemaker with a high school degree. There were two other children, ages 13 and 9, in the family.

The family heard about the home care project through an acquaintance, the mother of another child with cancer. When normal cure-oriented treatments were exhausted the patient's mother contacted the staff herself, and the patient entered the program sooner than might otherwise have been the case. Initial contact by a project staff nurse was made a few days before the patient was discharged from the hospital. The patient was scheduled to return to the hospital weekly for 3 weeks to receive a new drug as an outpatient.

The project staff spent an afternoon telephoning nursing agencies near the family's home to locate a home care nurse. A public health nurse with a bachelor's degree who lived 30 minutes from the family's home agreed to serve in that capacity. The local county public health agency agreed to provide a back-up nurse. This was the first such case for the primary home care nurse. An explanation of fundamental issues pertinent to the case was given to her by the home care staff over the telephone. Written materials concerning home care, medications, and cancer were then mailed to her. While this was a suboptimal way to recruit and inform the nurse, such procedures were often made necessary by the rural character of Minnesota. This nurse proved to be resourceful; for example, she sought out and read books on death and dying and contacted other nurses she knew or the project staff when she was unsure of the best approach. She later reported, however, that her experience with home care had demanded a great deal of her energies, given the uniqueness of the situation for her.

The patient's mother was a competent woman; however, she had a need to talk at some length. This latter attribute was expressed over the course of the home care in an unusually large number of long telephone calls to the nurse. The first problem the mother telephoned the nurse about occurred the second day the child was at home. It concerned difficulty getting her to take her pain medication since swallowing was difficult. The nurse made some suggestions; however, this problem resolved itself since the girl managed to swallow the medication even without efforts to make it easier. When the patient went home from the hospital, she was suffering some pain and had been taking a combination of meperidine hydrochloride (Demerol), hydroxyzine pamoate (Vistaril), and acetaminophen (Tylenol) with codeine. These, as well as an antiemetic, and been sent home with the family. Provision for obtaining morphine in liquid form from local sources was explored should the need arise.

One week after the child went home the nurse made her first home visit. She examined the girl and instructed the mother in techniques for making the child's sore feet less irritated. The patient was spending the days on the living room couch and moving to her bedroom at night. In talking privately with the mother, the nurse determined that the mother seemed to understand the gravity of her child's condition—that is, she had begun to think about her child's funeral arrangements. She was, however, uncomfortable using the word *cancer* in conversation; she referred to "that six-letter word."

A few days after the home visit, the mother called the nurse and reported that the patient was vomiting and experiencing increased pain. The nurse recommended administration of the antiemetic that was in the home and called the project staff for their recommendation concerning how to handle the pain. The project staff nurse, following consultation with the physician, recommended an increase in dosage to the home care nurse, who related this to the mother. It should be noted that one or another of the project staff nurses was available for consultation with the home care nurse 24 hours a day. In other cases the child's physician might be contacted, or the home care nurse would use her own judgment within ranges that had been recommended by the physician in deciding on dosage changes. Another involvement of project staff in this case was recommending that the child's primary hospital nurse telephone the home care nurse. She did so and they discussed the child's past nursing care and current treatment. The hospital nurse contact with the primary home care public health nurse was almost always a source of helpful information and support.

Frequent telephone contact with the mother and home care nurse continued. In one telephone call from the mother the patient's sore feet were discussed further and the home care nurse arranged for a sheepskin pad to be delivered.

After 3 weeks of the new drug treatment, which was not successful, the child's physician explained to the patient and the family that while there might be other drugs they could try, there was a poor chance they would be effective. The patient herself then made the decision to stay home rather than seek further treatment. In her own words from a letter she wrote to her friends at school, she stated:

> They have other drugs that could be tried, but with about the same percentage of success. So I have made my decision—no more drugs. It gets very discouraging when there aren't any more veins left to start IV's in. I want to spend my time at home with my family and my pet.

At that point, inclusion in the home care project would normally have been offered if the mother had not initiated the contact already. The mother's initiative had resulted in inclusion 3 weeks earlier. In staying home with no further cure-oriented treatment, the mother looked forward to caring for her daughter as long as possible, but anticipated that her daughter would eventually enter and die in their local hospital.

This family was very religious, and their minister was an important source of support during the patient's illness. The home care nurse called the minister, introduced herself, and brought him up to date on the patient's condition and prognosis.

Telephone contact between the mother and home care nurse continued at the rate of about one call every other day. The mother was doing a good job caring for her daughter, with her husband and two other children providing only a small amount of direct assistance. Neighbors and nearby relatives were very good about bringing in meals and also doing the laundry.

The patient at that time was having trouble voiding urine, and the home care nurse suggested to the mother methods of encouraging urination as well as ascertaining the need for incontinence pads. A few days later, she made her second home visit. She instructed the mother in the Credé method of voiding. The patient's condition had continued to deteriorate. She had lost much weight and moved very slowly. She was not in much pain, however.

The nurse contacted the child's local physician regarding his signing of the death certification when necessary. Also about this time, this is, 1 month after the termination of cure-oriented treatment, a meeting took place at the request of the minister between the parents, the home care nurse, and the minister himself. He talked to the parents about their anxieties and grief. They began planning the funeral service, which he would conduct.

The patient continued to get weaker. She now spent all of her time on the living room couch rather than going to her bedroom at night. She was unable to drink from a glass without spilling and began to take liquids from a baby bottle. She was extremely slow at everything she did, but she still asserted her independence by feeding herself or changing her gown. The mother found this very trying but let her daughter continue even though it consumed a great deal of time.

On the third visit to the home, the nurse dropped off pressure pads for bedsores. By this time, the patient had lost a great deal of weight. She was asleep during the visit, and the nurse talked with the mother. Such conversation, as well as most telephone calls, continued to provide comfort and reassurance. The nurse also imparted technical information on the use of medication.

Over the next 2 weeks, telephone contacts between the mother and nurse occurred almost daily. The nurse had an emesis basin delivered to assist the mother in her daughter's mouth care. The patient was groggy much of the time and no longer received visitors. She was not in much pain, and pain medication had been greatly reduced.

About 2 months after the end of cure-oriented treatment, the mother called the nurse to tell her the patient had died. The girl had displayed slower breathing the night before. In the morning her mother observed that the girl's breaths were shallow. The mother was making breakfast in the kitchen, and when she returned to the living room she discovered her daughter had stopped breathing. It had been a quiet death, with no one present in the room though all family members were in the house and awake. The mother called the nurse about 1 hour after the death. She did not wish the nurse to come to the home; this case was atypical in that regard. The mother had already contacted the minister and the mortuary. The nurse then contacted the local physician and the oncologist, as well as the project staff. Four days later, the nurse attended a memorial service for the patient and talked briefly with the parents. The parents volunteered the information that they were very happy their daughter had died at home with the rest of the family. The parents reported that all members of the family openly cried when the girl died. The father was pleased that his son did so, since he had been worried that the boy had been "holding back" his feelings about his sister's condition too much. Sporadic telephone contacts with the mother were made by the home care nurse for several months following the death. This mother did not seem to need much support from the nurse at that time.

Both parents adjusted well to the death of their daughter. When interviewed at 1 and 6 months after the death, they reported no lasting sleep disturbances or other psychosomatic complaints. Both talked openly about their daughter and about cancer. As we have noted, the mother had in the past been reluctant to use the word *cancer*. Both parents had, at 6 months after the death, resumed almost all their former work and social activities. Their minister and their faith continued to be a great source of support for them.

PRACTICE THEORY

The general means for successful home care of the dying child that evolved from the research just reported can be divided into four aspects:
1. Encouraging parental control
2. Limiting uncertainty .
3. Giving priority to comfort
4. Providing an integrating matrix.

Encouraging parental control as a general principle for effective care is recommended only with limiting uncertainty as a precondition. This enables the assumption of parental control to be effective. Giving priority to comfort concerns the setting of goals for care given to the patient, providing an integrating matrix refers to the nurses' role in coordinating health care delivery, and acting as a consultant to the parents.

It soon became obvious from the research that "home care" and "care in the home" are two different things. Home care is not merely a transfer of place for doing the care; it involves a complete reordering of perspective and priorities for nursing. The role and function of the nurse in home care needs to be redefined. By encouraging parental control we mean encouraging parents to assume as much control of the patient's care as possible, with the nurse providing needed supervision, guidance, and support. What led to this concept was necessity (the nurse could not be there 24 hours a day), and, after experimentation, the discovery that parents were not only able but eager to assume the role of care giver. Our experience led us to change our concept of the roles and functions of the nurse and of the parents in the provision of home care to the child.

What then are some of the important functions of the nurse in this role? In working with the family, the nurse must teach the parents whatever they need to know not only to feel that they are in control of the situation, but actually to be in control. What the nurse must teach includes not only explaining how the child may physiologically die but also, what the feelings are that can go along with this. The nurse must sift through past clinical experiences and educational background to identify everything that it is necessary to teach the parents so they can effectively assume control.

The second aspect of the means, limiting uncertainty, evolved out of the need to encourage parental control. To apply this principle, the nurse posits a particular eventuality (for example, hemorrhaging), states the extremes (from massive hemmorrhage to slight or temporary bleeding), and then specifies a few points in between, which represent the more likely eventualities. At the time of referral, parental uncertainty is most likely to involve concern as to whether or not they will be able to provide the necessary care and handle whatever emergencies may arise. During the time the child is home, the uncertainty on the part of the parents is most often centered on the daily needs of the child—the physiological needs of nutritional intake, regularity of void-ing and bowel movements, sufficient activity for proper functioning, turning to prevent bedsores, and so forth. At the time of death, there is most often uncertainty regarding changes that may take place in the child, such as Cheyne-Stokes respiration. Almost all parents need preparation for such changes. Immediately after death, many parents are uncertain as to whether specific authorities have to be called in, at what specific time to summon them, and in what order (for instance, should the physician or funeral home be called first?). Following the child's death, parents often wonder if the feel-ings they are experiencing are normal.

Therapeutic care and comfort are not quite the same thing. Traditionally, nursing care assigns a higher priority to the patient's long-range needs and comfort than to his short-term wants and immediate comfort. For example, a patient with mouth sores is traditionally discouraged from eating spicy foods. Comfort care, in contrast, sets more immediate priorities defined more by the immediate wants of the patient than by supposed long-term needs. For ex-ample, comfort care would dictate that if the child with mouth sores wants to eat spicy foods, the child should be allowed to do so. It is proximity to the time of dying that justifies giving priority to comfort care, which is based on the principle of acceding as much as possible to the wants of the patient.

If parental control is to be effectively realized, it is necessary that health care resources be available to them when and as they are needed. This is made possible by providing an *integrating matrix* of complex interactions involving a variety of factors. As death draws near, the patient's medical needs often progressively lessen, while needs of other kinds progressively increase. Relations within the family may become very complex at this time, and the nurse must be able to find the resources that are necessary for the family to maintain maximum functioning without undue fatigue. For some families the clergy member or the spiritual leader may play a very significant part, while in others the help of grandparents is an asset. For some families the nurse needs to make possible the conditions that will give the family the privacy they desire. Almost invariably the nurse has some interaction with and coordinates the desires of the funeral home personnel, the primary phy-sician, and the coordinator for the home care services. Without the nurse providing these integrating functions, parental control would not be possible and home care would simply become care in the home.

The proposed nursing practice principle may be summarized as follows: when caring for the family of a child who is dying at home, the nurse should teach the parents how to give basic nursing care to the child, help them cognitively structure what changes to expect, and assist them in obtaining needed resources at various critical illness points. This will lead to a reduction of parental uncertainty and an increase in perceived parental control, which will in turn promote patient satisfaction, comfort and security, and family adjustment to the death of the child.

Practice guidelines

In a manual developed for delivery of home care services for children dying of cancer, specific guidelines for nursing care were included, based on the general principles just stated. The guidelines divide the responsibilities into time segments including time of referral, the interim phase, the point when the child is no longer responding to curative efforts, the period of dying, death itself, and the period after death.

At the time of referral, one thing the parents must know is how to reach the nurse at all times through use of a beeper or by telephone. The nurse's role should be that of facilitating the care and guaranteeing that quality care is being provided, with reassurance to the family that this is in fact so. She should constantly observe the family, assess their situation, and act accordingly. The nurse should be alert to such things as How tired are the parents? Do they need additional short-term help such as a home health aide, a relative coming in to sleep one night, or possibly even the nurse herself staying overnight? The nurse should look at the resources for equipment and supplies, know where oxygen can be obtained if necessary, know how to get drugs and to make sure that at night and on weekends adequate medication will be available, know what is available from the American Cancer Society, such as hospital beds (although these have not been as important as we would have thought), Chux, wheelchairs, and so forth. Other available resources should be identified, such as equipment, rental agencies, ambulance services, and homemaker services, as well as various financial and support resources. (We have found that Candlelighters, a national organized support group for parents of children with cancer, is helpful.)

During the interim (or maintenance) period, the families will perhaps need a weekly visit from the nurse to observe their child's nutrition, changes in appetite, taste, and eating habits. While it is desirable to try to provide high-calorie foods or high-protein supplements, the nurse should encourage the parents to permit the child to eat more or less what he wants. The nurse should be alerted if problems such as nausea, weight loss, anemia, or constipation arise. It is important that constipation be prevented, since enemas may be contraindicated. It is important that parents keep a record of bowel movements. Even with a limited food intake, a bowel movement every 2 or 3 days or the child's normal pattern should be maintained.

Major emphasis should be given to pain control. We have found that methadone is extremely helpful. Long-acting pain control, such as medications that only need to be given every 8 hours, will be effective for most of the families involved. Adequate sleep is essential for the parents, as well as the child, to prevent fatigue on the part of the primary care givers.

With regard to physical care, parents should be taught to prevent skin breakdown, to perform mouth care, to administer medications, and to use technical skills. Parents have been taught to give injections, to change IV bottles, to suction, to monitor oxygen, and to irrigate catheters. Procedures should be demonstrated to the parent and then the nurse should observe as the parent performs the technique. Close supervision may be needed, but parents have been able to learn such techniques and keep accurate records.

Another area the nurse should encourage is maintenance of family life. Parental decision making should be supported. Parents should also be informed of the possibility of bleeding, high fever, respiratory difficulties, and seizures, if there is a possibility they may occur. In preparation for the death, parents should be encouraged to express their feelings and to talk about the availability of the nurse and other support persons, the behavioral changes that may occur, and perhaps, funeral arrangements.

Near the time of the death, it is important for the nurse to teach the families about the physiology of dying. Parents should be told there is a great deal we do not know but told about the expected manner of death for the type of disease and the complications involved. It is important to be sure the parents understand that as the dying process occurs there is not too much they can do wrong. Parents should be told to check temperature and pulse. Respiration changes often frighten parents, and they should be encouraged to understand Cheyne-Stokes respiration as well as central nervous system involvement and possible actions. If parents ask how much longer it will take their child to die when no one knows definitely, they must be listened to by the nurse and their questions answered to the best of her ability. We have found that if a family does want to know, the nurse's best judgment should be used, even though it may be in error. Frequently the health professional is embarrassed by predicting 3 days when the child lives 2 weeks. This does not seem to bother the family as much as the health professional; a time framework seems to be helpful to parents even if it is later proved incorrect.

At the time of the death it is important to support family members. After the physician has been notified, the physician is perhaps the best one to notify the county coroner or medical examiner. The mortician should be told which physician to call as well as the phone number so that difficulties regarding removal of the body from the home will be avoided. In most areas dying at home is not the expected thing, and it is important to avoid any difficulty with authorities. If the nurse can arrange for removal of equipment and supplies immediately it is often of help to the family.

After the death it is usually desirable for the nurse to maintain contact with the family, but the amount of contact that is appropriate does vary. Some families feel they do not need much nurse contact after the child's death; others greatly appreciate a rather close follow-up by the nurse involved.

From our data, it is difficult to say which kinds of families can and cannot care for their child at home. We have found that, regardless of their socioeconomic status or educational level, most families have been very capable of giving quality care. It is important, however, that there be support from the nursing staff.

Institutionalization of home care

This study began without institutional support or legitimation, since such a "home care for a dying child with cancer" alternative system had not, to our knowledge, been previously developed. However, while home care is health care in a noninstitutional setting, this does not mean that it cannot be institutionalized as a legitimate alternative. The study would not have been complete unless the general feasibility or nonfeasibility of institutionalizing home care as an alternative health care delivery system was tested. This, of course, raised a whole new set of questions, and, in some cases, obstacles.

The institutionalizing phase of the program began 6 weeks before the end of the second year of the 3-year grant received from the National Cancer Institute, but the planning for this implementation phase began long before that. In fact, in the beginning of 1973, after I had worked with several families, I made an appointment with the director of the University of Minnesota Hospitals to discuss the possibility of the hospital carrying out such a program. His advice at that time was to contact Blue Cross of Minnesota. After attending a management-level meeting at the headquarters of that organization, I wrote a letter requesting payment for nurses involved in this type of care. They responded with a letter in which they refused to cover such costs, but encouraged me to submit a grant for the research and development aspects. After receiving considerable help from the Blue Cross organization, I developed a grant proposal and submitted it to them for possible funding. The grant was neither approved nor disapproved; however, I received a letter expressing regret that no funds were available for this endeavor. I then made a decision to submit a proposal to the National Institutes of Health. These contacts with the University of Minnesota Hospitals and the insurance company were part of the necessary preparation for institutionalization.

Of additional crucial importance was the development of the University of Minnesota Hospitals' Home Health Services Department. When direct care services were stopped at the third year of the grant, the transition to the University of Minnesota Hospitals' Home Care program proceeded with only a minimum of difficulty. Six months after the transition, we were unable to identify any children dying in the hospital who had not been offered the alternative of home care. Four children died in the hospital under active, cure-oriented treatment.

The second agency to implement home care was St. Louis Park Medical Center, under a nurse coordinator who worked with two pediatric oncologists. By the end of a 6-month period she had worked with two families, one involving a public health nursing agency, the other a part-time hospital RN, and successfully coordinated the effort. She was experiencing minimal difficulty.

The third agency to implement home care was the Children's Health Center of Minneapolis. The director of nursing for the Children's Health Center has participated on the Home Care Research Grant advisory committee since the beginning of the federally funded program. With her leadership, a coordinator position was funded and a two-phase program for home care was developed at the institution. At the end of 6 months, referrals began to be made to the department and relationships were being established throughout the Health Center. Both the Health Center and the University Hospitals received strong administrative support so that the remaining difficulties were in establishing the necessary relationships and providing for the flow of referrals.

A fourth group was the public health nursing agencies throughout the state of Minnesota and the surrounding states who have almost without exception provided home care for children in their areas. They did this in spite of limited personnel and resources.

Issues and future directions

One potentially prohibitive issue in providing home care for the dying child is cost. While it may seem less expensive to avoid hospitalization, some have raised the objection that conventional cost analyses ignore such factors as the cost of work days lost by attending parents.

We consider only such costs as charges for professional services, overhead, supplies, equipment, and so forth in our cost data, since that is the system used by home health agencies, hospitals, and third-party payers. The more sophisticated analyses, such as that done by Lansky (1979) on the broad-ranging costs of childhood cancer, (child's wardrobe, restaurant meals, missed employment, and so forth), are interesting but beyond the scope of the present project except insofar as hidden costs of home care would be an unusual burden to the family. While the cost of food, linen, laundry, and heating while a child is in the hospital is part of the hospital bill, we do not consider such items in the child's residence in the cost of home care, since, though they are real, they are (1) part of a normal healthy child's expenses and (2) not covered by third-party payers. It remains to be seen if lost employment costs are greater for home care than for parents of children who die in the hospital, since it is common for parents to take time off to be with dying child whether the child is at home or in the hospital.

A question may be raised concerning the motivations of the parents who enter the study. Perhaps the reason that the families studied did so well is the result of self-selection or selection by physicians. It is not clear that we will ever know for sure why the choice was made in many cases. Parents, when asked, will give an answer but closer examination complicates the picture. Often there is no one reason. The mother and father of the same child may give different reasons. Some parents place trust in the counsel of their physician who suggests the home care; others tell their physician they want home care before the physician brings it up. Thus the parents, the child, the physicians, nurses, and others become intermeshed in the decision-making process in a manner difficult to untangle after the fact.

The attitude of health professionals toward the home care program has changed over time from one of general uncertainty to one of general acceptance. Individual differences among physicians still inject uncontrolled selection factors. Some physicians refer almost every patient whose death is anticipated. Other physicians apply their own criteria of appropriateness based on their subjective appraisal of the parents' abilities or the child's condition. Some physicians refer later than others so that for some home care is considered so late that the child dies within 1 or 2 days, often never leaving the hospital.

Clearly, random assignment to home versus hospital care or random offering of the alternative to only some families would be preferable to avoid selection bias in evaluating the effects of home care of the potential dying child. However, random assignment or any limitation of the parents' and child's freedom of choice would be viewed as untenable or unethical by the vast majority of referring physicians we work with. Therefore the subject selection bias remains in the design.

In the future the child's physician's clinical opinion will always be a factor, and it is reasonable to expect physicians will continue to have individual attitudes in this as in other elements of care. We are not arguing that all dying children must or even should die at home. Rather, we wish to look at the viability of home care as an alternative for those who desire it. We have had a broad range of ages, cancers, and family situations, so we can show that home care may be viable for diverse, if self-selected, individuals.

An indication of the magnitude of selection is given by an examination of all deaths of University Hospitals childhood cancer patients for the first or second years of our research. In the first year, 32 patients died with 12 (37.5%) participating in home care. In the second year 30 patients died, with 19 (63.3%) participating in home care. The large increase in the second year is an indication of the acceptance of the program by University Hospitals physicians. The second-year rate is approximately the same as the third-year rate. In rare instances, we know of parents who were offered home care but chose not to have it. In other cases home care was talked about but no decision was made before the child died. In some instances the physician did not mention home care for some reason, and in others home care was never indicated, for example, the child died unexpectedly. Based on medical record review, the proportion of children not appropriate for home care (such as those receiving treatment that required hospitalization or those who died unexpectedly) is 20%; appropriate children who did not participate, 15%; and children who participated, 65%.

Another issue that may be raised concerns staff satisfaction with the project, since there was attrition in the project staff. For the core group of 58 children in the first and second years we used (coincidentally) 58 different nurses as primary or coprimary home care nurses. Geography made it unusual to use the same nurse more than once. Nurses were recruited from local communities, and in most communities only one child involved in the project died. In the Minneapolis-St. Paul area, nurses were more likely to be used repeatedly. Within the project staff, individuals who had repeated contact with families in either providing or coordinating the care or conducting research interviews were subject to a high turnover.

The high turnover rate is cause for concern. It is common in other settings, for example, hospices and pediatric ICUs, and therefore we should not be surprised to observe it in our research project as well. Freudenberger (1975) uses the term *burn-out* to describe the phenomenon of fatigue, psychosomatic complaints, and often resignation that occurs in individuals who work in high-demand situations such as walk-in crisis centers. In general his notions may be relevant to our situation. In any case it must be recognized that support for staff who work day in and day out with dying children must be available, either from the staff person's own resources (such as spouse, friends, or colleagues) or as a built-in part of the project itself (such as having discussions to air frustrations, ensuring recognition for staff efforts, or having a staff member's time partly assigned for staff support). We have examined the support systems in the cooperating institutions and stressed the need to help staff cope with the stresses attendant to the nurse coordinator's job. However, it is unlikely that this problem of attrition and burn-out will be resolved easily.

A final issue is how home care delivery compares to a hospice program and whether it is a viable alternative to such a program. We provide the majority of our services in rural areas. For this reason, our program has dealt primarily with dying at home when hospice programs are not available. An integral part of the hospice notion is formal intervention by chaplains, social workers, volunteers, and so on, to help the family cope with grief. In our program we have nothing of the sort other than the follow-up provided by the community nurse and coordination with a multidisciplinary team. This is primarily because of geographical constraints. Beyond nurse visits after the death of the child, formal, nondemand, supportive follow-up of families is not part of our services, as it is not part of the services of local hospitals in which a child might die. We exploit the resources available in the child's community, but they are usually few and not always useful. Family, neighbors, and friends may supply informal volunteer help. The clergy may become involved if the family desires, and sometimes the nurse coordinator contacts local social workers.

Our program has allowed children to die at home even when their home was hundreds of miles away from a regional treatment center and in a sparsely populated area. The total population density of the county that includes Minneapolis and the University Hospitals is 1724 persons per square mile. This county holds approximately one fourth of the entire population of the state. Formal hospice programs for adults now exist there. However, we study home care services provided to children who live in counties with total population densities of 10 persons per square mile or even fewer. It is not practical to transport a specialized team of care providers hundreds of miles, nor is it practical to have such specialized teams located throughout such sparsely populated areas.

With society's demand for home care increasing, the importance of alternative models of health care delivery is being acknowledged. The research questions for the future are questions of even broader scope than those we have addressed here. Can we develop the community services necessary to make home health care work? Are we really willing to let the consumer assume the major care-giving role? What are the significant factors involved in the parents' recognition of their ability to be the primary care giver to their dying child? What has precipitated the parents' dependence on health care system professionals if in fact the professionals are not needed? How can the health care system be both responsible to the needs of society and flexible in meeting those needs?

The "comfort care" concept and its physical, psychological, sociological, and cultural implications must be identified more clearly. It is hoped that others will continue investigations into this area. There is much to learn.

REFERENCES

Freudenberger, H.J. 1975. The staff burn-out syndrome, Washington, D.C., Drug Abuse Council, Inc.

Lansky, B. 1979. Childhood cancer: nonmedical costs of the illness, Cancer 43:403-408.

Martinson, I.M., et al. 1978. Home care for children dying of cancer, Pediatrics 62:106-113.

Martinson, I.M., 1979. Home care for children dying of cancer. In American Cancer Society, editors. Care of the child with cancer, September 11-13, Boston.

BIBLIOGRAPHY

Aguilera, D.C., Messick, J.M., and Farrell, M.S. 1978. Crisis intervention: theory and methodology, ed. 3, St. Louis; The C.V. Mosby Co.

American Cancer Society. Ca—a cancer journal for clinicians 28(1): 18-22.

American Nurses' Association. 1975. Research in nursing: toward a science of health care, Pub. No. D-52.

Ayer, A.H. 1978. Is partnership with parents really possible? The American Journal of Maternal Child Nursing, pp. 107-110.

Baker, L. 1976. You and leukemia: a day at a time, Philadelphia, W.B. Saunders Co.

Barton, D. 1977. Dying, death and bereavement as health care problems. Barton, D., editor. Dying and death: a clinical guide for caregivers, Baltimore, The Williams & Wilkins Co.

Benoliel, J.Q. 1972. The concept of care for a child with leukemia, Nursing Forum. 11:194-204.

Binger, C.M., et al. 1969. Childhood leukemia: emotional impact on patient and family, New England Journal of Medicine 280:414-418.

Bluebond-Langner, M. 1978. The private worlds of dying children, Princeton, N.J., Princeton University Press.

Bluebond-Langner, M. 1974. I know, do you? A study of awareness, communication, and coping in terminally ill children. Schoenberg, B., et al., editors. Anticipatory grief, New York, Columbia University Press.

Bradtke, L., et al. Hospital, Milwaukee, Milwaukee Children's Hospital.

Burton, L. 1975. The family life of sick children. London, Routledge & Kegan Paul, Ltd.

Cornwell, J., Nurcombe, B., and Stevens, L. 1977. Family response to loss of a child by sudden infant death syndrome, The Medical Journal of Australia, April 30, 1977, 656-658.

Diers, D., 1979. Research in nursing practice, Philadelphia, J.B. Lippincott Co.

Dingle, J.H., Badger, G.F., and Jordon, W.S. 1964. Illness in the home, Cleveland, The Press of Case Western Reserve University.

Edwards, A.L. 1954. Manual for the Edwards personal preference schedule, New York, The Psychological Corp.

George, J.A., and Stephens, M.D. 1968. Personality traits of public health nurses and psychiatric nurses, Nursing Research 17:2:168-170.

Glezen, W.P. and Denny, F.W. 1973. Epidemiology of acute lower respiratory disease in children, New England Journal of Medicine 288:10:498-505.

Greer, K., and Martinson, I.M., producers. 1979. Time to come home, a documentary, Minneapolis, University of Minnesota School of Nursing.

Hollingshead, A.B. 1957. The two-factor index of social position, author published, 1957.

Karnofsky, D.A. 1953. Experimental cancer chemotherapy. In Physiopathy of cancer. Honburger and Fishman, editors. New York, Holber & Harper, pp. 783-830.

Isles, J.P. 1979. Children with cancer: healthy siblings' perceptions during the illness experience, Cancer Nursing, October, pp. 371-377.

Lentz, E.M., and Michaels, R.G. 1965. Personality contrasts among medical and surgical nurses, Nursing Research 15:43-48.

Martinson, I.M. 1978. Evaluating nursing care: home care for the child with cancer. In The Proceedings of the Nursing Mirror International Cancer Nursing Conference, September 4-8, London, England.

Martinson, I.M. 1978. Home care: a manual for implementation of home care for children dying of cancer. Minneapolis, University of Minnesota, School of Nursing.

Martinson, I.M., et al. 1980. Home care for the child with cancer. Final report, grant #CA 19490, Washington, D.C., Department of Health and Human Services, National Cancer Institute.

Moldow, D.G., and Martinson, I.M. Home care for dying children: a manual for parents, Minneapolis, University of Minnesota School of Nursing.

CHAPTER 5

GROUNDED THEORY AND QUALITATIVE DATA
the socializing influences of life-threatening disease on identity development

Jeanne Quint Benoliel

Knowledge about the social impact of life-threatening disease on individuals and families has relevance for nursing both scientifically and practically. Yet gathering systematic knowledge about this phenomenon is not easy because it deals with people undergoing transition. To understand the meaning of life-threatening disease in the personal and social lives of individuals and families requires a conceptual framework and a method that takes account of the sociocultural context affecting human responses to disease as well as the responses themselves. This chapter reviews the origins of research designed for developing a theory concerning chronic disease in adolescence and describes the chronological process whereby selected conceptual and theoretical perspectives influenced my decisions about the types of data needed and the methods chosen for producing them.

The study took place between 1966 and 1969. Secondary analysis of field notes, analytical memoranda, manuscripts, and other research materials developed during that period provided the data on which the chapter is based. I have made an effort to show how the research plan evolved in the first year and how the study came to be implemented in the second and third years. I have given detailed consideration to the interrelationships of theory and qualitative data processing during the implementation of one phase of the research—a study of the social process whereby young people aged 10 to 16 years develop identities as persons defined as having juvenile-onset diabetes mellitus. I then examine the implications of this research for the creation of social theory and the practice of nursing.

ORIGINS OF THE RESEARCH

My thoughts about conducting research into the meaning of chronic disease in adolescence were stimulated during my participation in a large study of dying patients and hospital personnel. Between 1962 and 1967 I served as a member of a three-person research team studying dying from a sociological perspective (Glaser and Strauss, 1965, 1968; Quint, 1967). In autumn of 1966 we reached a decision to collect some data about the impact on families of terminal illness in children. Participant observation in several pediatric clinics that offered services for different types of life-threatening and chronic diseases contributed to my subsequent decision to study chronic disease in adolescence. The identification of a specific problem and the selection of a method,

The ideas presented here are based in part on a study of dying patients and hospital personnel supported by PHS Research Grant NU-00047 from the Division of Nursing, DHEW, and on a Special Nurse Fellowship (5F4-NU-10,227-02) awarded by the Division of Nursing for study of the social consequences of chronic disease in adolescence.

however, were also influenced by previous experience in research and by concepts, ideas, and findings reported by other investigators.

Previous and related research

Historically my interest in the impingement of disease and treatment on human behavior began with clinical observations on the effects of mutilating surgeries on patients and questions about the adaptations that these major changes imposed on them in their everyday lives. Eventually that interest led to an exploratory study of the processes whereby women adjust to radical mastectomy and learn to live with a status that carries negative values within society (Quint, 1963, 1964, 1965). That study provided the means for my introduction into the intricacies of using participant observation for research purposes, and I was fortunate to have the ethnomethodologist Garfinkel (1967) as consultant to the project. His guidance played a major part in the process whereby my thinking shifted from the action-oriented perspective of a nurse viewing people as patients in need of help to the more reflective perspective of a scientific investigator viewing people as persons undergoing major transitions in living with important personal and social consequences.

Consultation with Garfinkel broadened my perspective on the problem I had chosen for study and my awareness of the influence of social context and social relationships on the women's perceptions of themselves and their adaptations to the change. Ideas influential to my thinking came from two other sources. Goffman's writing (1959) on the presentation of self in everyday life stimulated my interest in the relationship of front stage and backstage operations to the playing of roles and the managing of expressions of emotions. Strauss' notion (1959) about the complex relationships of face-to-face interaction and transformations of identity provided a framework for examining changes across time. In fact, his concept of *turning point* was used in the analysis of the mastectomy data with mastectomy viewed as an incident serving as a significant turning point in the lives of the women and their families. Goffman's later work (1963) on the relationship of information control to the development of personal identity provided another conceptual perspective for examining the mastectomy experience, particularly as it was influenced by the words and actions of family, friends, physicians, and nurses (Quint, 1965).

The mastectomy study also provided opportunities for learning research methods. The experience validated the importance of sponsorship as a strategy for gaining access to the desired set of informants and respondents. The experience highlighted the conflicts between the role of nurse and the role of observer in patient care situations and pointed to the need for explicit methods and procedures to offset the bias of emotional involvement and selective perception in research about delicate and sensitive matters in human affairs (Benoliel, 1975a).

Interest in interactional processes as they influence human behaviors in response to negatively valued experiences continued during a study designed to describe how, when, and where student nurses encounter death and dying while being socialized as nurses (Quint, 1967). Concepts of awareness context and dying trajectory developed from the earlier study of dying patients and hospital personnel influenced my thinking about socialization processes and the relationship of knowledge to expectations and outcomes. Thoughts about changes in behavior over time were also influenced by Becker's studies (1963) on deviant behavior and his use of the concept of *career* for developing sequential models of various kinds of deviant behavior. These efforts combined led eventually to an interest in *status passage* as a concept useful for viewing the meanings that individuals attach to themselves and to their experiences as persons defined as chronically ill (Glaser and Strauss, 1971).

Preliminary fieldwork: process and outcomes

The study of chronic disease in adolescence came into being as a direct outgrowth of the dying patient study. In fact, my decision to study terminal illness in children was an extension of the original investigation and was designed to make available comparative information about dying trajectories observed in children with different types of terminal illness. The idea of dying trajectory as a form of status passage had already been developed, based primarily on data about dying adults. The choice of comparision groups by type of disease and type of setting (hospital, clinic, home) for children with life-threatening diseases was to provide data for judging similarities and differences in patterns of dying observed in children and adults. Under the rationale for theoretical sampling (Glaser and Strauss, 1967) comparison groups were selected on the basis of categories of interest to the theory such as types of settings and the desired scope of population—for instance, one hospital was chosen instead of many. The concept of dying trajectory was based on analysis of data from comparison groups at several levels.

The period of data production began with a decision to talk with families of children with cystic fibrosis using the outpatient department of a university medical center as the starting point for making contacts. For a period of roughly 9 months, I collected data by a combination of participant observation and interview in pediatric clinics that provided services for children with three major long-term diseases: cystic fibrosis, diabetes mellitus, and bronchial asthma. A considerable amount of time was given to interviews and conversations with children and parents in the clinics and in their homes.

Detailed field notes were written following each observation or interview, and duplicate copies were made available to all members of the team. Weekly meetings were held for review of these data, identification of theoretical categories and properties, and discussion of methodological questions and concerns. Memoranda describing and outlining the major outcomes of these discussions were prepared and kept as analytical references. In addition, each member of the team kept a personal set of analytical references including memoranda based on the coding of fieldwork data using the constant comparative method of qualitative analysis (Glaser, 1965). In my case these memoranda also included ideas about various categories and relationships among categories, thoughts about comparison groups, personal reactions to events and people, and concepts of interest from the work of other investigators.

Comparative analysis of these data led to identification of some salient properties of the three diseases as social phenomena. Variations in the interactional patterns between staff and patients, as well as between parents and children, helped to clarify some crucial differences in the types and degrees of social impingement imposed by each disease and its treatment regimen. Comparison of these differences pinpointed the relative importance of such matters as awareness of prognosis, effectiveness of available medical treatments, social visibility of the disease, and anticipated course of the disease. The selection of *social visibility* as a major category was based on analysis of fieldwork observations and exploratory interviews. It was deemed sufficiently significant to serve as a theoretical starting point.*

The preliminary fieldwork also led to decisions about the relevance of other variables for selecting the groups to be compared. The need for closer scrutiny of the effects of the different diseases on family processes was recognized. Thus the comparison groups were projected to include families of different socioeconomic status and families with different household characteristics. The logic of including different types of groups (in this case, families) made possible comparisons at different conceptual levels of analysis— families with the same type of chronic disease, families with different types of chronic disease, and finally, families with different types of chronic disease and from different social classes. The scope of the evolving theory and its limits were to be determined by the conscious and deliberate choice of the groups to be included (Glaser and Strauss, 1967).

The preliminary observations and analysis also pinpointed the relevance

---

Social visibility is a conceptual category that refers to the "obviousness," the salience of overt signs, of a given disease in terms of public awareness. A disease with low social visibility is one that is relatively invisible to laypersons much of the time though not necessarily to medical and other specialists who have been trained to see certain cues as carrying special significance.

of age, sex, and age at onset of disease as key variables influencing the behavior of young people with chronic disease. Thereby evolved another set of
comparison groups. A preliminary decision was reached at this time to limit
the proposed investigation to individuals between 10 and 16 years of age, the
period of transition into adolescence.

The experience of performing participant observation with these children
and their families also provoked a great deal of thinking about data production
as an interactional process. The processes of entree into the clinics and of
making contact with respondents depended on my ability to negotiate a reasonable role or set of roles with the significant persons concerned. To achieve
successful outcomes in these matters, I had to be aware of the importance of
reciprocity in human exchanges and to allow claims on my time and energy
as well as to make claims on the time and energy of others. My ideas about
reciprocity in performing fieldwork were greatly influenced by the writings of
Wax (1960) about her experiences in the field and of Olesen and Whittaker
(1967) about the special problems of sustaining roles in research that continues for several years. By its very nature, the negotiation of roles in the field
was an ongoing interactional process heavily dependent on my sensitivity to
factors such as timing and mood.

When the subject at hand carried a high degree of threat, as was so in
some of the interviews, the need for flexibility of approach became readily
apparent. This flexibility included readiness to shift roles with relative ease—
for instance, to avoid an unnecessary or disturbing scene or to initiate a new
contact when old ones had outlived their usefulness. At times my experience
as a nurse came in handy for recognizing in advance certain areas of potential
conflict—particularly with staff. Flexibility also meant a willingness to move
into new and untested roles in which my own emotional life might be stimulated in ways that could cause painful personal involvement. Yet the outcomes of the research seemed at times to depend on an ability to engage in
reciprocal activities that are not ordinarily expected of persons engaged in
research. In retrospect, it seems to me that a willingness to listen to the often
painful stories of the various people concerned—staff as well as families—is
a salient characteristic for the fieldworker who is dealing with subject matter
(such as the meaning of life-threatening illness) that carries a high degree of
personal threat.

In a sense, being a nurse provided prior training in the practical aspects
of listening to people at times of crisis and change but limited experience in
analyzing systematically the sources of bias deriving from personal involvement, anxiety, and selective perceptions. In the latter activity I was strongly
influenced by the suggestions of Schwartz and Schwartz (1955) for systematic study of problems of bias in participant observation.

The theoretical framework

During the period of preliminary fieldwork, time was also devoted to review of the current literature on theories and research pertaining to families, adolescence, chronic illness, and socialization processes. The theoretical framework for the study of chronic disease in adolescence was based on three perspectives on human behavior.

Underlying the research was an assumption that human behavior is a complex process involving interplay between conscious and unconscious forces. The approach chosen for the study was based on the symbolic interactionist perspective on human nature and was concerned mainly with the conscious elements that influence the formation of an inner identity. This perspective views an individual as living in a symbolic environment—a "named" world— that is created in the mind out of interactions with other people. The theory had its origins in ideas formulated by George Herbert Mead (Strauss, 1964). The assumptions and propositions underlying the interactionist perspective were taken initially from the writing of Rose (1962) and later from the conceptualizations offered by Blumer (1969).

This perspective on human behavior sees human beings as creatures who define and classify situations—including themselves—and who *choose* ways of acting toward and within them. The individual is perceived as being in a continuing state of emergence; he both influences and is influenced by other individuals with whom he interacts and the situations in which he finds himself. Particularly influential to my thinking were the ideas of Olesen and Whittaker (1968:ix) that people exist simultaneously in three modes of being:

1. The environmental world as defined by institutions and social structures of society
2. The world of social relationships in which interaction with others is central
3. The inner world that deals with ideas of the self.

According to symbolic interactionism, the definitions and choices an individual makes in any situation are closely tied to an inner definition of self. The notion of a complex and differentiated self composed of many discrete identities came from ideas developed by McCall and Simmons (1966) and Stryker (1968) and stimulated new thinking on my part about the development of identity.

My thinking about the meaning of identity was also fostered by Erikson's (1963) theories that the development of ego identity in childhood and adolescence takes place by stages and is a function of a culture identity. His ideas that personality develops through the mastery of developmental tasks at different periods of the human life cycle (Erikson, 1968) provided a perspective for conceptualizing the special tasks faced by adolescents with chronic ill-

ness. His perspective on development also implied the importance of understanding the influence of social relationships and cultural context on developmental processes. In other words, the incorporation of a new identity and
the learning of relevant patterns of behavior takes place by means of socialization.

According to Shibutani (1962), any group whose outlook serves as a frame
of reference for a person in organizing his perceptual world is a *reference
group*, and groups with high power in this regard are those in which primary
relationships and direct experiences take place. In childhood, members of the
family serve as significant others for initial formulations of identity. This reference group is of singular importance because it indoctrinates new members
into the ongoing culture of society. In searching for the meaning of chronic
disease in the lives of young people, it was judged necessary to look at the
impact of the disease on the ongoing and shifting worlds of their families and
to understand the modes of coping with the change used by families. The
perspective on families selected as suitable for the proposed investigation was
the conceptual orientation of Hess and Handel (1959) who make the claim
that families are changing social groups and that each creates an individualized pattern of relationships and interactions through mediation with the wider
society.

Mediation with the wider society required a perspective for analyzing the
influence of cultural values on the behaviors of individuals and families. Coleman (1961), Gottlieb and Ramsey (1964), Simmons and Winograd (1966),
and other investigators of the adolescent experience pointed to the subculture
of the American urban adolescent as an increasingly powerful socializing force
in society through its particular values and systems of social reward. The
influence of peer society as a reference group was considered a necessary
ingredient of the projected study.

THE RESEARCH PLAN

In the spring of 1967 a research plan was devised for studying the social
consequences of chronic disease in adolescence. The concept of status passage was used as an organizing framework within which to examine the
changes introduced by life-threatening disease. The original statement of the
problem follows.

The research problem

Being informed of having a chronic disease can be thought of as a critical
juncture in the human life cycle. It marks the starting point for a transition

from one status to another—from "normal" person to "nonnormal" person by ordinary social standards. The status—person with chronic disease—is assigned by the physician to whom society has delegated responsibility for making distinctions between wellness and illness, thereby legitimating the status. Furthermore, movement into the status is directed by the physician and his associates, who provide a set of generalized rationales for what to expect and how to behave. In the physician's view, the status carries with it a relatively well-defined set of rights and duties for playing the role that accompanies the status. The individual, however, lives in many social worlds—family, church, and neighborhood to mention a few. Each of these worlds has its values, norms, social structure, social roles and role sets, and patterns of social interaction. The fate of the emerging status and the status passage itself are determined by interplay between the complexities and requirements of these many social worlds.

When the diagnosis of chronic disease is established in late childhood, the status passage becomes very complex because the individual is about to enter adolescence, the crucial period of transition from childhood to adulthood. Studying the interaction between two simultaneously occurring and highly important status passages affords an opportunity to learn more about adolescence in general and to understand with greater clarity both individual and family adaptations to chronic illness. In this regard, the study has significance for social science, medicine, and nursing.

The study proposed focused on the *social and behavioral outcomes* of living with a chronic disease during a crucial period in the human life cycle—a time during which the development of adult work and sex roles is a primary social task and an alteration in parent-child relationships is a usual associated phenomenon. The broad aim was to understand how a chronic disease and its recommended treatment regimen influence the social behaviors of the person undergoing transition, the members of his family, and other significant people in his life.

The study was limited to the effects of chronic disease with *low social visibility* on the social roles and role relationships of young persons, especially with their parents and peers, during the period from preadolescence into adolescence. The selection of social visibility as a central theme to guide the research is directly related to the principal concerns experienced by adolescents in modern society. Marked by internal physiological alterations and external changes of the body, adolescents show a high degree of concern with physical appearance. Under most circumstances, it is a period of shifting away from primary relationships with members of the same sex toward primary relationships with members of the opposite sex. Physical appearance "as a man" or "as a woman" is very important in these matters. According to Muuss

(1962), the importance of *body* and *social life* is either explicit or implicit in the development of all theoretical positions on adolescence.

In addition, changes within society have decreased the influence of the family as a primary socializing institution and have increased the importance of the peer group as *the* influential reference group. It has its own subculture and value system, and there is undoubtedly more than one such subculture in large metropolitan settings. Because of the relative importance of physical appearance and acceptance by peers, social visibility is seen as a critical variable during the transition into adolescence. It is also viewed as a central variable influencing the health behaviors of individuals with diseases that "make them different," and chronic disease falls into this classification. A study of adolescents with chronic disease provides an opportunity to understand the relative importance of social visibility as a determinant of behavior.

Specific objectives in the original research plan

Within this broad framework, the research was to be concerned with three distinct but interrelated problems:
1. The *management of social visibility* by the individual concerned at different chronological points in the transition from preadolescence toward adulthood
2. The *meaning and management of chronic diseases* by different types of families
3. The effects of disease and treatment differences on the *enactment of social roles* by the young person with disease, by family and friends, and by health professionals.

The study had as its long-range goal the development of a theory of chronic disease in adolescence, and the original proposal identified the need for comparative data based on type of disease, type of family, and adolescent perspectives on the social visibility of disease. These decisions were influenced by various theoretical positions on the variables at issue as well as the analysis of the preliminary data.

Types of chronic disease

Unlike acute disease with its limited time span of incapacitation, chronic disease is marked by the continuous nature of its effects and required treatments—thus by an ongoing impingement on social roles. Some chronic diseases, such as cerebral palsy or blindness, are both physically and socially restricting and generally are readily observable to the world at large. Other chronic diseases are characterized by low social visibility and thus allow the person to appear "normal" much of the time. For comparative purposes, four chronic diseases meeting the criterion of low social visibility were chosen for the study:

1. *Cystic fibrosis*, a disease in which the recommended treatment regimen requires extensive and active participation by the parents in terms of *time* and *effort* each day, but in which treatment is ultimately a palliative measure in that the child is unlikely to live beyond 21 years, if he lives that long.
2. *Diabetes mellitus*, a disease in which success of the recommended treatment regimen depends on a daily routine with a high degree of temporal regularity and restriction on diet and requires a high degree of *self-control* and *self-maintenance* by the adolescent himself.
3. *Bronchial asthma*, a disease in which the recommended treatment regimen requires some modification in the home environment, often including changes in the diet, but with variable *temporal* or *daily participative* demands compared to diabetes mellitus and cystic fibrosis. It is a condition characterized by seasonal variations and by abrupt exacerbations, often requiring emergency medical treatments.
4. *Chronic pyelonephritis*, a disease in which the recommended treatment regimen (long-term medication, high fluid intake, sometimes salt or protein dietary restriction) tends to be *periodic* and *variable*. It is a condition with few observable symptoms other than fatigue, except for acute exacerbations during which the individual "looks and feels sick."

These conditions were selected because the diseases themselves and the recommended treatments vary in two general ways: (1) they make different kinds of social demands on the adolescent and the family, and (2) they carry different degrees of social acceptability within the value system of American society.

These variations were thought to provide a rich opportunity to study the following:

1. The *development of awareness* (knowledge about the disease, its treatment, and its controllability) in chronic diseases with different degrees of social acceptability
2. The effects of *different states of awareness on the strategies used* by medical and nursing personnel, the individuals with disease, and their families to achieve their various purposes
3. The effects of different types of *continuous treatment demands* on the adolescent and his family

It was hypothesized that open awareness about disease and treatment between physician and parent, between parent and child, and between physician and child could be directly related to the *social acceptability* of the disease, and conversely that awareness would be closed or partial when the disease carried a *social stigma*. It was also hypothesized that the type of awareness instituted by the adolescent with his peers would be directly related to the social value attributed to the disease. Support for the position that socially discrediting conditions contribute to partial awareness was given by Davis (1963) in his study of polio victims and their families who received incomplete diagnostic and prognostic messages about the state of the handicap even though physicians and other hospital personnel knew that full recovery of function was not possible. The frequency with which dying patients were placed by others in a context of closed awareness of forthcoming death was additional evidence that a nonacceptable status would interfere with open communication about its true dimensions (Glaser and Strauss, 1965: 29-46).

Yet awareness of the meaning of an ascribed state is not a static entity, and definitions of the situation change as new cues are provided and people live through different stages of illness (Davis, 1963; Quint, 1964). The study was centrally concerned with understanding the effects of the selected chronic diseases on the social roles and role relationships of the diagnosed individuals—with parents and other significant persons—during the period of transition into adolescence. For completeness of understanding, the study was also concerned with the modes of adaptation used by the families to cope with the continuous and emerging demands imposed by the disease and treatment.

Type of family

Because parents are generally expected to serve as control agents for managing the disease, the study was designed to examine similarities and differences in parental roles in families with different socioeconomic backgrounds. In this regard the study was concerned with understanding the management of chronic disease in families with somewhat different values and styles of living. Evidence from studies by Handel and Rainwater (1964), McKinley (1964), Miller and Riessman (1964), and Pearlin and Kohn (1966) indicated that parental values and child-rearing practices of middle-class and working-class families differed, particularly with respect to techniques for socializing the child toward "right" behavior. On this assumption *social class* was selected as a key variable for comparisons of parental and adolescent roles. The comparison was expected to consider such phenomena as the management of two types of parental control (upbringing of the child and enforcement of medical directives); division of labor between the parents; variations in parental expectations and control strategies on the basis of age, sex, and position in the family of the child; the impingement of the recommended treatment regimen on the parents' lives; and its effect on family cohesiveness and lifestyle.

The study was also formulated to compare other characteristics of the family such as household composition, number of parents at home, family mobility pattern, and religious practices. In combination, the research aimed to understand how chronic disease was managed under different sets of structural conditions and how the types of management affected the course of the disease and the future of the child. (It should perhaps be noted that understanding the impact of chronic disease on individuals and families also required rather extensive knowledge about the physical and physiologic effects of each disease, the rationales for medical treatments, anticipated outcomes of medical treatments, and contingencies affecting those outcomes. Reference to that literature has not been incorporated into this discussion.)

Since social class and other family characteristics determine a family's financial and social resources, these variables were assumed to influence accessibility to health care services and attitudes toward seeking medical care. Another area for study concerned the onset of the disease and the use of health facilities. Phenomena of interest here included the time of the condition's discovery by the parents; the time of diagnosis by the physician; variations in perceptions of what is important by physician, parent, and child; types of crisis states associated with disease and their controllability; degree of congruence among interactants as to what constitutes a "crisis"; family history and prior experience with the disease; parental expectations and disappointments in health care services; and kinds of medical advice received and followed or not followed.

Although the study was primarily designed to contribute ideas toward the development of theory in nursing (most likely one or more social theories of chronicity), the research also had pragmatic goals. It was concerned with identifying *critical junctures* and *temporal features* that form essential elements of status passage for persons with chronic disease—as a basis for building toward explicit help for the chronically ill person and his family.

The adolescent and social visibility

A decision was made to provide for comparisons of adolescent behaviors on the basis of four variables: age, sex, position in the family, and age at which the diagnosis was established. For each disease the management of social visibility depended on several factors, including how well the treatment regimen was followed and what the adolescent learned about preventing the disease from being visible to other people. Yet there were always unexpected events that even the physician could not predict, and thus control of visibility could never be absolute. The problem faced by the individual with disease was to learn ways of minimizing the possibility of unwanted or undesirable social consequences and conversely to develop strategies for making the disease visible if openness achieved a necessary purpose.

Within the overall framework the investigation was concerned with understanding the influence of social values and norms, emerging roles and role expectations, social interaction and interaction tactics and strategies, and the timing of critical events. It was hypothesized that openness with peers about the disease would be an age-graded phenomenon, that is, as the child moved into adolescence, a tendency to keep the disease hidden was expected. It was also hypothesized that adherence to medical directives would be strongly influenced by the frequency of crisis states, their visibility to other people, and the ease with which they could be controlled or prevented.

This part of the research required a broad understanding of adolescence. The review of the literature included publications about normal physical growth and development as discussed by Tanner (1963) and Gustafson and Coursin (1965), development of thought processes in childhood and adolescence (Inhelder and Piaget, 1958), characteristics of the subculture of youth (Coleman, 1961; Gottlieb and Ramsey, 1964; and Stone and Church, 1968), the language of adolescence (Schwartz and Merten, 1967), development of ideas about masculinity and femininity (Pitcher, 1965), and parental influences on adolescent self-esteem and behavior (Pearlin and Kohn, 1966; Rosenberg, 1965; and Sebald, 1968). Updating of information in these and related areas continued throughout the investigation.

The choice of diabetes mellitus

The selection of juvenile-onset diabetes mellitus for the first phase of intensive study of chronic disease and family life was not a random choice. The atmosphere observed in the diabetic clinic reflected an emphasis on teaching people facts about the disease so they could be responsible for themselves. In contrast to other clinics, there was open talk among the families about diabetes and their experiences in living with it. The overall tone of the clinic was hopeful—quite in contrast to the subdued atmosphere in the cystic fibrosis clinic and to the tensions observed among family and staff in the allergy clinic.

By the autumn of 1967 I had come to recognize the importance of having access to data from all members of the household to study chronic illness as a family process. Contacts with siblings were viewed as crucial for developing a valid image of the social impact of each disease. An important contingency on the matter of willingness to talk about the illness related to the "death expectations" carried by the disease and the timetable of dying likely to be involved (Glaser and Strauss, 1968). During the preliminary phase of the study, there was considerable evidence suggesting that parents of children with cystic fibrosis might be resistant to the idea that siblings be interviewed. Stated in theoretical terms, parental efforts to create and maintain a context of closed awareness about certain realities of the disease (and perhaps also about the family) posed problems of strategy for the investigator in gaining access to certain kinds of data.

The decision to begin intensive study with diabetic families was essentially guided by two realities. Families who were accustomed to an atmosphere of open talk about the disease and treatment were seen as more openly receptive to being studied than were those in which a closed pattern of talk was prevalant. The choice of diabetes was seen as a relatively easy way of making the transition to the next phase of the research. In addition, I recognized a personal need for time away from the intensive interviews with families in which cystic fibrosis and bronchial asthma were the diseases of concern.

A STUDY OF JUVENILE-ONSET DIABETES IN ADOLESCENCE

The core of the research now became centered on the process of becoming diabetic and on the meanings of this experience during the transition from childhood into adolescence. That adolescence is a time of life when the psychological problems and difficulties of diabetes control are exacerbated had long been known. Two elements identified as primary contributors to the difficult problems associated with the period are (1) the physiological changes resulting from growth spurts and physical maturation and (2) the psychological and behavioral changes associated with a shift toward independence from parents and other authority. Rather extensive literature on emotional and social problems associated with childhood diabetes had accumulated, and it pointed to some very complex relationships among the physical, psychological, and social factors involved. The bulk of this literature does not bear directly on the subject matter of this chapter but was considered in the original research report (Quint, 1969a).

The research problem restated

The importance of social visibility as a primary conceptual category had already been established, and questions that at an earlier stage were posed about chronic disease in general were now posed with specific reference to diabetes mellitus. The study now focused on: (1) the *meaning of being diabetic* at different chronological points in the transition from preadolescence to adulthood, (2) the meaning and management of diabetes by *different types of families* and (3) the effects of the disease and recommended treatments on the enactment of social roles by the person with diabetes, by family and friends, and by health professionals.

Juvenile-onset diabetes mellitus commonly makes its appearance during childhood or early adolescence. It is a form of chronic disease characterized by a low social visibility except when the disorder exists in a labile form referred to in the literature as *brittle*. The low social visibility of diabetes, however, is dependent on the diabetic's ability to follow a treatment plan that blocks the appearance of telltale signs. On a day-by-day basis, this means living in such a way that episodes of *insulin shock* (hypoglycemia) and *diabetic coma* (ketoacidosis) are minimized through a proper balance of insulin, food, and exercise. Without cooperation in maintaining a balanced regimen of treatment, the person with juvenile-onset diabetes is prone to exhibit such peculiarities of behavior as irritability, mental confusion, lethargy, and, in extreme cases, convulsions or loss of consciousness.

The success of the recommended treatment regimen depends on the availability of *replacement therapy* in the form of insulin and on a daily routine of considerable temporal regularity and restrictions on eating. "Success" in the study referred to the individual's ability to control the signs that told other people about his unusual status and not the medical definition of success, which has more to do with control of the metabolic effects of the disease and the prevention of complications. Success in keeping the signs invisible requires a high degree of self-control and self-maintenance by the diabetic himself and, presumably, depends on a reasonable knowledge of the disease, its treatment, and its controllability.

In addition, diabetes mellitus produces internal physical changes that tend to be progressive in nature. It is treatable but not curable, and there are severe social consequences tied to the more remote physical phenomena. The reality is that the diabetic's future is limited in terms of time. Perhaps even more relevant, he can know with greater precision than many persons how he is likely to die. It is no secret that a person with diabetes is prone to develop arteriosclerosis that affects especially the kidney and heart and is a likely candidate for retinal hemorrhages and circulatory problems. He has a physical disorder that without continuous daily treatment leads to an early death.

The treatment is characterized by a *transfer of medical responsibility* from the doctor to the patient and family. For parents the delegated role of treatment agent is temporary. For the child with diabetes the role of treatment agent becomes a life-long enterprise.

From a sociological perspective the person with diabetes undergoes a process of socialization whereby he learns a new identity. Central to this process is the matter of how he develops awareness of what he needs to do and for what reason. A central concern of the investigation was the production of data that would help to clarify two questions: (1) How does the child or adolescent with diabetes learn what is involved in being a diabetic? (2) How does he behave in response to this knowledge?

Research design

Ideally, a longitudinal approach with a team of investigators collecting data from selected families for a protracted period of time would have provided more complete and sensitive data about the process of becoming diabetic. Such research is costly, and it asks of those being studied as well as the researchers a tremendous commitment of time and energy, sometimes involving psychological as well as fiscal costs (Benoliel, 1975a). It was not a practical approach in this case, and an alternative approach—that of studying different families at different stages of development or change—was used.

The choice of cross-sectional design was heavily influenced by matters of accessibility and economy of personal resources and was aided by the suggestions of Richardson, Dohrenwend, and Klein (1965: 21) for evaluating alternative methods in planning a piece of research. The reality of asking people to donate their time and energy to the interviewer with no guarantee of personal help or recompense was perhaps not too much to ask for a short span of time. For them to agree to multiple contacts was perceived as unlikely. I did not have an unlimited supply of time, and the option of seeing many families on a one-time basis was in keeping with this fact. It was also compatible with the research orientation of using multiple comparison groups in terms of their relevance for the development of grounded theory (Glaser and Strauss, 1967: 48-55).

In making this choice I necessarily set the stage for collecting data at a more superficial level than would have been possible had there been sequential contacts with the participating families. In a sense the decision placed me in the role of observer-as-participant, which, according to Pearsall's definition (1965: 38) offers little opportunity for any deep involvements with the people being studied. It does have the advantage of the position of "outsider," which in this case seemed to trigger some of the respondents to talk openly about many sensitive issues with relatively little encouragement on the part of the investigator.

The sample

Unlike research in which homogeneity of cases is desirable so that hypotheses can be rigorously tested, the selection of participants in this study was guided by the deliberate choice of comparison groups that were unlike each other on the basis of selected characteristics. The selection process had to take account of two sets of criteria—those pertaining to the family and those descriptive of the diabetic child. For very practical reasons the choice was also limited to persons living within a reasonable distance of travel to the city in which the study was centered.

The importance of socioeconomic status and household membership for selecting types of families had already been established. Household member-ship was limited initially to the two patterns of one-parent and two-parent households, with variations in numbers of siblings as well as the child's ordi-nal position in the family left to chance. About 6 months after the study began a third comparison group came into being with a decision to seek out families in which one of the parents was diabetic. Fortunately for me, the services offered through the diabetic clinic were available to families with a range of social and financial resources. Though it was more fortuitous than deliberate, the nine families that comprised the final sample were representative of three different socioeconomic levels and the three major religious groupings found in the United States. Three families had more than one person with overt diabetes living in the household and six did not.

The criteria for choosing the principal subjects were age, sex, and age at onset of diabetes. With so many variables at issue, it was not possible to obtain exact equivalence by age and sex in combination with the desired character-istics of the families. Also, two families of participating subjects resisted being in the study so the data from these two families were incomplete though still useful for other types of comparison. The final sample of young people with diabetes consisted of 13 individuals who ranged in age from 5 to 19 years. Of the 8 girls and 5 boys, 9 fell between ages 10 and 16 years. The earliest age of onset among these was 18 months and the latest 12 years. The sample contained 1 person who had had diabetes for only 2 months and at the other extreme one who had lived with the disease for 11 years.

As the study progressed the need for additional comparative data from young adults with diabetes was recognized—primarily to broaden the per-spective on being diabetic in terms of its effect on other statuses. Subse-quently, semistructured interviews were conducted with two young men and three young women who were selected because they were diabetics known to be knowledgeable (or had at least been exposed to a high degree of knowl-edge) about the disease and its treatment.

Some limiting factors were clearly established. All of the participants were individuals and families who had contacts with medical specialists in juvenile-onset diabetes mellitus. The study was also limited to white families and was not designed to examine the impact of being diabetic on those from different racial and subcultural backgrounds. These decisions limited the scope of the developing theory and the generalizability of the findings.

Data sources

The data came from several sources. The bulk of them came from semi-structured interviews with young diabetics and their families, most of whom were clientele of a diabetic clinic associated with an urban medical center. With the consent of attending physicians, contacts with the families were made either by face-to-face meetings in the clinic or by telephone, and arrangements for participation were made by contractual agreement. (Approval of the forms and the procedures to be followed had been granted by the Committee on Human Experimentation of the university in which the study was done.) Whenever possible, the interviews were conducted in the homes of the participants, thereby making possible the inclusion of observational data of the family in its usual context.

The records of the clinic were used as sources for two kinds of data. Because they provided a running account of the physicians' contacts with these families, they were used as checks against the data collected by interview and proved to be quite valuable. Record data were used for building an image of the overall pattern of diabetic control (by medical standards) shown by each of the young participants, for comparison with their own versions of the state of their diabetic control.

Other data about young diabetics and their families were obtained by participant observation in the diabetic clinic and at a diabetic camp located in the nearby mountains. For obtaining a broad perspective on the meaning of diabetes, a variety of resources proved useful as supplementary sources of information. Formal and informal interviews were conducted with physicians, nurses, dietitians, and other personnel at the medical center. Attendance at four of the open educational meetings sponsored by the local Diabetes Association provided additional data about the diabetes specialist's perspective on juvenile-onset diabetes and on the diabetic individual's perception of what constitutes a problem. Information about the activities of two diabetes-centered organizations in the community was obtained through informal contacts with the office staff as well as from written materials provided by each organization.

Data production

The process of data production took place over a period of 18 months beginning in the summer of 1967 with 2 weeks of participant observation at a camp for diabetic children. The decision to study only diabetic children and their families was made in November, and the interviews began in February 1968.

Participant observation at camp

Before attending the camp, I had attended several planning meetings held for the staff and had also participated in a work weekend at the camp before

its opening for the 1967 year. By request, I was assigned to a living arrange-
ment with a group of girls 12 to 13 years of age. In addition to performing the
expected functions of a camp counselor (which provided entree to the camp),
I allocated blocks of time for making observations in different functional areas
of the camp so as to learn something about its social structure and patterns
of social relationships. By so doing, less time was available for producing data
on the young diabetics' perspectives and behaviors.

The major sources for data were the eight girls and six women counselors
who shared time and space together on their assigned sleeping deck. There
was little opportunity for direct observation of what happened to the boys at
camp except during the coeducational activities of eating, sharing in field
sports, and attending campfires, folk dances, and other social gatherings. This
deficit was remedied later when interviews were conducted with two of the
men counselors who provided indirect data about the activities and behaviors
of the diabetic boys. Contacts with the girls in other age groups were also
somewhat limited primarily because social activity at camp tended to follow
closely an age-graded pattern.

Throughout the period at camp I chose the role of participant-as-observer
and made no effort to do explicit interviewing but relied instead on informal
conversation and a careful eye for unexpected and unanticipated events. Field
notes were kept on a daily basis for analysis at a later time. A memorandum
written in January 1968 dealt with the subculture of the camp and included
descriptive and interpretive comments about the camp staff and the properties of the camp, including its program of activities, ratio of staff to campers,
daily routines of living, instructional programs, and philosophy of diabetic
medical treatment. These data provided information for understanding the
socializing influence of the diabetic camp on various young people who participated as regular campers each year.

The interviews

In the literature on chronic illness in families relatively little attention had
been focused on siblings. Except for the work of Crain, Sussman, and Weil
(1966), little information could be found on the effects of diabetes on the
brothers and sisters of diabetic children. The decision to interview the entire
family was stimulated by the work of Hess and Handel (1959), who had studied families as living groups, and by Seeley, Sim, and Loosley (1956), who
had studied families within the social context of suburban life. In both instances families were seen as totalities—though from somewhat different
perspectives—and siblings as well as parents served as sources for the reported findings. The decision to interview entire families was made on an

assumption that data from all members of the household would give a more valid image of the social meanings of diabetes than could be obtained from restricting the interviews to parents and the diabetic child.

Before making contact with any family, an interview guide was prepared based on ideas that evolved out of the ongoing analysis of data. The principal sources of information about the effects of diabetes on parents came from observations and conversations with 16 partial families in the clinic. (The term *partial family* meant that contact had been made with the diabetic child and one parent and thereby only fragments of information about the effects of diabetes on the family as a whole had been obtained.) From these data the major topics to be covered in the interviews were determined and written into a schedule of questions.

The schedule was given a trial run with one family, but it proved to be inadequate for determining differences in perspective of the principal informant, the parents, and the siblings, or other family members. Subsequently, three interview schedules were developed and used for the remainder of the study. The topics included on the interview schedules are given in Table 2.

The format for the interview would probably be classified as the nonschedule standarized type, which, according to Richardson, Dohrenwend, and Klein (1959:52), is most appropriate for dealing with sensitive topics when the respondents are heterogeneous. The schedule included topics that were basic to each interview, but the interviewer was free to word questions so that they were meaningful to each respondent and also to shift the sequence of topics if such a change were in keeping with the readiness and mood of the person being interviewed. In actual practice the interviews combined a nonstandardized approach with a standardized and semistructured format, a procedure made possible because the investigator conducted all of the interviews and was completely familiar with its conceptual framework.

The interviews took place over a period of 12 months. For the most part they were done in the homes of the informants, but a few took place elsewhere to accommodate the personal interests and time schedules of some individuals. The interviews varied in time from 30 to 90 minutes, and about 2 to 6 hours was required for typing each interview into a usable manuscript from notes taken during the interview itself.

Actual face-to-face contact with the nine participating families varied depending on how much time they were willing to give and on how many family members were available to be interviewed at a given time. In size the families ranged from four persons to eight. The actual contacts with the nine families varied between two and five. The number of interview hours per family ranged from four to nine.

TABLE 2 ▪ Topics on the interview schedules for principal subjects, parents, and siblings

Principal subject	Parent	Sibling
History of onset	History of onset	Origins of disease
Insulin administration	Treatment management and schedule	Food management
Urine testing	Diet management and food	Treatment regimen
Diet and food management	Reactions and illness	Talk about diabetes in family
Effect on what allowed to do	Effects on family as a whole	Reactions and illness
Effect on total family	Effect on child with disease	Discipline
Effect on subject	Effect of disease on spouse	Reactions of parents
Reactions and illness	Effect on yourself	Concerns about diabetes
Understanding of diabetes	Effect of disease on siblings	Other events in family
Effect of disease on mother	Sources of help	
Effect of disease on father	Talk about diabetes in family	
Effect on siblings	Family history	
Other children with diabetes	Major change in family as result of diabetes	
Sources of help for subject		
Sources of help for others		
Perceptions of medical care		
Major change for subject in having diabetes		

Data production as a process of negotiation

All methods in science involve a relationship between the investigator and the subject being considered. Where human behavior is at issue, the relationship is exceedingly complex in that both researcher and researched create data through interactions that meet their personal and collective needs as human beings. This point, particularly as it pertains to the experimenter's expectations coming to fruition in behavioral research, was made by Rosenthal (1966) and Friedman (1967) and earlier by Bridgman (1959) in relation to the human element in the so-called "pure" sciences. In essence, the crucial instrument for measurement and assessment in all research is the investigator. Criteria of validity, reliability, and objectivity are of necessity relative to a chosen frame of reference. For instance, Bruyn (1963) identified some basic differences between the operational approach and the sensitizing approach to the study of human behavior. Denzin (1977:28-56) detailed the importance of reciprocity in the logic of naturalistic inquiry derived from the symbolic interactionist perspective.

In this study the concept that best describes the process of data production is negotiation. The term implies a *reciprocal relationship* that involves the giving and receiving of favors. The concept of reciprocity has been used by a number of writers (Schwartz and Schwartz, 1955; Wax, 1960) for describing the working interactions that take place between researchers in the field and those providing the data.

Making contact: negotiation for access to data

Initially negotiation took the form of making contact with the physician in charge of the diabetic clinic as a first step toward meeting the young diabetics and their families. The initial encounter took place in the physician's private office, away from the medical center, where agreement was reached that the investigator would be free to come to the clinic to meet with the patient and family. Any arrangements with the families for participation in the research were to be made by direct agreement between them and the investigator.

Throughout the period of investigation no family was selected without previous consultation with the medical staff. This matter of keeping the channels of communication open was a form of exchange used for the specific purpose of minimizing the chances of misunderstanding and for preventing loss of face through lack of being informed—both for the physicians who were medically responsible for the participating families and for myself. In a sense the strategy might be viewed as a form of preventive *face-work* to lessen the possibility of incidents that could interfere with the collection of relevant data. According to Goffman (1967), face-work refers to actions used by individuals to avoid, minimize, and counteract threats to the images of self (the face that one presents to others) in interactions with others. In no instance was an effort made to block the participation of families selected as potentially desirable informants.

Once entree had been secured, the next phase was making contact with the families themselves. Initially the roles that seemed most appropriate were those of listener, uninformed outsider, and observer. The waiting room for the clinic was a conference room in which the parents sat together around a table and talked with the diabetic intern about food or compared notes among themselves on how to manage diabetes at home. Sometimes the young people entered into these conversations, but often they were busy playing or reminiscing about their experiences at camp. The spatial and social arrangements fostered a good deal of group interaction, and many interesting data were obtained simply by assuming the role of interested bystander.

In approaching the parents directly, I generally assumed the role of a member of a research group at the center interested in their lives and the complexities of having a child with diabetes. These semiprivate conversations always took place within the waiting room, a situation not conducive to asking for details about delicate matters. A number of mothers were anything but secretive in the presence of the group, though there were individuals who were reticent and kept pretty much to themselves. For the most part, there was a rather constant flow of conversation from which to pick and choose that which appeared to be conceptually relevant at the time.

The conditions were not optimum for talking with the young people themselves, primarily because of a lack of private space. Though there was opportunity to initiate further contacts with the families at this time, the choice of moving in that direction was delayed when the thought came to mind that spending time at the diabetic camp was a more appropriate way for establishing personal contacts with the young diabetics.

During this early period I wanted to obtain a general picture of the effects of diabetes on families. The social and spatial arrangements were such that these data were available with a minimal amount of direct negotiation. The conditions of the situation were such that the establishment of a workable contract was an easy matter. The atmosphere encouraged people to talk openly about the problems of diabetes. In addition, I imposed no demands on them for extra time but instead offered to be an interested listener during a rather lengthy period of waiting. In exchange for information, I was giving something—whether it was relief from boredom, the opportunity to express grievances, or the chance to express deeply felt emotions.

During the period at camp the situation was almost the reverse, and the utmost in tact and diplomacy was needed to gain access to the data known only to the young diabetics themselves. A good deal was available by simple observation, but the inner thoughts of the 12- and 13-year-old girls were not that open to the outside world. I accepted at the outset that the information available to me by direct exchange in conversation would be limited by the realities of sex similarity combined with age difference. As a woman equivalent in age to their mothers, I was a member of the older generation—the "other" group—and thus I was suspect until proven otherwise. According to the Group for the Advancement of Psychiatry (1968), early adolescence is a period marked by withdrawal from adults and from their values. From Sebald's sociological perspective (1968), the behavior of adolescents in Western society can be attributed to a crisis produced by a discontinuity of statuses with the intergenerational conflicts and problems of communication closely tied to the rapidity of social change.

In this setting I did not push for the facts but instead allowed time for the establishment of trust. Negotiation was marked by an air of caution and restraint, and respect for the young diabetic's right to privacy took precedence over the desire to be verbally aggressive in a search for understanding. In the end few data were obtained in verbal form, but relationships were established that facilitated asking for participation in the study at a later time.

Family contacts: negotiation for consent

Making arrangements for participation was complicated by the reality that two agreements had to be negotiated—one with the young diabetic, and the other with the parent(s). For legal reasons parental consent would have been necessary even if the interviews had been restricted solely to the young people. In this case there was the added matter of requesting time to talk with all members of the household, and the parents were the gatekeepers with power to block access to these sets of respondents. The problem of getting consent was far from easy to solve. It involved making both social and psychological contact with at least two people, each of whom might perceive the whole enterprise as a serious threat. It required offering an explanation that was motivationally stimulating to each. It meant obtaining specific agreements as to time, place, and willingness to participate.

The request for participation was designed to be both simple and straightforward. It consisted of a brief explanation of my interest in learning how families live with diabetes, and it emphasized the confidentiality of each interview. The approach to both child and parent was one of asking for help, and the point was made that participation in the project was not going to help them personally. Although an introductory conversation about the study sometimes involved the mother first, agreement was always obtained from the young diabetic before the parent was asked to give consent.

With 4 of the families arrangements were made by telephone. For the other 5 the initial contact was made face-to-face at the clinic. In appearance I aimed for a subdued effect through the use of inconspicuous colors and style of dress. In demeanor I aimed for a quiet and friendly approach, but both dress and manner of speech in later contacts with families varied depending on my assessment of the family's own style of living. The deliberate use of an inconspicuous appearance and mild manner during these introductory maneuvers was seen as a necessary step for negotiating the social identity of interviewer with persons whose own styles of dress and behavior were unknown quantities. According to Stone (1962:101), through his appearance the individual announces his identity and shows his values, moods, and attitudes for others to see. McCall and Simmons (1966:146) believe that appearance plays a critical part during the introductory phase when individuals are negotiating to establish mutually compatible social identities.

Negotiation for consent with the young diabetics encountered few obstacles; the young people were quite responsive to the interest shown in them. Negotiation with parents was a relatively easy process in seven of the families. In two families efforts to obtain total family participation was effectively blocked by the mothers, and in both instances there was evidence of an undercurrent of tension about diabetes within the family. On two occasions negotiation with the young diabetic was successful, but negotiation with the parent was not. In one case I talked first with the mother in the clinic, but on the follow-up telephone call to the home permission was refused on the basis that the father was not interested. This refusal served as a reminder that other investigators such as Bell, Trieschman, and Vogel (1961) had reported difficulties in gaining access to working class families when they used the mother as intermediary with the father. That working-class persons resist participating in research projects had been reported by several investigators, and in this study I became aware that more work would be required to obtain consent from the working-class families than from those in the middle class. However, the reasons for acceptance or rejection were undoubtedly influenced by a complexity of factors that could not be fully ascertained. The presence or absence of tension about diabetes seemed to be one factor of importance, with low tension concomitant with a willingness to participate and high tension generally associated with resistance.

I preferred face-to-face contact for negotiation primarily because of the broad range of interactional cues that were available. Yet telephone conversation did not appear to be a major deterrent to successful negotiation. It did place me at a disadvantage for pursuing negotiations that were tentative, and it placed those who were inclined toward refusal in a position of considerable power. Ball (1968) pointed out that the telephone gives certain advantages to those who in other circumstances would have little power to control. The most important single element that appeared to foster a positive response was the parents' personal and affirmative reactions to the interest and concern shown for their problems. As the study continued, I realized that a major element contributing to my own sense of ease or difficulty during the interactional processes was related to my feelings of comfort and adequacy when talking with individuals whose educational and social backgrounds were similar to my own.

The interview: a continuous flow of negotiation

As had been pointed out by Garfinkel (1967) and Cicourel (1964), the meaning of any data produced by human interacting with human must take account of the reality that the investigator relies on common-sense knowledge and everyday language when he selectively notices certain events and makes certain choices about their relevance, including a determination that they are "measurements" of some kind. Schutz (1955) suggested that man gives meaning to objects, facts, and events by interpreting them on the basis of four types of orders (marks, indications, signs, and symbols), but he tends to substitute one for the other in everyday life quite unknowingly and thereby tends to confuse his levels of abstraction. Stated differently, the process of interviewing involves human beings with all of their idiosyncratic, situational, and cultural variations coming into play so that bias and selective interpretation are built-in features. The problem for the investigator becomes one of explaining within the limits of his knowledge how the properties of the situation and the aims and styles of interviewing can influence the kind and character of the data obtained.

The collection of data by single interviews depends on the investigator's ability to negotiate effectively and purposefully within a role system of short duration; there are no second chances for data as occur with multiple contacts across time. The kinds and amounts of data in this study varied a good deal in part because the respondents represented a range of viewpoints by age, sex, and relationships with one another.

As negotiator for information from a heterogeneous group of respondents bound together in a network of primary relationships, I faced a complex and difficult task. In each case I had to make a "good fit" between the general role of interviewer and the complexity of other roles that come into play during ongoing interaction with the goal of obtaining selected information for later use in constructing a coherent story of the world of the young diabetic.

The bargaining process was heavily dependent on flexibility—both in creating an atmosphere conducive to open discussion and in shifting easily from one role to another as the occasion demanded. The interviews were easiest to perform when the respondents were women as I could identify readily with the roles they were playing. Conversely, the process of bargaining was more difficult with the children, especially young ones who shifted easily from one role to another without benefit of politeness or decorum. In this regard the young children had not yet been socialized into what Gouldner (1960:171) termed "the generalized norm of reciprocity" used by adults in social exchanges.

The strategies used were determined by the character of the information that was desired. The fundamental goal of each interview was to ask for accounts of selected events and topics *in the respondent's own words*. Thus the "tell me about" question was a frequent opener followed in turn by questions that made use of the respondent's own phraseology. In taking notes during the interviews every effort was made to capture the key words and phrases. In addition, I tried to be sensitive to the gestures and verbal cues indicating that a given topic or event carried significant meanings for the respondent. Yet in talking about sensitive matters conversational devices were used to offset the possibility of loss of composure, and no effort was made to force the respondent to talk about an emotionally distressing topic. The requirement of paying almost constant attention to the two interacting factors of verbal messages and nonverbal cues resulted in characteristically high stress for me.

During the interviews there were occasions when I had to deal with unexpected and unwanted contingencies—such as maintaining my "cool" while talking with a suspicious youngster or deciding how to answer a personal question about my private life. When disruptive or interfering roles appeared, as occasionally happened with the preadolescent children, I had to shift into an appropriate counterrole until such time as the interaction could again be centered on the matter of data production. (According to McCall and Simmons [1966:148-61], all interactions involve an exchange of gratifications, and both parties engage in bargaining—using power and social skill to achieve their ends.) These events were at times upsetting and irritating, but they interfered only minimally with the goal of obtaining information about the effects of diabetes on the family. Events of this nature were recorded and transcribed along with the other data that comprised the final report of the interview.

The completeness of the data was dependent on the structural conditions governing the interviews. To begin with, the contractual arrangements concerning the confidential nature of each interview prevented certain topics from being readily available to the interviewer for open discussion and clarification with other respondents. I took the position that it would have been a deliberate misrepresentation on my part to use privileged information from one interview to enter the private domain of another member of the family unless an invitation to do so was extended by that person. Commenting on disguised observations, Erikson (1967) suggested that a beginning point for an ethical position by sociologists might be on the issue of deliberate misrepresentation. As a result of the ethical position taken certain data were more limited in detail than was desirable for completeness of understanding.

Another factor influencing the kind and amount of data obtained was the sequence in which individuals in a family were interviewed. Although the young diabetic was generally the first to be seen, the other interviews did not follow a set pattern but were scheduled on the basis of availability of the respondents. As to whether the data were more complete or less complete when a particular sequence of interviewing was followed is a difficult matter to appraise, and it could not be answered by these data. Certainly sequence does make one fundamental difference in that the data brought to attention first serve as direction-setters for the development of thoughts and ideas about the sum of findings. Also, as Richardson, Dohrenwend, and Klein (1965:79-81) pointed out, sequence can make a great deal of difference in the success of a study when a bad experience for one respondent has an adverse effect on other respondents. However, sequence of interviewing in this study was thought to be less important overall than the securing of interviews with as many respondents as possible.

Completeness of the data was greatly influenced by the numbers of interviews done at any one time. I learned very quickly that my recall and efficiency were diminished when more than three interviews were scheduled in an evening. To avoid the interfering effects of multiple interviewing, efforts were made to spread the interviews over a period of time. This approach was not always in keeping with the interests of the family, however, and in one case the entire family was interviewed in 1 day. In consequence, the data from the families were somewhat variable in quality and detail. It was assumed that data obtained under less pressured and less tension-producing circumstances also suffered less from the effects of fatigue and interference with recall.

A fourth condition that interfered with the completeness of the data had to do with my difficulties in making interpretations and judgments about the relevance and meanings of certain words, phrases, and actions. The difficulty seemed most apparent in interpreting what was said and done across the boundaries of age. The problem of making judgments about the meanings of data obtained from young people in particular had its origin in psychosocial and semantic differences. These problems of interpretation could be traced to generational differences related to age-graded subcultures in modern society (Sebald, 1968; Stone and Church, 1968) as well as to differences in thought processes and semantics associated with childhood and adolescence (Inhelder and Piaget, 1958:334-50).

The data transcribed from the notes were of several kinds. One type consisted of incidents, events, or descriptions dealing directly with substantive issues—for example what the informant said about the giving and taking of insulin injections. Another class of data contained the observations or verbatim reports that said something about the perceived social relationships in the family; an illustration is the comment made by a 13-year-old girl as her mother walked into the next room, "She'll probably listen. She usually does," meaning that her mother regularly eavesdropped on our interviews. Descriptive notes about the residence, style of living, patterns of dress and demeanor, and any observed interactions among the family were also included. Transcripts of the interviews, including comments about any subjective reactions, were made as soon as possible after the interview to offset the effects of memory loss.

A severe limitation of these data was the lack of a checking device, such as a tape recorder, for analyzing the complexities of interaction that took place during the interviews. In this regard the data suffered not only from lack of detail and loss of memory but also from a lack of precision in knowing exactly how data were created through the process of negotiation. Cicourel (1964:73-104) argued that the interview needed to be studied as a form of social interaction involving common-sense interpretations by both interactants, and he questioned the assumption followed by investigators such as Hyman et al. (1954) that investigators could be trained to produce scientific measurements. Given the limitations in this study, however, the data did prove to be useful for understanding something about the social world of the young diabetic. The key to the analysis was found in the comparative value of total family interviewing.

Data analysis

The preliminary phase of the study made use of theoretical sampling in combination with the constant comparative method of joint coding and analysis. Out of this analysis came the development of a general schema for viewing chronic disease as a social phenomenon. A vocabulary of terms for describing and explaining these processes appeared, including the concepts of social visibility, disease trajectory, awareness management, and control agent. With the selection of diabetes for intensive study, the analysis began to shift in emphasis. Consultation conferences with other investigators studying different forms of chronic illness and the analytical memoranda written earlier provided the conceptual categories that served as a broad framework within which to work. The early analysis led to the identification of at least two types of families—child centered and parent centered—but a more explicit framework was needed for comparing the data on families as a whole.

The second phase of the analysis began with the development of analytical schedules to be used for coding and comparing the data from the interviews. The first schedule was devised in June 1968 for analyzing the stages of adjustment to disease. The topics selected for inclusion on this protocol came out of the symbolic interactionist perspective in combination with ideas identified in several studies of socialization. Direction for organizing the schedule came from Strauss' ideas (1959:44-131) about the transformation of identity, Hill's analysis (1965) of the generic features of families under stress, and Davis' report (1963) on the definitions of time and recovery of children handicapped by poliomyelitis. The schedule was fundamentally concerned with the process of change—time, critical points of disjuncture, crisis states, significant persons, and significant events. The seven areas incorporated into protocol I were as follows:

1. General background of family at time of onset
2. Recognition of "something wrong"
3. Contact with medical personnel
4. Period of impact
5. Assumption of treatment responsibility by parents
6. Key events and people in the learning process
7. Turning points

Several months later a second schedule was designed for analyzing the present meanings of diabetes and treatment for the family as a whole. Its development was influenced primarily by the conceptual system formulated by Hess and Handel (1959:1-19) for understanding and explaining the social and psychological complexities of ordinary family living. Of particular help in this analysis were their ideas about the existence of family themes in the established modes of interaction and the patterning of social relationships in terms of age and sex. An outline of the topical areas included in protocol II is contained in Table 3.

The analysis at this point was centrally concerned with understanding the impact of diabetes on the family as a social group. Review of the available data was influenced by several other theoretical perspectives on families, including differences between middle-class and working-class parents' attitudes about children (Rainwater, Coleman, and Handel, 1959), different types of family organization (Farber, 1962), stages in the family life cycle (Chilman, 1968), social networks of families (Bott, 1957), cultural variations in the value systems of families (Kluckhohn, 1968), conceptual differences between primary and secondary socialization (Berger and Luckmann, 1966), and lay alliances of families with handicapped children (Meadow, 1968). As the interviews with each family were completed, they were coded for inspection as a unit, and the analysis began with a search for the common elements of experience. A second goal at this time was to identify the structural features of the families that influenced how the commonalities of experience were incorporated into the different styles of living. A final purpose was to understand when and how the health care system intersected with and influenced the family during the transition that followed the diagnosis.

TABLE 3 ■ Analysis protocol II

Effects of diabetes on family life

Some properties of the family
Estimate of socioeconomic status

Membership of household
Extended family—location and
relationships
Length of time since onset of
diabetes
An estimate of family
relationships

*Management of diabetic treatment
at home*
Administration of insulin—who
does what
Urine testing—who does, how
used
Dietary management and food
Precautionary measures
Parents as treatment agents

Some consequences of the diabetes
Reactions and illness—frequency,
management
Parents as control agents
Sources of information about
diabetes

Special meanings of the diabetes
For mother—at first, now, any
change
For father—at first, now, any
change
For child with diabetes
For each sibling

*Special meanings for the family
as a whole*
Major disruptive influences rising
from disease
Cohesive influences associated
with the disease
Influence of genetic factor
Participation in diabetic network

The rather cautious approach used in handling these data came from the investigator's perception of their many limitations. In addition to the issues of selectivity in observation, interpretation, and recording already mentioned, the data from each family were in reality very small slices of information taken from a prolonged sequence of life space and time. For some of the families, even these data were incomplete.

During this period the importance of total family interviewing as a research method was confirmed. An understanding of the social history and particular familial meanings attributed to the diabetes increased in proportion to the number of informants who participated. More than that, however, the singular importance of siblings as informants for understanding the impact of diabetes on the family was a constant finding, no matter how different in structure the family might be.

As sources for comprehensive data, the interviews were of value in several ways. Most obviously, when the same events were described by several members of a family, they gave corroborative evidence of the relative importance and meaning of those events. In addition, the interviews provided evidence of discrepancies in viewpoint about the same event, and they often contributed new and significant information directly related to the individual's position in the family constellation. The data from each member of the family were distorted by his personal bias, but in combination they provided a useful means for constructing two realities—a chronology of the illness and an image of its present meanings. Stated differently, the variations in perceptions and perspectives of the parents and children when compared contributed to a systematic understanding of the influence of diabetes on the ongoing and changing group known as a family.

One other important finding about the usefulness of these interviews had to do with events that were omitted from discussion. Information not offered by a respondent about himself but offered by one or more members of his family tended to relate to events or experiences that were intensely meaningful (and often emotionally loaded) to that individual. For example, siblings reported on parental behaviors at the time of the diagnosis quite differently than did the parents themselves. The diabetic's description of his own behaviors was not always in keeping with the stories told by others in the family. It was by pulling the stories together that a meaningful collage began to take form.

The analytical procedures at this time moved simultaneously in two directions. Each family was analyzed as a unit while at the same time there was a comparative analysis of each family with all of the others. This coding and intrafamily comparison resulted in two analytical profiles for each set of interviews—one concerned with the process of change, and the other descriptive of the present meanings of diabetes in the family. The cross-family comparative analysis produced other memoranda of a more general nature. Among the topics covered in these memoranda were some properties of juvenile-onset diabetes, some notes on how families assimilate and use information about diabetes, the transfer of diabetic treatment from physician to family, properties of families who have trouble with diabetes, and ways by which diabetes can contribute to disruption of social order in the family.

After the collection of the data was completed, the third phase of the analysis began. Heretofore the family had been the core of the analysis, and relatively little attention had been focused on the personal meanings of being diabetic. For this purpose, a third analytical schedule was created, with the concepts of status passage and role-identity as its theoretical underpinnings.

Taken from the work of McCall and Simmons (1966:67-71), the concept of *role-identity* refers to the imaginative view an individual holds in his mind about himself *"as he likes to think of himself being and acting* as an occupant of that position" (italics by McCall and Simmons). According to this conceptualization, the role-identity serves to guide actual performance by functioning as a source for plans of action and by providing criteria for evaluation of performance. Since role-identity exists only in the mind of the individual, it cannot be measured directly; its characteristics must be judged on the basis of indirect evidence. The topics that were incorporated into analytical protocol III are listed in Table 4.

The process of reviewing and analyzing the data from the young diabetics was also influenced by a number of other perspectives on socialization processes and identity development. Among those whose ideas made a major impression were Lindesmith and Strauss (1968:233-295), who discussed the relationship of the development of language to role-playing processes; Pitcher (1965), who noted the early influence of primary socialization on children's expectations about manhood and womanhood; Becker (1963), who conceptualized the learning consequences of movement into a special subculture; Douvan and Adelman (1966), who studied the different meanings of physical appearance to adolescent boys and girls; and Turner (1956), who explored in some detail the relationship of role-taking to reference groups.

Again the analytical procedure took a two-pronged approach. The data from each diabetic were analyzed within the social context of his family relationships, and they were also used for cross comparisons with other diabetics in the sample. In this way the commonalities of the experience of becoming

---

TABLE 4 ■ Analysis protocol III

The meaning of being a diabetic

General background	Expected and unexpected
The label and the transition	consequences
Taking daily injections	Social contacts with confirming or
Doing urine tests	negating effects
Restrictions attached to food	Talk about diabetes—usual inter-
Exercise	action pattern
Experiencing the insulin reaction	Contacts with other diabetics
(hypoglycemia)	Future orientation
Gaining some control over insulin	Characteristics of role-identity
reactions	(at this time)
Episodes of sickness	

diabetic were highlighted, but also the many variations in personal meanings and experience were made evident. Concerning the common elements of experience, the analysis pinpointed those events and experiences that serve as markers for the young diabetic by giving meaning to his new identity. As for variations in experience, the analysis was mainly concerned with the socializing influence of the family, to some extent with the influence of physicians as direction-setters, and finally with the relative importance of contacts with other diabetics.

The actual process of analysis took place by using the field notes on each subject as a basis for creating an analytic descriptive profile of the meaning of being diabetic (based on the topics in protocol III). Thus the final comparisons were based on the derived and interpreted data comprising these profiles and not on the field notes themselves. The final comparisons were also facilitated by the many analytical memoranda created during the ongoing process of data analysis.

Throughout the study the typed interview notes and analytical memoranda were reviewed systematically by the senior investigators who supervised the research. In a sense they provided the main mechanism for establishing the validity of the conceptual categories derived from analysis of empirical data. The interview data were not coded independently by blind reviewers, as is commonly done in hypothesis-testing studies for establishing some measure of reliability. Rather, reliability depended on the investigator's reliance on multiple sources of data, selection of behavioral indicators representative of the conceptual categories identified as necessary to a proposed social theory of diabetic identity development, and conservative approach to the interpretation of the findings (Denzin, 1977).

A final word may be in order about my personal experiences that contributed in an unforgettable way to an understanding of the social consequences of diabetes. One such episode occurred during the summer at camp; being suddenly wakened by the screams of a child suffering a severe hypoglycemic reaction made quite an impression. The meaning of what it must be like to be the parent of a child with diabetes was forcefully brought home by the emotional impact of that unexpected emergency in the middle of the night. The event served as a kind of reality shock, and it had a sensitizing effect that was far-reaching in its influence—both in guiding the collection of the data obtained from parents and in drawing conclusions about its relevance.

The experience was a cogent reminder of the gap that often exists between describing an event and experiencing an event. It delivered a telling message that getting a good night's sleep may be an extraordinary event in the life of a parent with a diabetic child. In fact, there is much in the treatment of diabetes that impinges on the ordinary experiences of living. As the analysis continued, the data came to reveal more and more that the core meaning of juvenile diabetes as a social phenomenon lies in the reality that the commonplace in living becomes uncommon (Benoliel, 1975).

Major concepts and findings

According to these data, the developmental and variable character of the emerging diabetic identity is its basic feature. The events and experiences that provide the defining terms for the diabetic child fall into two broad categories. The first set consists of the physical and social changes that are a direct result of the metabolic processes and/or treatment procedure and that cause the individual to experience pain, embarrassment, fear, or social restriction by virtue of being different from other people. Secondary to the first set are the derived experiences imposed by the actions and choices of other persons with whom the diabetic interacts.

Parental style as agent of diabetic control

To judge from the data, the attitudes and actions of parents are by far the most important elements affecting the social environment in which the young person begins to understand the personal and social implications of being diabetic. Of great importance in this matter of socialization is the parental style of functioning as an agent of diabetic treatment. The four styles identified in the analysis—protective, adaptive, manipulative, and abdicative—created different kinds of socializing environments and thereby fostered differences in the self-perception and diabetic role performance of the child, as has been reported (Benoliel, 1970). My interest in parental style as agent of diabetic treatment was stimulated by Hadley's conceptualization (1966) of three patterns of parent-child relationship—protective, rejective, and adaptive—for examining differences in the relinquishment of the "sick role" by children who had successful corrective surgery for congential heart conditions.

The study also showed that parents of diabetic children had to modify their lives in three important ways:

1. Adopt a time-scheduled pattern of living in keeping with the requirements of the diabetic regimen.
2. Manage "food as treatment" and cope with the effect of this requirement on the family's established eating habits.
3. Assume clinical management of the diabetes and monitor diabetic signs and symptoms in their roles as the delegated agents of medical treatment.

These demands impinged heavily on the adaptive capacities of the families, and the analysis showed two general patterns of accommodation. Five of the families had incorporated the diabetic regimen into a way of life that was reasonably stable and yet flexible to the changing needs of the young diabetic. The other four families had developed a diabetic subculture that was characterized in one way or another as a situation of recurring crisis events.

The five families that were able to fit the diabetic regimen into a way of life that was reasonably satisfying had some common characteristics. There were two parents in the home, and they were in reasonable agreement on the development and enforcement of rules of conduct and other matters pertaining to the diabetes. In addition, both parents were actively involved in socializing the young diabetic. The other four families had not achieved a stable pattern of accommodation, and the diabetes persisted as a source of tension and strain. More than that, conditions of living were such that three of the young diabetics were using a type of diabetic role performance that was keeping them in a rather consistent state of poor diabetic control—a physical state known to lead to early complications and death. These findings not only had theoretical implications, but also implied the need for health care services designed to assist families during their early adaptations to living with diabetes. Some recommendations to this effect were published in 1977 (Benoliel, 1977).

A diabetic role-identity

The data also served as a basis for some theoretical considerations about the emergence of a new identity. With my findings as a starting point, I began with the assumption that being a diabetic is an unwanted and undesirable status and that the incorporation of good diabetic habits into a way of life requires the transformation of a negatively valued status into a self-image that has a positive value. The question that can then be posed is what kind of experience contributes to the development of a positive self-image as a diabetic? Conversely, what type of experience leads to the development of a negative self-image and to negligent performance? Although the answers are not observable directly, the diabetic role-identify does demonstrate itself indirectly through the person's role performance as a diabetic.

Despite the abruptness of movement into the diabetic career, the creation of a diabetic role-identity is a gradual process. It emerges out of the child's experiences with a variety of events that function as personal reminders that he is diabetic, and the reminders take many forms: procedures that must be performed; restrictions on activities; feeling states that tell him he is "high" or "low" (referring to blood sugar levels); and visible effects that he may or may not be able to control. It emerges also out of interactions with other people who by their actions and reactions convey messages about their definitions of diabetes. To judge from these findings, the most important influence on the emerging diabetic role-identity is derived from interactions within the family, and the socializing approaches and activities chosen by the parents set the tone and direction that it will take.

The development of a particular role-identity can be viewed as an amalgamation of at least two basic components. There is the *cognitive component*, which consists of a system of concepts and ideas organized in the thoughts to give meaning to the notion of having the identity of diabetic. The concepts and ideas include a set of expectations about self and others, an awareness of the salience of certain events on the enactment of the role, and an idea of the consequences of certain actions. These cognitions have their origins in fact and in fantasy, and they can be viewed as having value attachments that fall on a continuum of desirable (positive) to undersirable (negative).

Also influencing the formation of this inner image is an *affective component* consisting of the feeling states, perhaps a system of feeling states, that come to be associated with the concepts, ideas, and events associated with the generalized notion of having the identity of diabetic. There are, however, particular feeling states that come to be associated with one or another aspect of the identity. In the case of diabetes there may be considerable variation in the feeling or affect that comes to be associated with different aspects of being diabetic. The origins of these feeling states are multiple and begin with an established general pattern of mood and reactions toward self and others and toward the world at large. Role experience that causes a certain feeling tone to emerge on a regular basis is one contributor—for example, the pain associated with taking shots or the fear tied to loss of voluntary control during hypoglycemic reactions. Interactions with other people provide the major means whereby a pattern of feeling states comes to be learned, and the actions of the significant persons in an individual's life are the primary direction setters. McCall and Simmons (1966:130-40) suggest that identities are "negotiated, legislated, and adjudicated" through interactions with others, and these procedures take place by means of cognitive processes (thoughts) and expressive processes (overt expressions or actions). In other words, identities are not imposed but are shaped out of bargaining experiences with others.

Assuming that choices concerning role performance are governed by both cognitive and affective forces, one can construct a set of categories for discrimination of four theoretical types of role performance. In the case of diabetic role performance, a standard for the cognitive component is based on the medical ideal (proposed by medical experts in diabetes) that the diabetic know everything possible about his disorder and its treatment. A standard for the affective component is conceived as a value attachment that has its origins mainly in feelings of self-esteem. By combining these dimensions and

| Value | Knowledge of valid facts | |
attachments	High awareness	Low awareness
High esteem	High conformity	Unintentional nonconformity
Low esteem	Variable conformity	Unconcerned nonconformity

TABLE 5 ■ Type of diabetic role performance

using compliance with medical treatment expectations as a measure, four types of diabetic role performance can be analytically distinguished, as shown in Table 5.

Underlying *high-conformity* role performance is the ideal type of diabetic role-identity characterized as both knowledgeable and high in self-esteem. That is, there are positive values attached to the status, and the performance itself is one of compliance without compulsion. The polar opposite, *unconcerned nonconformity*, derives from a role-identity that is lacking in knowledge and low in self-esteem. Where *unintentional nonconformity* exists, the choice is based on lack of information. *Variable conformity* derives from a role-identity in which knowledgeability and low self-esteem engage in something of a tug-of-war for control.

In lieu of the term *esteem*, the value attachments might alternatively be described in terms of high and low access to social rewards. By using the term *esteem*, emphasis has been given to the invisible self-image that governs the selection of actions, whereas use of the social reward concept would have emphasized interactional influences.

The importance of self-esteem in the creation of the diabetic role-identity became increasingly evident as the data were analyzed and the role performances of the 13 young people were compared. The meaning of being diabetic for each came out of interactions in which combinations of cognition and affect came together, and there were several categories of interaction that functioned as influential socializing experiences. Through these types of interaction, examined in detail in the final report of the study (Quint, 1969a), knowledge and esteem came to be bound together to form a framework for the initial formulations of the diabetic role-identity.

The category of interaction that had the greatest impact on the character of the emerging diabetic role-identity was the pattern of day-by-day interaction that developed in the family for dealing with the regular events and untoward experiences that were part and parcel of living with diabetes. Differences in parental styles of coping with the diabetes affected the transmittal of information to the child as well as expectations about his ability to take over as principal agent of diabetic control. The cognitive element of the diabetic role-identity was retarded in its development when protective or abdicative styles were prominent, and one result was a tendency toward diabetic role performance that was either unintentional or unconcerned nonconformity. The cognitive element was nourished by the adaptive style if the parent had access to sound and up-to-date information about diabetes, and role perform-ance in the direction of high conformity was stimulated. The manipulative style did not noticeably prevent access to information, but it created an emo-tional climate that interfered with its effective use and thus fostered a diabetic role performance of the variable conformity type.

Admittedly, making judgments about the effects of daily interaction on the affective component of the diabetic role-identity is highly conjectural, and the comments that follow are offered in this light. It is proposed that basic family themes and parental styles of functioning create learning fields for the inter-nalization of patterned feelings that, in turn, enhance or inhibit the young diabetic's choice of role-performance in the direction of high conformity. Stated in a somewhat different way, the young diabetic's sense of self-esteem is di-rectly related to the emotional climate that is part of his everyday living, and moral judgments about his worth are conveyed mainly through the expres-sive processes used by his parents. Family patterns that promoted high con-formity in diabetic role performance were remarkably similar to the parental patterns of behavior described by Coopersmith (1967) in his study of the an-tecedents of self-esteem in preadolescent middle-class boys.

A theory of chronicity

The findings of the study pointed clearly to the sequential and shifting nature of chronic disease and to the multiplicity of conditions that influence the process of becoming diabetic during childhood and adolescence. The data also showed that awareness is an element of considerable importance in the development of theory about chronicity because the effectiveness of treat-ment at home lies in the hands of the individual and his family. *Awareness* refers to knowledge that serves as a *determinant for action* regardless of whether it is correct or incorrect from the perspective of ideal therapy.

A theory of chronicity must also take account of explicit ways by which a disease or other infirmity creates conditions in need of attention. Chronic metabolic disorders, of which juvenile diabetes is one, are characterized by the properties of *permanency, progressivity,* and *periodicity.* There is no cure, though there may be periods of apparent remission, and the individual must plan on the use of *replacement therapy* for the remainder of his life. As time goes by, the diabetes causes or is associated with internal derangements that impair his ability to function as a socially normal being and may lead to loss of vision, to chronic disability at an early age, or to an early death. Finally, the disorder manifests itself by acute episodes or *crisis states* that can be controlled mainly by adopting a *self-disciplined style of living.*

The matter of periodicity is of singular importance in the day-by-day life of the diabetic who must take insulin to survive, and two kinds of acute episodes can bring havoc to his life if they are not controlled. Insulin shock reaction, or hypoglycemia, can be a very frightening experience for the diabetic and it can bring an unwanted side effect of being labelled in an undesirable way. To offset the possibility of these reactions, the diabetic can never forget about time. In fact, time must become the ruler of his life.

The other significant crisis state in diabetes does not come on abruptly as does hypoglycemia. Rather the signs of ketoacidosis may be subtle enough that the individual can function with reasonable social competence in a relatively poor state of diabetic control. By living under these circumstances, however, he increases the chances of early physical disability as compared to living in a state of reasonably consistent diabetic control. Prevention of this complication depends heavily on the disciplined use of food and physical activity. *Regularity of schedule* is probably the single most important factor contributing to consistency in diabetic control.

The meaning of chronicity is a learned phenomenon that is in a continuous state of revision as the individual moves from status to status through his experiences in the human life cycle. The development of awareness about what is involved in being diabetic begins during a period of transition when the individual is introduced to certain events and experiences that come to function as reminders of his special status. These reminders come in several forms: activities to be performed regularly; primary and secondary social restrictions; direct experience with crisis states; and events that serve as reminders of stigmatizing concomitants.

In matters of daily living the effects of chronic disease are socially disorganizing at those points where the disease overlaps with usual and ordinary activities and where the salience of other statuses is at issue. The question of disclosure of the label to other individuals increases in proportion to the negative social consequences ascribed to the disease. The data in this study indicated that as the child with diabetes moved into adolescence a pattern of openness with peers about the disorder gave way to a *selective openness*— usually with special and trusted persons only. This practice served the important function of creating a corps of backstopping agents, people who knew what to do if a crisis state accidentally took place in a public place and the individual missed the warning cues or ignored them.

Just as chronicity is a process of change for the individual, so does it produce alterations in the pattern of family relationships. The influence of chronic disease begins with a reorganization of family structure and style during the period of transition, but the structure of the family continues to undergo modification as new phases of being diabetic appear. The disorganizing effects of chronic disease tend to appear whenever there is a major shift in the family life cycle.

The refinement of performance as diabetic takes place by a trial-and-error process in which danger periods are identified and special precautions put into effect. Sources for learning come through crisis incidents that serve as reminders of the controlling demands of time and food, and through exchange of information within a network of diabetic families. The potential shortening of the life cycle of the child acts as a constant undercurrent of tension and reaches a high pitch for the agent of treatment whenever a crisis state appears. The disruptive influence of diabetes (as one form of chronicity) occurs within the family principally when the requirements of the diabetic regimen interfere with child-rearing practices in general and with already established patterns of eating and uses of food.

The individual's style of performance in response to the expectations of medical treatment is affected by a multiplicity of circumstances. Performance in the direction of conformity with the "diabetic rules" is directly affected by the opportunity to obtain valid and complete information about diabetes, but consistent performance in this direction requires more than exposure to facts. The type of role-performance selected is directly related to the processes of legitimation and adjudication provided to the individual through interaction with the principal agents of socialization: physicians and members of the family. Points of disjuncture occur for the individual when a crisis state is not amenable to control, but such events may or may not be perceived as having serious consequences for the future. As direction-setters for the future, both sets of socializers are influential through their advice and their methods of offering role support. *Future directions* are also affected by the frequency and type of contact with others in similar circumstances, and continuity of contact with a special subculture of diabetics is a factor of some importance in giving special meaning to the experience of being diabetic.

These thoughts contain some of the elements that are fundamental to the creation of a social theory of chronicity. No effort has been made to organize them into a coherent system of concepts, properties, and relationships, although the ideas have been published in preliminary form (Quint, 1969b). They do provide the basis for a limited social theory about juvenile diabetes as one form of chronicity in adolescence.

IMPLICATIONS FOR NURSING

The creation of social theory grounded in empirical data about health-related crises and major transitions has important implications for nursing practice and nursing science. The position taken here is that nursing practice fundamentally takes place by means of social transactions between practitioners of nursing and those who are receiving nursing services. The creation of social theory that clarifies the social impingements of critical changes and the conditions affecting how individuals and groups adapt to them can provide concrete direction for identifying circumstances of high risk, structural defects in the available health services system, and needs for assistance not yet met by the system. Some implications drawn from this research about juvenile diabetes and the health care system illustrate these points.

Juvenile diabetes and health services

The findings indicated several family types that appeared at greater risk than others of not assuming the responsibilities of the diabetic regimen in a manner that provided the child with reasonably good diabetic control and the opportunity to have some productive years as an adult. The diabetic regimen made tremendous demands on a family's resources, and any family that was deprived in social, psychological, or economic resources could be judged a high-risk candidate. Families from the lower socioeconomic levels of society had a high-risk potential because they lacked funds to implement the treatment in an optimum way, their systems of values and beliefs did not fit well with those that dominate the present system of health services, and parents were not prepared by training or experience to take over the complicated position of agent of diabetic treatment as expected by the physician. The findings showed clearly that the child's adaptation to diabetes was made easier when both parents participated actively as socializing agents—a pattern found in the middle-class families (Rainwater, Coleman, and Handel, 1959; Sebald, 1968) In a sense the life-style of working-class families makes them a high-risk group for assimilating the diabetic regimen into an adaptive pattern geared to the teaching and socializing needs of the young diabetic.

The findings also showed that even families with the best of social resources found themselves in conditions of high risk at the time of initial diagnosis. In addition, they shared the common experience of dealing with a system of health care deficient in services designed to help families deal constructively with the serious interpersonal problems, cultural conflicts, and structural modifications precipitated by having a diabetic child. This problem was directly related to structural conditions determining how the delivery of health services to persons with chronic illness was to take place.

At the time of the study the crux of the problem was that the system of health services was not well equipped for the teaching and socializing functions necessary at the time the physician delegated medical responsibility for diabetic management to the family. A particularly significant gap was the lack of specific services to help families make explicit plans for the transition from hospital to home. The extent to which referral to visiting nurse services provides this kind of assistance is a problem in need of study. At the time of the research there was reason to think that the services offered by nurses through such agencies were geared more toward traditional teaching activities associated with diabetes than toward the gamut of teaching and counseling needs implied by the findings.

The need for intermediary services to help the parents of diabetic children make the transition from hospital to home was quite apparent. Since the study was done, the diabetic clinical specialist has appeared; but much remains to be learned about how effective these new services are in helping families make positive adaptations to chronic illness at home. Recognition of the need for transition services to assist diabetic children and their families (as well as people with other chronic diseases) was an outcome of this research, and some specific recommendations about the essential ingredients of these services have been offered (Benoliel, 1977; Quint, 1969a).

Social theory and nursing science

The creation of social theory grounded in empirical data is a necessary step in the development of systematic knowledge that can properly be called the province of nursing science. Social theory should not be confused with sociological theory; the former is grounded in data that cut across the traditional fields of scientific knowledge and combine perspectives from more than one field. It provides a theoretical basis for the study of nursing practices by clarifying the *process* or *context* in which intervention is proposed. Systematic study of interventions by nurses is of limited scope without a theoretical perspective on the social situation in which an intervention is proposed and a clarification of the concepts or variables that are critical to the situation.

Research of the type described in this chapter provides one means of conceptualizing the interacting influences of personal characteristics, social processes, and cultural circumstances as they bear on the adaptation of individuals and groups to crisis and change. Such research leads to speculation about theoretical relationships among variables that can be refined and tested through additional scientific investigation. As a practice-oriented discipline, nursing must be concerned with the influence of social interaction on health-related attitudes, beliefs, and behaviors. Theory based on the empirical world of people undergoing health-related crises is essential to the creation of scientific knowledge in nursing.

REFERENCES

Ball, D.W. 1968. Toward a sociology of telephones and telephoners. In Truzzi, M. editor. Sociology and everyday life, Englewood Cliffs, N.J., Prentice-Hall, Inc., pp. 59-75.

Becker, H.S. 1963. Outsiders, New York, The Free Press.

Bell, N., Trieschman, A., and Vogel, E. 1961. A sociocultural analysis of the resistances of working class fathers, American Journal of Orthopsychiatry 31:388-405.

Benoliel, J. 1970. The developing diabetic identity: a study of family influence. In Batey, M. editor. Communicating nursing research, vol. 3. Boulder, Colo. Western Interstate Commission for Higher Education, pp. 14-32.

Benoliel, J. 1975a. Research related to death and the dying patient. In Verhonick, P., editor. Nursing research I, Boston, Little, Brown & Company, pp. 189-227.

Benoliel, J. 1975b. Childhood diabetes: the commonplace in living becomes uncommon. In Strauss, A., editor. Chronic illness and the quality of life, St. Louis, The C.V. Mosby Co., pp. 89-98.

Benoliel, J. 1977. The role of the family in managing the young diabetic, The Diabetic Educator 3:5-8.

Berger, P.L., and Luckmann, T. 1966. The social construction of reality, New York, Doubleday & Co., Inc.

Blumer, H. 1969. Symbolic interactionism: perspective and method, Englewood Cliffs, N.J., Prentice-Hall, Inc.

Bott, E. 1957. Family and social network, London, Tavistock Publications, Ltd.

Bridgman, P.W. 1959. The way things are, Cambridge, Mass., Harvard University Press.

Bruyn, S. 1963. The methodology of participant observation, Human Organization 22:229-233.

Chilman, C.S. 1968. Families in development at the mid-stage of the family life cycle, The Family Coordinator 17:297-312.

Cicourel, A.V. 1964. Method and measurement in sociology, New York, The Free Press.

Coleman, J.: 1961. The adolescent society, New York, The Free Press of Glencoe.

Coopersmith, S.: 1967. Antecedents of self esteem, San Francisco, W.H. Freeman & Co., Publishers.

Crain, A.J., Sussman, M.B., and Weil, W.B., Jr. 1966. Family interaction, diabetes and sibling relationships, International Journal of Social Psychiatry 12:35-43.

Davis, F. 1963. Passage through crisis, Indianapolis, The Bobbs-Merrill Co., Inc.

Denzin, N.K. 1977. Childhood socialization, San Francisco, Jossey-Bass, Inc., Publishers.

Douvan, E., and Adelson, J. 1966. The adolescent experience, New York, John Wiley & Sons, Inc.

Erikson, E.H. 1963. Childhood and society, ed. 2, New York, W.W. Norton & Co., Inc.

Erikson, E.H. 1968. Identity: youth and crisis, New York, W.W. Norton & Co., Inc.

Erikson, K.T. 1967. A comment on disguised observations in sociology, Social Problems 14:366-373.

Farber, B.: 1962. Types of family organization: child-oriented, home-oriented, and parent-oriented. in Rose, A., editor. Human behavior and social processes, Boston, Houghton Mifflin Co., pp. 285-306.

Friedman, N. 1967. The social nature of psychological research: the psychological experiment as a social interaction, New York, Basic Books Inc., Publishers.

Garfinkel, H. 1967. Studies in ethnomethodology, Englewood Cliffs, N.J., Prentice-Hall Inc.

Glaser, B.G. 1965. The constant comparative method of qualitative analysis, Social Problems 12:436-445.

Glaser, B.G., and Strauss, A.L. 1965. Awareness of dying, Chicago, Aldine Publishing Co.

Glaser, B.G., and Strauss, A.L. 1967. The discovery of grounded theory, Chicago, Aldine Publishing Co.

Glaser, B.G., and Strauss, A.L. 1968. Time for dying, Chicago, Aldine Publishing Co.

Glaser, B.G., and Strauss, A.L. 1971. Status passage, Chicago, Aldine Publishing Co.

Goffman, E. 1959. The presentation of self in everyday life, New York, Doubleday & Co., Inc.

Goffman, E. 1963. Stigma, Englewood Cliffs, Prentice-Hall Inc.

Goffman, E. 1967. Interaction ritual, Chicago, Aldine Publishing Co.

Gottlieb, D., and Ramsey, C. 1964. The American adolescent, Homewood, Ill., Dorsey Press.

Gouldner, A.W. 1960. The norm of reciprocity: a preliminary statement, American Sociological Review 25:161-178.

Group for the Advancement of Psychiatry. 1968. Normal adolescence, New York, Charles Scribner's Sons.

Gustafson, S.R., and Coursin, D.B. 1965. The pediatric patient 1965, Philadelphia, J.B. Lippincott Co.

Hadley, B.J. 1966. Becoming well: a study of role change, Ph.D. dissertation, Los Angeles, University of California.

Handel, G., and Rainwater, L. 1964. Persistence and change in working-class life style. In Shostak, A., and Gomberg, W. editors. Blue-collar world, Englewood Cliffs, N.J., Prentice-Hall Inc., pp. 36-41.

Hess, R.D., and Handel, G. 1959. Family worlds, Chicago, University of Chicago Press.

Hill, R. 1965. Generic features of families under stress. In Parad, H., editor. Crisis intervention: selected readings, New York, Family Service Association of America, pp. 32-52.

Hyman, H.H., et al. 1954. Interviewing in social research, Chicago, University of Chicago Press.

Inhelder, B., and Piaget, J. 1958. The growth of logical thinking, New York, Basic Books Inc., Publishers.

Kluckhohn, F.R. 1968. Variations in the basic values of family systems. In Bell, N. and Vogel, E. editors. A modern introduction to the family, New York, The Free Press, pp. 319-330.

Lindesmith, A.R., and Strauss, A.L. 1968. Social psychology, ed. 3. New York, Holt, Rinehart & Winston.

McCall, G.J., and Simmons, J.L. 1966. Identities and interactions, New York, The Free Press.

McKinley, D.G. 1964. Social class and family life, New York, The Free Press.

Meadow, K.P. 1968. Parental response to the medical ambiguities of congenital deafness, Journal of Health and Social Behavior 9:299-309.

Miller, S.M., and Riessman, F. 1964. The working-class subculture: a new view. In Shostak, A., and Gomberg, W. editors. Blue-collar world, Englewood Cliffs, N.J. Prentice-Hall, Inc., pp. 24-36.

Muuss, R.E. 1962. Theories of adolescence, New York, Random House Inc.

Olesen, V.L. and Whittaker, E.W. 1967. Role-making in participant observation: processes in the researcher-actor relationship, Human Organization 26:273-281.

Olesen, V.L., and Whittaker, E.W. 1968. The silent dialogue, San Francisco, Jossey-Bass Inc., Publishers.

Pearlin, L.I., and Kohn, M.L. 1966. Social class, occupation, and parental values: a cross-national study, American Sociological Review 31:466-479.

Pearsall, M. 1965. Participant observation as role and method in behavioral research, Nursing Research 14:37-42.

Pitcher, E.G. 1965. Male and female. In Roach, M. and Eicher, J., editors. Dress, adornment and the social order, New York, John Wiley & Sons Inc., pp. 214-216.

Quint, J.C. 1963. The impact of mastectomy, American Journal of Nursing 63:88-91.

Quint, J.C. 1964. Mastectomy: symbol of cure or warning sign? General Practitioner 29:119-124.

Quint, J.C. 1965. Institutionalized practices of information control, Psychiatry 28:119-132.

Quint, J.C. 1967. The nurse and the dying patient, New York, Macmillan Publishing Co., Inc.

Quint, J.C. 1969a. Becoming diabetic: a study of emerging identity, Doctor of Nursing Science dissertation, San Francisco, University of California.

Quint, J.C. 1969b. Some thoughts on a theory of chronicity. In Norris, C., editor. Proceedings of the First Nursing Theory Conference, University of Kansas Medical Center Department of Nursing Education, pp. 58-67.

Rainwater, L., Coleman, R.P., and Handel, G. 1959. Workingman's wife: her personality, world and life style, New York, Oceana Publications Inc.

Richardson, S.A., Dohrenwend, B.S., and Klein, D. 1965. Interviewing: its forms and functions, New York, Basic Books, Inc., Publishers.

Rose, A.M. 1962. A systematic summary of symbolic interaction theory. In Rose, A. editor. Human behavior and social processes, Boston, Houghton Mifflin Co.

Rosenberg, M. 1965. Society and the adolescent image, Princeton, N.J., Princeton University Press.

Rosenthal, R. 1966. Experimenter effects in behavioral research, New York, Appleton-Century-Crofts.

Schutz, A.: 1955. Symbol, reality, and society. In Bryson, L., et al., editors. Symbols and society, New York, Harper & Row, Publishers Inc., pp. 150-156.

Schwartz, G., and Merten, D. 1967. The language of adolescence: an anthropological approach to the youth culture, American Journal of Sociology 72:453-468.

Schwartz, M.S., and Schwartz, C.G. 1955. Problems in participant observation, American Journal of Sociology 60:343-353.

Sebald, H. 1968. Adolescence: a sociological analysis, New York, Appleton-Century-Crofts.

Seeley, J.R., Sim, R.A., and Loosley, E.W. 1956. Crestwood Heights: a study of the culture of suburban life, New York, Basic Books Inc., Publishers.

Shibutani, T. 1962. Reference groups and social control. In Rose, A., editor. Human behavior and social processes, Boston, Houghton Mifflin Co., 128-147.

Simmons, J.L., and Winograd, B. 1966. It's happening, Santa Barbara, Ca. Marc-laird Publications.

Stone, G.P. 1962. Appearance and the self. In Rose, A., editor. Human behavior and social processes, Boston, Houghton Mifflin Co., pp. 86-118.

Stone, L.J., and Church, J. 1968. Childhood and adolescence, ed. 2, New York, Random House Inc.

Strauss, A.L. 1959. Mirrors and masks, Glencoe, Ill. The Free Press.

Strauss, A.L. 1964. George Herbert Mead, on social psychology, Revised ed., Chicago, University of Chicago Press.

Stryker, S. 1968. Identity salience and role performance: the relevance of symbolic interaction theory for family research, Journal of Marriage and the Family 30:558-546.

Tanner, J.M. 1963. The course of children's growth. In Grinder, R., editor. Studies in adolescence, New York, Macmillan Publishing Co., pp. 417-432.

Turner, R.H. 1956. Role-taking, role standpoint, and reference-group behavior, American Journal of Sociology 61:316-328.

Wax, R.H. 1960. Reciprocity in field work. In Adams, R. and Preiss, J., editors. Human organization research, Homewood, Ill., Dorsey Press, pp. 90-98.

CHAPTER 6

LABORATORY AND FIELD EXPERIMENTATION
development of a theory
of self-regulation

Howard Leventhal
Jean E. Johnson

We want to tell you of our collaborative effort to use nursing and psychological theory and laboratory and field experiments to contribute to the development of a model of self-regulation under stress. Before doing so we would like to raise a more general question that was first raised more than a decade ago by the sociologist Edward Rogers (1968): "What can health professions ask of behavioral theory and behavioral research?" Addressing the Medical Sociology Section of the American Sociological Association, Rogers argued that the practical output of sociological (behavioral) studies "ought to be improvement in programs of disease control." He also stated that "one of the most striking things about the large number of studies . . . is the virtual impossibility of transforming the study findings into public health program form."

This conclusion seems somewhat surprising when we look at the problems facing public health (health professions) today. Infectious disease is no longer a major issue for public health; epidemics have long been controlled by various public health measures, such as draining swamps, water purification, and waste disposal (Saward and Sorenson, 1978). Securing public participation in inoculation programs is a continuing problem (Leventhal et al., 1960) that seems to be growing more severe as parents fail to inoculate their children and update their own inoculations against scourges such as measles, polio, diphtheria, and tetanus (Mortimer, 1978). Thus many of the public health problems in infectious disease control are behavioral.

Chronic illness also confronts us with a host of behavioral problems. The identification and modification of risk factors related to cancer or heart disease focus on behavioral problems such as diet and weight control (Winikoff, 1978), cigarette smoking (Leventhal and Cleary, 1977), and a host of problems in so-called compliance with medical treatment (Sackett and Haynes, 1976). Given these problems, it is astonishing that so negative a judgment could be made of the contribution of behavioral research to public health. Yet Rogers' judgment was probably correct, and it still has the ring of truth some 15 years later (Leventhal and Cleary, 1979).

Why have sociological and psychological research made such a meager contribution to the solution of public health problems? While moderate funding has undoubtedly restricted the quantity and quality of research and thus the growth of knowledge, we believe there is a more fundamental reason for the lack of contribution. The questions addressed by much behavioral research, psychological as well as sociological, do not provide answers relevant to the solution of health problems. It is all too easy to misunderstand this statement. We do not mean that most behavioral research fails to answer practitioners' questions by being too abstract or theoretical. On the contrary, we believe much behavioral research fails to suggest answers to critical practice questions because it merely describes the characteristics of the situations and persons involved in specific health problems and pays little attention to the reasons for the relationships between variables. Thus as Rogers (1968) suggested, sociological studies of health care problems merely identify who is distressed and who is at risk, their ethnic and social characteristics such as education and income (Dohrenwend and Dohrenwend, 1970), their personality characteristics and family membership (Croog, 1970; Fox, 1978), and their recent life events (Hinkle, 1974; Holmes and Masuda, 1974). Findings of this sort are useful in identifying potential target groups for intervention— that is, they can identify the types of persons who have unmet health care needs—but they are not particularly useful in telling us how to intervene to meet these needs. Because the studies do not address the specific factors most closely related to disease, they do not help us design disease control programs (educational or otherwise) that " . . . can be focused clearly and directly, with a minimum of involvement with remote events, attention to which tends to reduce program effectiveness" (Rogers, 1968:159; see also Mechanic, 1974).

If descriptive data are useful primarily for knowing who is at risk, then what do we need to know to change behaviors so as to reduce risk and improve the delivery of health services? In our opinion the first requirement is to understand the process underlying the behavior we wish to change. Whether the behavior is smoking (Leventhal and Cleary, 1974; Lichtenstein and Keutzer, 1971), lack of successful accomplishments (McClelland, 1978), anxiety (Lang, 1968; Wolpe, 1958), or pain and distress (Hilgard, 1973; Johnson, 1975; Leventhal and Everhart, 1979), our chances of altering it are greater if we understand the process by which situational and personal factors exert control over the behavior.

But how do we come to understand the underlying process? There seem to be two critical steps. First, we try to formulate a conceptual model of the process. The model directs our attention to particular features of behavior and to particular features of the environment. It also leads us to expect relationships between different specific behaviors and particular environmental events. Second, we attempt to test the model. We can do this (1) in observational studies in which we examine the frequency of behaviors in different environments and the association between behaviors in specific groups of persons or (2) in experimental studies where we prepare specific stimulus conditions, educational programs, environmental arrangements, social contexts, and so forth, and observe the consequences of these environmental conditions on designated behaviors. Compared to the observational or correlational method, the experimental method has distinct advantages. It permits us to control the temporal order of events so that we know that particular environmental variables preceded specific behaviors. It also allows us to vary the makeup of the environment so that we can better identify the specific environmental ingredient essential for the appearance of the behavior. The only way of ruling out the possibility that an association between situational and behavioral events is because of unmeasured characteristics of the persons or of the preference of different persons for different environmental situations is to use an experiment with random assignment to conditions.

In this chapter we will attempt to show how experimental methods can be used in laboratory and health care settings to help develop a model of self-regulation. The aim of our research was two-fold: (1) to increase understanding of the processes underlying self-regulation of responses during threat and (2) to generate procedures useful for self-regulation by patients undergoing treatment. Developing initial hunches, elaborating a total model, deriving and testing specific hypotheses, refining and revising theory, and crystallizing alternative views of the outcomes and attempting to tease out which is closer to the truth and which explains a wider range of behaviors were all part of our research effort. This is the stuff that adds spice to what might otherwise be the pallid pursuit of "objective facts." The traditional view that science is the accumulation of objective fact and gradual closing in on "truth" is a false one (Hempel, 1966; Kuhn, 1970). Phrases such as "the joy of groping," "the joy of grappling," and "dashes of insight in the midst of seas of confusion" more aptly describe the process of developing theory through research. Putting together successive theoretical inferences and insights increases the depth of our understanding of the problems and enlarges our view of human behavior. Employing a variety of research strategies stimulates the formation of insight into new methods of attacking other behavioral problems. It takes considerable time and energy to learn about the kinds of processes we are studying, and the research and theory-building activities we will describe do not fit the idealized, orderly model of scientific endeavors found in many texts.

There is one final feature of the research endeavor that must be mentioned. The work has been influenced by conceptualization of the nature and purpose of health care and the role of the practice of nursing. A guiding theme has been that nursing focuses on the total functioning person—that is, on the patient's *motivation* or desire and efforts to act; his *cognition*, or perception and interpretation of his body and his situation; and his *emotion*, or his subjective feelings and overt expressions of emotion. From this perspective nursing has three functions:

1. *Technical,* such as the giving of medication and the treatment of wounds
2. *Educational,* such as providing information, models, and guidance relevant to illness and treatment, information concerning feelings and the similarity of feelings among patients, and information important for self-

management and participation in treatment for chronic and acute conditions

3. *Supportive*, that is, being there and caring

Respect for the rights of patients and the belief that the patient must be self-regulating are central to our view of nursing specifically and health care in general. Our views of health care have influenced our theoretical and empirical pursuits; sometimes the influence was purposeful and specific and other times it was intuitive and vague. Perhaps the major impact of using a nursing focus was that its emphasis on *doing* led us to phrase behavioral concepts and questions in an action framework rather than to be satisfied with a descriptive framework. Of course, the relationship was reciprocal; as our view of the process of self-regulation became enriched, our view of the foundations of nursing practice became more specific. But it was the interplay between views of the role of nursing in health care and views of psychological processes that made us conclude that the most fruitful connection between practice and research is at the level of theory and that nursing research must conceptualize psychological variables within an action framework to contribute to practice.

In the sections that follow we will lay out the history of our research programs. We will try to show the interplay between theory and data and between laboratory research and field research conducted in natural settings. We begin by presenting a general model of behavior during taxing or threatening situations and an exploratory study that examined the usefulness of the model. Next the model will be examined further through a series of experimental studies focusing on a particular type of intervention. Each author then presents theoretical interpretations of the research, which differ in significant ways.

THE RESEARCH PROGRAM
Background to the program

It is difficult to reconstruct precisely how we began to work on distress reductions through psychological preparation, but we shall try to do so. A very strong impetus came from nursing theory and practice. Jean Johnson's years in surgical nursing persuaded her that psychological factors played a key role in the patient's health and illness behavior and his postoperative recovery. Observations of patients convinced her of the significance of anxiety and distress and also convinced her that coping was a complex process involving psychological factors that could be influenced by nurses. A physician might have conceptualized the problem somewhat differently, leading to a different practice impact of the research program. For example, physicians are trained to diagnose and prescribe so as to cure disease or retard its progress. Thus it is not surprising that physicians interested in behavioral research tend to focus on problems of patient compliance or on creating procedures to increase patients' conformity to physicians' prescribed regimens. These studies usually focus on didactic education (Sackett and Haynes, 1976) and problems in organizing information to enhance patient understanding and memory (Ley, 1977). Consistent with their medical orientation, physicians often treat emotional responses with drugs. By contrast, nurses focus on the person with a health problem. The nurse attends to patients' perception of their illness, the impact of illness on patients' lives, and the response strategies used by patients to cope with these experiences. The nurse's orientation recognizes the patient as an active problem solver and attempts to enter his problem-solving domain to provide corrective information, models, and support where needed, so the patient can achieve more accurate understanding and more effective regulation of his illness and treatment. The psychological processes of the patient are as central to nursing as is the didactic physiological orientation to medicine.

A second impetus came from psychological theory. Howard Leventhal had been investigating emotional behavior for several years. After many studies on the effects of fear-arousing communications on beliefs and behavior, he had come to a major revision in his thinking about the nature of emotion and its relation to adaptive activity (Leventhal, 1970). His experiments on fear-arousing communications had been designed from the frame of reference of emotional drive theory. Drive theories assume that some kind of drive, such as hunger, thirst, sexual arousal, or fear, must be present if an organism is to behave and to learn. Psychoanalysis (Freud, 1926) and traditional behavioral theories (Dollard and Miller, 1950) share this viewpoint and argue that a person can be instructed to believe or act in a particular way, but he will neither believe nor behave as instructed unless some drive is present. Drive is necessary for motor activity, and the person will not learn a new belief or behavior unless the new behavior is drive reducing. Therefore the model argues that the arousal of fear is an essential antecedent to performance, and the reduction of fear by specific behavior such as rehearsing a particular belief (smoking is dangerous) or engaging in specific practices (throwing away cigarettes) is necessary if these behaviors are to be "learned."

The drive model was simple and seemed reasonable (Miller, 1951; 1963). It also had the didactic quality of the medical model, since the communicator was using fear-arousing information to compel the recipient to comply. But experiments did not support the drive model deductions. Subjects did alter their beliefs and their behavior in response to fear communications, but these changes did not appear to depend on a process of fear arousal and fear reduction. Instead, it appeared that presenting a fear communication to a subject created an occasion for active problem solving or "information processing," which could proceed in either (or both) of two directions. First, the subject could process the information in a way that led to fear behavior. Second, the subject could process the information in a way that led to the perception and interpretation of the presence of danger. Both the creation of fear and the perception and interpretation of danger affected attitudes and intentions to take protective action; but their impact varied depending on their relative strength, which differed by person and by time. For example, once the threatening material was removed, the fear began to decline. Within a few days all that remained was the individual's knowledge of danger. If this knowledge included a plan for action, that is, if the individual had thought through and rehearsed specific protective behaviors, he was likely to take protective action (Leventhal, Singer, and Jones, 1965). Thus subjects who were exposed to threatening messages on the dangers of tetanus were intent on obtaining tetanus shots but they obtained shots only if they had thought about their daily schedules and planned a particular time to go for shots. If the subjects did not plan or rehearse the behavior, they did not act. Both components, the knowledge of danger and the plan for action, were essential for behavior. The likelihood of action was no greater, however, if the threatening information was strong and aroused much fear or if the threatening information was mild and aroused little fear! Any level of threat combined with a self-generated plan of action led to the same frequency of protective action. The fear aroused by intense threat messages had only a short-term effect in increasing *intentions* to act immediately after exposure to the messages. But these emotionally induced intentions were not durable. This new model, called the parallel response model (Leventhal, 1970), gave much greater weight to the problem-solving activities of subjects—the nursing orientation described earlier.

Our initial study in a health care setting
Background

How did our two backgrounds interact in our first investigation in a health care setting? What was the product of the combination of the parallel response model (derived from attitude-change research) and the nursing theory and years of clinical experience of a skilled nurse-practitioner? The first investigation was a nonexperimental study conducted with James Dabbs (Johnson, Leventhal, and Dabbs, 1971). The study examined the factors related to postoperative fear. Indications of postoperative coping from two different perspectives: (1) the drive model and (2) the parallel response model. Since the predictions of the two models conflicted with one another, this nonexperimental study had the characteristics of a *strong experiment* (Chamberlin, 1965): if it came out one way it would support the drive model, and if it came out the other it would support the parallel response model.

According to the drive model, patients who were extremely fearful before surgery were expected to continue to manifest high levels of fear postoperatively and to show a poor postoperative recovery (Janis, 1958). High levels of fear are more intense than magnitude of the danger warrants; a high level of fear is neurotic because it reflects earlier (childhood) fears and it is not susceptible to reassurance because there is nothing in the current situation that can realistically alleviate imagined dangers based on earlier (childhood) happenings. The drive model also predicts that low levels of preoperative fear will lead to poor postoperative recovery. When patients are not frightened, they will not be driven to engage in preparatory behavior. According to the drive model, the patients who will perform best postsurgically are those who are moderately frightened before their surgery. A moderate fear level is high enough to drive the patient to prepare for the postoperative experience, but not so high as to disrupt his adaptive capacities. In summary, the drive model predicts a curvilinear relationship between preoperative fear levels and postoperative adjustment. It predicts that patients who are highly fearful presurgically will continue to manifest high fear levels postsurgically, since they are not open to reassurance and cannot cope with fears that are not grounded in reality. On the other hand patients who are not fearful at all before surgery will lack the motivation to engage in mental work. Thus it is the moderately fearful who will fare best; they will not be angry postoperatively, they will need the least medication, and they will actively cope and be rehabilitated most rapidly.

The parallel process model posits that fear behaviors and behaviors for coping with danger can vary independently of one another. It is important, therefore, to distinguish between emotional or fear behaviors and instrumental or coping behaviors. Fear behaviors include reports of subjective emotional states (reports of fear, tension, irritability, fright, depression, anger, and so forth), reports of worry and pain, expressive reactions (facial responses indicating fear, surprise, or excitement), postural changes indicative of tension (body swinging, muscle tension, and so forth), various psychophysiological reactions (increases in rate and variability of cardiac response, skin sweating, and so forth), and reactions that are facilitated or amplified by psychophysiological changes (such as gagging, vomiting, and other forms of gastrointestinal distress). Coping behaviors would include reactions to control a stressor (such as deliberately swallowing a camera tube, obtaining a preventive inoculation to avoid a disease threat, seeking medical care for a symptom), and asking for help and assistance from medical authorities (such as requesting an examination, asking for medication, deciding to stay in the hospital to be close to the source of care). There are two points worth making about this distinction. First, the emotional behaviors are generally seen as automatic and involuntary reactions that are expressive of fear, while the coping or instrumental behaviors are generally seen as deliberate, volitional reactions designed to regulate either the environmental agent causing the emotion or the emotional behavior itself. Second, the distinction cannot be drawn hard and fast, as it is partly dependent on underlying process, that is, on whether the behavior is automatic or deliberate; and partly dependent on function, that is, on whether the behavior is expressive of emotion or an instrumental attempt to cope with emotion. For example, an expression of fear may be an automatic reaction to threat and be permitted or amplified by voluntary action, and it may both be expressive of emotion and be an instrumental effort to cope by calling for help.

Fear behaviors stem from the perception of threats in the situation and concerns about the adequacy of coping resources (Lazarus, 1966, 1968; Withey, 1962). If fear is strong preoperatively, it is likely to be strong postoperatively; if fear is weak preoperatively, it is likely to be weak postoperatively; and if fear is of intermediate strength preoperatively, it is likely to remain so postoperatively. In summary, the parallel process model predicts a linear relationship between preoperative fear levels and postoperative fear if no special efforts are made to change the underlying process.

Coping, on the other hand, stems from the perception and evaluation of specific targets as dangers and from the availability of resources and skills to manage these targets. Everyone confronting surgery will perceive at least some experiences that they view as dangerous and/or taxing their abilities to cope. They will experience the need to act to regulate pain, nausea, fatigue, restlessness, boredom, and so on. While all surgical patients may be aware of the need to engage in coping behaviors, the critical factors influencing their actual ability to cope with postoperative recovery will be their available resources and coping skills. According to the parallel process model, factors such as the subject's belief in his ability to control his environment (Rotter, 1966) should be a key predictor of coping behavior. Fear behaviors may interact with or affect coping if the level of fear is sufficiently great, since very high levels of fear tend to disrupt ongoing coping activity.

Study design and procedure

A total of 62 women were interviewed the evening before surgery, interviewed briefly the morning of surgery, and reinterviewed on each morning of the 4 following days. A final interview took place the evening of the fifth day after surgery. The patients had all been admitted for elective abdominal surgery—44 for hysterectomy and 18 for cholecystectomy.

The important predictors (independent variables) of postoperative fear behaviors were preoperative fear level (measured with a set of five adjectives that the patient checked off as representative of her emotional state on three-point scales—not at all applicable, somewhat applicable, very applicable), a three-item worry scale, and nine items from the Taylor Manifest Anxiety Scale (Taylor, 1953) to measure trait anxiety or anxiety as a personality predisposition. Nine items from the Rotter (1966) Internal-External Control Scale were used to measure internal resources for coping (the items were worded so that the subject could respond to each on a seven-point Likert scale) and to reflect the subject's personality predisposition toward active control of her environment. We also recorded the patient's order of birth in her family since this factor had been shown to relate to fear level in threatening situations (Schachter, 1959).

Results

There were simple linear relationships between preoperative measures of fear level and postoperative measures of fear and other postoperative moods. Subjects low in preoperative fear were low in postoperative fear, depression, lethargy, and anger and were high in postoperative measures of well-being and happiness. Patients high in preoperative fear were high in postoperative fear, depression, lethargy, and anger and low in postoperative measures of happiness and well-being. The patients moderate in fear level preoperatively were between the other two groups but were closer to the low-fear patients than the high-fear patients. Postoperative fear and postoperative pain ratings varied with birth order and trait anxiety level; patients high on trait anxiety tended to report more fear and more pain. Those born later in their family tended to report less pain and fear after surgery than did firstborns. The combination of the two individual difference factors produced an additive impact; the women born later in their families were low in trait anxiety and tended to report the lowest levels of fear and pain.

There were no significant relationships between the two measures of postoperative coping, number of doses of analgesic requested per day of postoperative stay, and preoperative fear level. But both measures of postoperative coping were related to birth order and to scores on the Internal-External Control Scale. Subjects high in internal control (patients who believed they could and should control their environments) obtained a greater number of analgesics from the staff than did the other patients. Those who scored high in internal control obtained an average of 9 doses of analgesic; those who manifested external control received 6.2 doses; and those in the middle, 5.1 doses. Days in the hospital varied by both internal-external control and birth order. The firstborns who were high in internal control stayed in the hospital 8.9 days on the average, which was over a day longer than later borns (7.2 days average) and more than 2 days longer than firstborns who were higher in external control (6.4 days average).

Discussion

The main findings of the study tended to support the parallel process model rather than the drive model. There was a strong linear relationship between preoperative fear and postoperative fear and pain, and trait anxiety and birth order accounted for an additional portion of the postoperative ratings of fear and pain. Thus the data suggested that emotional responses in stressful situations are generated by relatively unchanging dispositions to interpret taxing situations as threatening. The amount of analgesia per days spent in the hospital (the coping indicators) were not related either linearly or curvilinearly to preoperative fear or trait anxiety levels. The key predictor of coping was the measure of internal control; patients high in internal control requested and received more analgesics and were hospitalized longer if they were firstborns. The latter finding was important as it suggested that the greater postoperative fear of the firstborns may have influenced the coping processes. Perhaps firstborns managed to obtain extra days of hospitalization because they were more fearful and felt more threatened by what they perceived as too early a departure from the safety of the hospital.

It is not immediately obvious whether internal control should lead to more or less use of analgesics or more or less rapid departure from the hospital. If the patients had been given preoperative instructions and practice in coping with postoperative conditions, one might expect internal control to relate to less use of analgesics and more rapid discharge. Thus if the environment provides the means for self-regulation and defines less use of analgesics and more rapid discharge as effective behavior one might expect individuals high in internal control to more readily meet these criteria. There were no such educational efforts in the hospital at the time these patients were studied and no clear indications as to whether early or late discharge indicated more or less effective coping behavior. One might speculate that as a consequence, those patients high in internal control may have defined coping in terms of taking analgesics and staying close to the authorities who could control danger.

The data in this study did not support the drive model, since the predicted curvilinear relationship between fear and postoperative coping was not found. (Similar conclusions were reached by Cohen and Lazarus [1973], Levy [1945], Sime [1976], and Vernon [1967].) Our conclusion from this study that the parallel process model represented the subjects' emotional processes better than the drive model was of more than academic significance. While neither the drive model nor the parallel process model specifically suggested how to go about reducing fear they pointed in very different directions. The drive model suggested that preparatory activities by nurses should attempt to generate fear in the nonfearful and reduce fear in the highly fearful in order to promote coping. The drive model states that fear is necessary for patients to engage in the mental work of preparation, though it fails to indicate what that mental work should be. The parallel process model suggests a need to attack the problem of fear reduction and the problem of coping through separate activities. It predicts that lower initial fear may be better and will not be worse than high or middle fear in promoting effective coping and reducing later fear. It also suggests that skill training might promote effective coping.

Psychological interventions and distress reduction

The study just described increased our confidence in the suitability of the parallel process model for the analysis of emotional behavior in stressful settings but its practice implications were implicit rather than explicit. One cannot readily alter birth order, and there is too little time (or money) to justify complex therapy to alter personality traits such as trait anxiety level and internal-external control, a factor that may be related to self-esteem (Ickes and Layden, 1978). Preoperative fear was the only independent variable studied whose effects suggested direct implications for guiding nursing practice. Even for this independent variable, the research did not provide direct information about the specific environmental events that could be manipulated by a nurse to reduce preoperative fear. In addition, the implicit cause-effect inferences we made in testing the models were weakened by the possibility that other variables that we did not investigate might account for the observed associations between variables.

Where could we find clues for how to generate environmental manipulations for varying fear and coping behaviors? There were three options. The first was to generalize from psychological theory and research. The second was to make use of nursing theory, research, and practice experience. The third was to make use of everyday common sense.

Leventhal and Cupchik (Cupchik and Leventhal, 1974; Leventhal and Cupchik, 1975, 1976) had conducted a number of studies on the effects of observing one's own laughter in humorous situations and they found that attention to laughter could disrupt the subject's pleasure. Their theoretical interpretation of these data was that the emotional response of laughter was a structured whole; that is, it consisted of perceptions and interpretations of stimuli (things that are funny) tightly linked to expressive reactions (facial expression and central motor reactions related to facial expression) and to autonomic responses (heart rate change, skin conductance, and so forth). Further, focusing attention on one of the component reactions (such as the expressive behavior) broke apart and disrupted the emotional experience. This theory suggested that one way of controlling fear might be to prepare the individual for his own component bodily reactions of fear before they occurred; by focusing his attention on these responses we might disrupt the organization of his emotional experience and thus undercut the intensity of the individual's distress from fear and pain. Preparing subjects to attend to the expressive and autonomic reactions associated with their emotions was effective in disrupting laughter (a pleasant emotional experience) but it was not clear that it would work equally well with fear (an unpleasant emotional experience).

A second option, suggested by past experiments on fear arousal and attitude change, was to develop some form of plan for actively coping with the threatening situation. An early study by Egbert et al. (1964) had found that informing the patient about impending surgery and rehearsing specific action plans for coping with pain and distress effectively reduced anxiety and enhanced effective coping with a fear-provoking setting. However, this study combined so many factors (reassurance, information, and coping skills) in its intervention package, including repeated postoperative contact with the experimental subject but not with the control group, that it was not clear which, if any, of the factors would be an effective intervention if manipulated alone.

Jean Johnson, drawing on nursing practice and psychological research and theory, was able to suggest a third alternative. In practice she had seen evidence that patients were better able to tolerate a stressful experience if they were informed about the treatment procedure before being exposed to it. However, the type or characteristics of information that helped people control their emotional reactions had received little attention. The classic experiment by Schacter and Singer (1962) had demonstrated that subjects who were told to expect the bodily sensations resulting from an injection of epinephrine responded with less emotion that those who were not told to expect these sensations. Extensions of Schacter's (1964) model of emotion attempted to demonstrate that when subjects believed their symptoms of physiological response were the result of a neutral aspect of their environment (such as noise or a pill) they would show less emotional response than when the symptoms were thought to be caused by a threatening aspect of the environment such as a shock (Nisbett and Schachter, 1966; Ross, Rodin, and Zimbardo, 1969). While the results confirmed this hypothesis, a careful reading of the reports revealed that the subjects who were led to believe the symptoms of arousal were caused by a neutral source were also given a description of the sensations typically experienced (such as rapid heart rate, shaking hands, and rapid breathing). We reasoned that the reduction in emotional response may have resulted from subjects being forewarned about the sensory experience rather than the aspects of the event they were led to believe caused the sensations. A study by Calvert-Boyanowsky and Leventhal (1975) strongly supported this interpretation.

Physicians and nurses often provide patients a description of the procedure about to be performed. Was a description of sensory information the same as what was usually provided patients? The usual information consists of a description of what will be done to and for the patients. We have labeled such information *procedural* because it describes how the procedure is done. On the other hand, sensory information describes the patient's perceptual experience—that is, it describes the sensations that can be expected. Sensory descriptions focus on what the patient will see, feel, hear, smell, and taste during an event. It focuses on the event from the vantage point of the person who will have the experience.

We thought that sensory information would be more effective than procedural information in reducing emotional response because the sensations perceived are the features that give rise to emotional reactions. If the sensations experienced were expected the person would not be confronted with an unexpected sensation and would feel less need to be "on guard" during the experiences. A well-informed person might be able to maintain a low emotional response or at least an emotional response well matched to the intensity of the sensation instead of exaggerated. Of course, we did not expect to eliminate completely reactions to unpleasant sensations.

Laboratory studies of sensory information
Background

We knew well that other explanations could be developed to account for the effects we attributed to sensory-perceptual information. Nevertheless it seemed time to test the effects of such information and to collect data on other possible explanations for the results we might observe. But was it time to study a patient population? There were two reasons why we thought not. First, we could not assume sensory information would have the expected effect without first testing it. We did not wish to expose patients to the risk of a negative effect from our intervention before we had some data that suggested the expected results would occur. Having positive findings in our first patient study was important not only to bolster our confidence but to increase the probability of securing a physician to collaborate in a patient study. Second, we felt we could not ask patients to answer a sufficient number of questions to rule out alternative interpretations of any effect we might find. For these reasons Jean Johnson (1973) turned to the laboratory and conducted three experiments on the effects of sensory information on ischemic pain.

Ischemic pain was selected for the noxious stimulus, as it was thought to provide a satisfactory stimulation of clinical pain (Smith et al., 1966). Also, the stimulus can be applied without harm for several minutes, allowing time for the operation of cognitive processes in pain reduction.

Johnson (1973) conceptualized pain as consisting of two components: one informational and the other affective or emotional. This conceptualization was congruent with that of other investigators in pain research (Beecher, 1959; Casey and Melzack, 1967; Melzack and Wall, 1965) and was also compatible with the parallel model, which separated emotional and informational processes. More important, many writers have argued that the primary sensory output from a painful stimulus need not have a one-to-one relationship to responses indicating distress (Beecher, 1959; Casey and Melzack, 1967). These assumptions led Johnson to the hypothesis that sensory information would reduce the experience of distress during ischemic pain but would have little or no effect on the experience of sensations from the noxious stimulus.

Design and procedure

Male undergraduates at the University of Wisconsin participated in these studies. They were told that the experimental procedure would be painful but not harmful. If the subject agreed to participate, he filled out a health questionnaire and a 25-item Mood Adjective Check List that measured five different mood states: well-being, fear, anger, helplessness, and depression.

Just before the ischemic pain procedure began the subject was given information about the procedure. This was the critical point for the introduction of the independent variables. In the first experiment there were two different experimental conditions and two different sets of instructions. The instructions were contained in a folder and were read by the subject. This procedure kept the experimenter from knowing the subject's experimental condition. The control group instructions provided procedural information; it said, "The sensations and discomfort you will experience are due to temporary ischemia of your arm (lack of blood in the arm). A tourniquet filled with air will cause high pressure on your arm. It is very unlikely that you have experienced discomfort of this kind before." The experimental group was given the sensation information that said, "You can expect to feel pressure and sensations such as tingling and aching, followed by numbness, very much like when your arm is 'asleep.' Your arm and hand will be temporarily very pale and blotched. This discoloration is typical when pressure is applied to the arm."

The ischemic pain procedure involved wrapping a standard blood pressure cuff around the upper arm and pumping it up to 250 mm Hg. The subject then squeezed a hand dynamometer 20 times to the 20-lb. marker. Each squeeze lasted 2 seconds and they were separated by 2-second pauses. This took about 1½ minutes, and the cuff was left on for an additional 3½ minutes, or 5 minutes in all.

Subjects reported the amount of distress and the strength of the sensations they felt on two separate scales. The scales were drawn as vertical lines similar to a thermometer, and the subjects were specifically told to think of the sensations and distress as two separate things. The timing of the judgments was controlled by prearranged signals played on a tape recording.

The second experiment (Johnson, 1973) was very similar to the first. This time, however, there were four groups, two given sensory information and two given procedural information. The subjects were treated identically to those in the first study; that is, they were told about the procedure, were given an opportunity to decline to participate, were exposed to the appropriate instructions (sensory or procedural), had their arm wrapped in the cuff, and were told how to make their ratings of sensation and distress. After the cuff was inflated and the subjects had made their first two ratings, half of the subjects in each condition were put to work on a set of multiplication problems. The other half of the subjects were given an attentional task consisting of instructions ("Look at and think about your arm and hand. Which of these sensations do you have now?") and checking yes or no to indicate whether they were experiencing any one of the sensations on a list of seven. The idea was to see if working at a distracting task versus paying close attention to the sensations would have any further effects on the subject's sensation or distress experience. The tasks were interrupted toward the end of the ischemic procedure to see if there were any marked change in distress as a result of the interruption.

Results

The results of the two studies can be reported together, as they were virtually identical. Subjects in the sensory information condition consistently recalled being told to expect specific sensations and reported they expected to experience the sensation; procedural subjects did not recall being told about sensations nor did they expect all of the sensations they experienced. This indicated that our attempts to manipulate the subjects' awareness of procedures and of sensations had been successful.

The subjects reported the intensity of their sensations and feelings of distress at 30- to 45-second intervals through the final 3 to 3½ minutes of the 5 minutes of exposure to ischemic pain. The first of these reports was 1½ or 2 minutes after inflation of the cuff. The sensory condition subjects generally reported lower sensation strength, but the differences were not large enough to have statistical significance. By contrast, both experiments showed clear differences for distress reports between the type of preparatory information groups. Subjects given sensory information reported substantially lower levels of distress than did subjects given procedural information. The results held throughout the rating periods, that is, from 1.5 to 2 minutes to 5 minutes after the application of the blood pressure cuff.

Discussion

The data supported the belief that sensory information reduced distress during noxious stimulation. The contrasting lack of effect on the sensation scale suggested that sensation information operated on the reactive (Beecher, 1959) or emotional (Leventhal, 1970) component of the pain experience. But how did sensory information work? Did it induce higher levels of fear before noxious stimulation, leading to preparatory worry and resulting in reduced distress during the painful experiences? This hypothesis is compatible with the drive explanation discussed earlier. On the other hand, did sensory infor mation arouse different expectations of being harmed; for example, did the subjects given sensory information feel there was little chance they could be injured? The procedurally informed subjects may have been less certain of their safety.

The subjects in both experiments were asked a number of questions before and after the removal of the tourniquet. Among these was a mood adjective checklist similar to that used in the surgical patient study, which was given to subjects before and after they received the information and after the cuff was deflated. Questions about expectations of danger were asked only at the experiment's end. The Mood Adjective Check Lists showed no significant changes in reported fear or other moods from before to after the delivery of either type of information. There was no support, therefore, for the hypothesis that different levels of fear were aroused by the sensory and procedural information that would lead to differential distress reactions during exposure to ischemic pain. The questions on danger showed no postexperimental differences, ruling out the hypothesis that sensory information reduced distress because subjects perceived they were in less danger than procedural information subjects. In fact, both groups of subjects accurately perceived that they were not in danger of injury.

The methods of these studies are presented in detail to show how much care and attention is needed to separate the affects of one theoretical process from those of another by experimentation. The protocol, what is said to the subject, the methods for producing distress, and so forth must be specified precisely or results cannot be replicated and one cannot go on to determine the constituents of the variation in preparation procedure that produced the difference between the groups. Care must be taken to ensure that the experimenter cannot influence the findings by knowing which condition the subjects are assigned to or by suggesting particular ways of answering questions. In both of the studies the subjects were *randomly assigned* to the treatment conditions. Random assignment is critical for eliminating alternative hypotheses relating to subject differences. For example, in the descriptive study by Johnson, Leventhal, and Dabbs (1971) one cannot determine whether the findings for preoperative fear level, birth order, and internal-external control are caused by these individual difference variables or by some other unmeasured characteristic of the subjects that happened to be associated with the three factors that were measured. In the later experiment, random assignment assures that the effects of individual difference factors are randomly distributed across the experimental conditions. When random assignment has been used, individual difference factors are unlikely to account for statistically significant findings.

Even when care and attention are used in design, there may be alternative explanations for the findings of an experiment. In this instance the alternatives examined involved expectations of harm and predistress levels of fear and anxiety. A critical reader may well question whether Johnson did an adequate job in ruling out these alternative hypotheses by using postexperimental questions. After all, the alternative hypotheses suggest that sensation information may have produced moderate fear or less severe expectations of harm *before* the subjects were exposed to the ischemic stress, and Johnson questioned her subjects about these factors *after* they had gone through the stress experience. It is possible that retrospective reports differ from prospective reports. To take account of this criticism Johnson ran a third study. Up to the point when the cuff was to be inflated the procedure was identical to that of the first experiment. At that point the experimenter stopped and asked the subject to answer a series of questions about his feelings and expectations *at that moment.* There were no significant differences between sensory and procedurally informed subjects with respect to the magnitude of anticipated strength of sensations or distress from the sensations.

Johnson's ischemic pain experiments persuaded us of two things: (1) giving sensory information is a viable method for controlling distress in situations of relatively prolonged exposure to noxious stimulation, and (2) the sensory information influenced the emotional component of the response system but had little effect on the informational and coping systems as reflected in ratings of intensity of physical sensations (see also Knox, Morgan, and Hilgard, 1974). Now we felt it was time to evaluate the applicability to clinical settings of the effects of sensory information on distress as observed in the laboratory setting by studying patients scheduled for a diagnostic procedure.

It is important to recognize what we expected to gain by extending our results to a health care setting. First, we did not expect to acquire a great deal of new information that would further elaborate basic theoretical processes. The primary goal was to see if sensory information produced significant effects in a clinical population. Naturally occurring threats differ in important ways from threats contrived in the laboratory. A diagnostic examination has the potential for greater impact than a laboratory experiment because laboratory subjects know that they cannot be exposed to dangers that have the potential for lasting effects. The diagnostic examination in and of itself is a threat and there also is the threat of what will be revealed by the examination. Subject characteristics and situational factors will vary greatly in naturally occurring threatening events. It is very difficult for the researcher to control all of the factors that could potentially influence the patient's response to the situation. However, if the preparatory information's effect was not strong enough to overcome the uncontrolled sources of variance, its usefulness to health care situations would be doubtful. A second possible gain from a clinical study would be to obtain nonverbal measures of distress. Only verbally reported data were obtained in the ischemic pain experiments. While we firmly believe verbal report a reliable and valid way to measure pain and distress, extending the evidence by obtaining behavioral data increases confidence in the finding. Replicating the laboratory experiment in a natural setting addressed ecological validity. The study was not designed to provide new theoretical insight.

Studies of gastroendoscopy
Background

A search was begun for a field setting to test the hypothesis that sensory information would reduce emotional distress by specifying the essential characteristics for such a setting:

1. It should be one where most patients experienced distress.
2. The patient had to be awake and able to experience and respond to the distressful circumstance.
3. It must be possible to develop a preparatory communication to describe the typical sensory experience.
4. The situation should last for a reasonable but not excessively long period of time so we could see distinct effects in more or less the same time frame we had used in the laboratory.

These requirements were more difficult to meet than we at first expected. For example, how can one be sure that a medical procedure or a laboratory procedure is stressful? And how does one go about determining the sensory experiences that patients or subjects have in a medical or laboratory procedure? With respect to whether an event is stressful, common sense is often our only source of information and it can be very wrong. The methods of identifying the sensory features and their appropriate labels were not well developed when the first clinical study was conducted, but we interviewed patients for the purpose of determining the nature of their experience.

Fortunately, we found a setting that met our criteria and one in which we could identify objective sensations: the gastroendoscopic examination. Gastroendoscopy is performed early in the morning; the procedure takes about 30 minutes. First, the throat is swabbed with a local anesthetic (which causes numbness), and the patient is asked to lie on an examination table and swallow a fiber optic tube (which causes sensations of gagging, of the flexible tube going down the throat, and so forth). Once the tube has been swallowed, the patient must occasionally reposition himself as instructed and lie still while the stomach is inflated with air (feeling of fullness) to permit examination of all parts of the stomach lining. The lights are dimmed (change in brightness) and the examination proceeds. The various measures of distress include signs such as the following:

1. Hand and arm tension, including pushing away the tube
2. Amount of tranquilizer (diazepam) required
3. Heart rate and heart rate changes from before to after the tube was inserted

Time to swallow the fiber optic tube and gagging while swallowing are considered measures of coping; the patient must deliberately act to swallow the tube and gagging is produced by this action.

Study 1

Design and procedure ■ The first of two investigations of gastroendoscopy was conducted with the collaboration of Dr. John Morrissey (Johnson, Morrissey, and Leventhal, 1973) and compared three conditions:

1. An experimental condition giving subjects an overview of the procedure and as detailed a statement as possible of the sensory experiences accompanying it
2. An experimental condition giving only an overview of the procedure (descriptions of the clinic, the equipment used, how the equipment functions, and statements about the occurrence of throat swabbing, intravenous medication, and so on)
3. A control condition where patients received no special information

Groups 1 and 2 received their information by listening to a 7½-minute cas-
sette tape recording and by looking at a booklet of pictures (11 in all) illus-
trating scenes from the procedure. There were 99 patients in the sample (35
control, 30 procedural, and 34 sensory).

Results ■ The results showed a reduction in amount of diazepam needed
for both the procedural and sensory groups in comparison to the uninformed
control group. Signs of arm and hand tension during the insertion of the tube,
recorded by an observer blind to the subject's condition, showed significantly
less tension for the sensory subjects than for either the procedural or the
control group; the latter two groups were virtually identical on this measure.
The observer also scored restlessness during the examination, and the patients given sensory information were significantly less restless. The sensory
group showed the smallest increment in heart rate as a result of tube passing
but the differences between groups were not statistically reliable. Forty-eight
percent of the patients gagged during the tube passage, and there were no
significant differences between conditions on gagging behavior.

Discussion ■ The results of the gastroendoscopy study suggested that
preparation with either procedural or sensory information reduced anticipatory distress as indicated by the amount of intravenous tranquilizer required
for sedation. However, only the sensory information group maintained low
levels of distress during the various steps of the examination. The indications
that the effects of the intervention could be demonstrated in a clinical setting
were most encouraging.

Study 2

Design and procedure ■ The second of the two studies investigated the
effectiveness of sensory information and the effectiveness of behavioral instructions for coping with the examination procedure. The sensory information was the same as that used in Study 1. The behavioral instructions were
designed to increase the patient's skill in coping with two specific parts of the
examination. The first component gave specific instructions for rapid mouth
breathing and panting to reduce gagging when the throat was swabbed with
local anesthetic. The second gave specific instructions on how to act while
the tube was being inserted and swallowed; the patient was told to make
swallowing motions with his or her mouth open and chin down. The patients
tried each of the actions while the tape played and were given additional
practice when the tape ended. There were no photographs accompanying the
behavioral message.

The hypotheses were as follows: Sensory information was expected to reduce distress (heart rate, tension, and so forth) in relation to the control group.
Behavioral instructions, on the other hand, were expected to have impact on

coping behaviors—gagging during tube swallowing and time for tube swallowing. The hypotheses were tested in a four-condition design:

1. An uninstructed control group
2. A group given behavioral instructions only
3. A group given sensory information only
4. A group given the combination of behavioral instruction and sensory information

Results ■   The data showed that patients who were given sensory information took less diazepam than patients in the other conditions. Patients in all of the prepared groups, sensation information alone, behavioral instructions alone, and the combination, showed slight declines in heart rate during the procedure while the unprepared control patients showed an increase of slightly over 10 beats per minute from before tube insertion to 15 minutes after tube insertion. Both of these findings fit our expectations, but in both instances the effects were modified by the age of the patient. The results reported held for patients under 50 years of age. For patients over 50, heart rates were lowest in the group given the combined preparation, and there were no differences between the groups for amount of diazepam. These older patients received much less diazepam, however, than did the younger patients, so the smaller dosages may have precluded observing a treatment difference. Finally, there were no differences for arm and hand movements. It seems that both preparatory messages reduced signs of distress, the sensory information more than the behavioral and the combination somewhat more than either component alone.

The two key measures of coping were gagging during tube passage and time for tube swallowing. Fully 9 of 10 of the patients in the control condition were observed to gag, as compared to only 4 of 11 in the combined condition. The sensory information group (6 of 13) and the behavioral instruction group (8 of 14) were in between. Time for tube passage produced very sharp differences between the conditions. Control patients took an average of 28 seconds to swallow the tube, behaviorally instructed took 29.6, and those given sensory information took 26.5. But the subjects given both sensory information and behavioral instructions took 43.0 seconds to swallow the tube!

Discussion ■   It can be concluded that preparation generally lowers indicators of distress. While the specifics of the data are less clear than one might like, it is clear that both sensory information and behavioral instructions reduced heart rates, tended to reduce the need for diazepam, and substantially reduced gagging—gagging might be seen as an indicator of anxiety and distress as well as an indicator of coping. The sensory information generally had somewhat stronger effect than the behavioral instructions. We do not know whether this difference was caused by a superiority of sensory information over behavioral instruction or by the characteristics of the two samples of information that we used. The sensory sample may have been a good example of the class of sensory information and the behavioral sample a poor example of the class of behavioral information.

The results do show, quite unequivocally, that the combination of the two types of information had the most effect, particularly on the coping indicators—gagging and time to swallow the tube. The combination substantially reduced gagging, with 53.6% fewer patients gagging in the combined group than in the control group. Also, it substantially influenced time to swallow the tube; in this instance, increasing the time from an average of 26 to 30 seconds in the other groups to an average of 43 seconds in the combined preparation group.

Why did it require both types of information to create the biggest impact on gagging and time for tube swallowing? And why did the combination *increase* rather than reduce the time it took to swallow the tube? We think the answers to these questions are simple, though they were not evident to us before we performed the study. Swallowing is typically an automatic or involuntary action. We do not think about swallowing our soup when we put a full spoon to our lips—the action is automatic. Swallowing a fiber optic tube, however, is quite a different matter. Here the patient must deliberately perform specific swallowing motions. When there is a transfer of control from automatic to voluntary behavior, we can expect the rate of performance to slow! It is clear the patients had control of their behavior; they took the longest but they gagged least. The combined information especially facilitated control of behavior. When patients were forewarned about the sensory experiences, they were less frightened, and when fear was low, the swallowing task was performed with little difficulty. In this instance fear behaviors and coping behaviors produce opposite reactions in the very same response system; that is, fear enhances the tendency to gag (See Dumas and Leonard, 1963), and the coping instructions are designed to enhance self-control over swallowing. By suppressing the fear reactions with sensory information the ability to cope was enhanced. If the two processing systems did not converge simultaneously on the same organ system at the same point in time we might not see the interaction between the two independent variables. Thus the interaction is situationally induced.

Extension of the research to other field settings

The findings discussed point to an expanded view of patient behavior in stressful settings by suggesting that a combination of forewarning about the sensations to expect and action instructions are important for self-regulation of emotional responses and coping behavior. The single factor of sensory information resulted in distress reduction in the ischemic pain laboratory studies, but in that situation the subject was limited with respect to the type of response that could be made. Coping required passivity and reduction in emotional arousal–enhanced passivity. Maintaining a low level of emotional arousal was sufficient to substantially increase the subjects' ability to cope with the painful experience.

In the endoscopy examinations the patient's task demanded more participation. On command the patient was to open his mouth, inhibit gagging, swallow the tube, and follow instructions for such behaviors as changing position during the examination. In this complex situation self-regulation had to be focused on controlling emotional and behavioral responses. The patient had to identify cues, interpret the cues, plan and execute emotional control strategies and coping behaviors, and evaluate the feedback from his internal state and the environment with respect to the impact of the self-regulatory efforts. No one strategy or method of self-regulation would be effective for every situation because situations vary in the type of demands made of people and in the criteria they specify for success.

The initial studies reinforced the notion that sensory information could be a useful intervention in practice settings and further study of the intervention could contribute to the understanding of response to threatening situations. But if those objectives were to be achieved, there was a need to attend to some basic issues. First, the intervention labelled "sensory information" in the gastroendoscopy studies differed greatly from the sensory information used in the ischemic pain studies. The definition of sensory information had to be refined before the specific factors responsible for the effects could be identified. Second, further exploration of how characteristics of situations might modify the effects of the intervention was required. Third, there was a need to know more about how a sensory information intervention and one that directed patients to engage in specific behaviors contributed to responses during threatening events. Those concerns were addressed by Johnson and her colleagues at Wayne State University in a series of studies in health care settings.

Orthopedic cast removal study

Background ■ The sensory information presented in the gastroendoscopic studies was a mixture of elements. We do not know which element or which combination of elements was responsible for the effects we observed. The information contained explicit references to nonthreatening experiences (such as the full feeling in the stomach compared to the feeling one has after eating a large meal) and the threat of the tube could have been greatly influenced by the photograph of the tube lying beside a thimble and a pencil. The photographs used with the sensory information showed people exhibiting calm behavior during various stages of the examination and personal pronouns were used in the narrative. The photographs used with the procedural information were void of people and no personal pronouns were used. Perhaps one or more of those elements of the intervention could have been responsible for the effects instead of the sensory information.

To find the answer to our question, "Was the description of sensations the primary factor responsible for distress reduction in the gastroendoscopic studies?" a clinical situation was selected that made demands on patients which were similar to those in the gastroendoscopic examination (Johnson, Kirchhoff, and Endress, 1975).

The experience of having an orthopedic cast sawed through and removed consists of many stimuli that can evoke fear as did the gastroendoscopic examination. The time for cast removal is much shorter than that for gastroendoscopy but holding still for a few minutes might be roughly as difficult to a child as holding still for 15 to 20 minutes to an adult. In both situations patients are expected passively to allow the physician to manipulate their bodies and to emit simple behaviors on command. By studying children the research was extended to another age group. Sensory information has its effect through activating cognitive processes, and children have not developed all of the complex cognitive skills available to adults. Perhaps the cognitive skills of the adult would prove necessary for the sensory information to be effective.

We prepared an intervention that closely adhered to a precise definition of sensory information. Basic to the definition of sensory information is the notion that information about the external and internal environment is conveyed through the special modalities of sensory perception. The products of sensory perception are what is seen, heard, felt, tasted, and smelled. It is those products that are given objective labels and used to describe the sensory experience. Sensory descriptions do not include interpretations of the sensations. That is, evaluative statements such as weak, distressing, and annoying are *not* included. To illustrate, let us consider the experience of eating chocolate ice cream. The sensory description would include such terms as cold, smooth, sweet, light brown in color, and solid turning to liquid in the mouth. The description would *not* include statements about how good or bad the ice cream tasted, because those are interpretations of the sensations and are influenced by experiences, associations from information stored in the memory, and so forth. Forewarning through information about the sensory experience allows the person to form a cognitive schema of the event. A schema is composed of the general properties of the experience and serves to guide behavioral sequences (Miller, Galanter, and Pribram, 1960). The schema gives structure to expectations about the experience at the sensory level; the information leads subjects to include in their schema what is and to exclude what is not part of the experience.

In addition to the sensations experienced, the cause of the sensations are described, be that cause neutral or threatening. For example, the sensory experience from a drug by injection includes the description of the injection. The parts of the experience are described in the order of occurrence, thus providing temporal orientation. The descriptions are identified as those that are typically experienced, thus suggesting that they should be expected as a normal part of the experience and cannot be avoided.

Although it is somewhat of a digression, an explanation of the methods we have used to obtain descriptions of the typical sensory experience may be helpful. The subjective sensations typical of an experience are identified from reports of people who have experienced or are experiencing an event. The first step is to identify by observation the potential sensation-producing elements in the situation. The next step is to ask people about their sensory experience in a semistructured interview. The respondents are asked to report their sensory experience for each element of an event. People often report their interpretation of the sensations such as "it tasted awful" or "it hurt a lot," instead of the actual sensations. Questions such as "What did it feel like?" or "How did it taste?" focus respondents on the physical sensations. As interviews accumulate, and after the free response is given, respondents can be asked about the adequacy of labels provided by others. When the event causes strong salient sensations, it is relatively easy to identify the labels to describe the typical sensations. We have defined typical sensations as those reported by at least 50% of the respondents. When the sensations are vague and not salient, the task is more difficult and a larger number of interviews will be required before one is confident that typical sensations and appropriate labels have been identified. Often more than one word will be used to describe a sensation because no one term captures the total experience. For example, burning and smarting might both be used to describe a sensation from a wound.

Design and procedure ■ Children 6 to 11 years of age who were to have an orthopedic cast removed were randomly assigned to one of three preparatory conditions. The control group received only the care offered to all of the children in the clinic; the procedural group listened to a 2½-minute tape. message that described the different rooms the child would go to, the instruments that would be used, and how the child would know when to go home; the sensory group listened to a 2½-minute taped message that included a few seconds of the noise of the saw and described such sensations as warmth, stiffness, and flying chalky dust. Both experimental messages included the reassuring statements that the saw would not cut skin and that there was no danger of being hurt.

The main indicator of the dependent variable, distress, was the child's behavior during the cast removal. An observer who did not know how the child had been prepared scored behaviors indicating distress (for example, kicking, hitting, pulling away, crying, or verbal resistance).

Results and discussion ■ The scores for behavioral distress were substantially and significantly lower in the sensory information group than in the control group, and the procedural information group fell in between and was not significantly different from either of the other two groups. First, the significant reduction of signs of distress by an intervention that included only a description of the context and sensory experience supports the interpretation that the results of the gastroendoscopy studies were caused by the sensory descriptions and not the other content of the intervention used in those studies. Second, the cognitive development of 6 to 11 year olds appears to be adequate for the cognitive processes activated by sensory information during noxious stimulation.

To explore children's individual characteristics and their reaction to having a cast removed we asked the children about their fear of having a cast removed while they were in the waiting room. Surprisingly, 56% of the children insisted that they had no fear of the impending experience. Only a few of the children reported more than a little fear. The children appear to have accurately reported their fear because those who said they were not afraid showed significantly fewer signs of distress during cast removal than those who admitted being at least a little afraid. Reports of fear during cast removal were also highly correlated with waiting room reports of fear. It is interesting to note that the children reporting no fear showed low signs of distress during cast removal regardless of their intervention group assignment, but there was a trend for both procedural and sensory information to further reduce distress behaviors. On the other hand, of the children who admitted some fear, only those who received sensory information showed few signs of distress during cast removal. It is unlikely that the sensory information helped the frightened children by reassuring them, as the fearful children reported that the sensory information was frightening.

Pelvic examination study

Background ■ The results of the orthopedic cast removal study caused Johnson and her colleagues at Wayne State to begin to question their assumptions about the mechanism underlying the behaviors we had observed during noxious experiences. Some of our theoretical interpretations of our earlier research implied that sensory information produced a reduction in emotional

responses (such as fear), which in turn prevented the disruption of cooperative behaviors. However, the significant effect of sensory information on behaviors during the procedure in combination with the absence of an effect on
reported fear raised questions about the relationship between emotional response and the cooperative behaviors we had observed. Comparisons of the
effects of an intervention believed to have a direct effect on emotional response with the effects of sensory information for a procedure in which the
threat is psychological instead of physical might help to clarify the relationship between the variables. The pelvic examination seemed to be such a procedure. During pelvic examinations patients experience physical sensations,
but the threat is predominantly psychological instead of physical. Sarah Sue
Fuller, a nurse and social psychologist, was primarily responsible for planning
and conducting the pelvic examination study (Fuller, Endress, and Johnson,
1978).

Design and procedure ▪ Young women 18 to 25 years of age were randomly assigned to one of four preparatory conditions, which were as follows:
1. A control condition in which subjects heard a tape-recorded message
   that emphasized the importance and necessity of routine pelvic and
   breast examinations
2. A sensory information condition in which subjects heard a recorded
   message that described the sensations to expect, the temporal order of
   events, and the duration of the examination
3. A relaxation condition in which subjects were instructed in a method
   of abdominal muscle relaxation to be used during the examination to
   maintain a low level of tension
4. A combined relaxation and sensory information condition in which
   subjects received both the sensory message and relaxation instruction

Subjects were questioned about their fear before and during the examination. Pulse rates were obtained before entering the examination room and
just before the physicians began to examine the subject. An observer recorded specific behaviors that could indicate distress (vocal utterances and
motor behaviors).

Results and discussion ▪ The only significant results were those associated with the sensory information condition. This group had reduced distress behaviors during the examination and low increases in heart rate from
before to during the examination. Relaxation instructions, particularly when
combined with sensation information, seemed to affect the subject's reports
of fear during the examination, but the relaxation instructions had no added
beneficial effects in reducing the level of overt distress behaviors. Thus the
subjects reported that relaxation helped even though it made no impact in

reducing their overt distress reactions or heart rates. It seems then that relaxation adds little to the subject's ability to cooperate passively during the examination but that it does suggest to the patient that she should feel better. The net result is to suggest a theoretical separation of distress indicators into two groups: overt distress behaviors that seem to respond to sensation information and behavioral instruction (as in the endoscopy study) and subjective reports of distress that, at least in the clinical setting, are reduced by a preparation procedure only when the procedure clearly suggests it is designed to be distress reducing.

The design of the pelvic examination study helped us to obtain more direct evidence about the relationships between variables and reinforced our doubts about the relationship between emotional response and passive-cooperative behaviors. The notion that sensory information resulted in a reduced emotional response, which then fostered the passive-cooperative behavior during the examination, may not be an accurate explanation. Even though we were less confident about why the effects occurred, the consistent effects of sensory information in situations that varied with respect to type of threat and with people who varied in age and gender were encouraging.

Surgical patient study 1

Background ■ The instructions about activities in the pelvic examination were designed to facilitate passive cooperative behaviors, not active participatory behaviors. The parallel response model presented earlier suggests that skill training is required if a person is to initiate behaviors and actively participate during the event. The pelvic examination study did not directly test that proposition. Surgery offered the opportunity to contrast the events we had so far studied, which had all been of short duration and posed limits on the types of behaviors subjects could display, to more severe and long-lasting stresses. The discomforts and interference with ongoing life activities as the result of surgery extend over weeks, and there are opportunities for patients to display active coping behaviors as well as emotional responses.

The parallel response model guided the design for a surgical study (Johnson et al., 1978a). The model predicts that emotional and coping behaviors will show some independence, that sensory information will reduce emotional responses during the experience, and that instruction in coping activities will facilitate coping behavior. The coping instructions were similar to interventions used in previous research (Egbert et al., 1964; Lindeman and Van Aernam, 1971; Schmitt and Wooldridge, 1973) that had been demonstrated to facilitate general recovery on measures such as reductions in length of hospitalization.

Design and procedure ■ The experimental design used two factors: one was information and the other instruction in coping activities. There were three levels for the information factor:

1. No information.
2. Procedural information, which provided a description of what would be done to and for the patient and the sequence of events over the preoperative and postoperative periods.
3. Sensory information, which in addition to detailing many of the procedures included descriptions of the typical sensations experienced with these events. For example, detail was given about the feel of the incisional pain and "gas pains," as well as sensations resulting from intravenous feedings and medications.

There were two levels for the coping factor: (1) instruction in postoperative exercises (for example, deep breathing, coughing, ambulation) that are believed to facilitate recovery and (2) no instruction in the coping activities (or exercises). Combining the two factors in a factorial design resulted in six conditions corresponding to all the possible combinations of the informational factor and the coping factor to which patients were randomly assigned. Cholecystectomy patients and herniorrhaphy patients were studied.

The main indicator of emotional response was scores on a Mood Adjective Check List that consisted of 15 adjectives describing five moods (well-being, happiness, fear, helplessness, and anger). Patients responded to the checklist the evening before surgery (preoperative measure) and the first, second, and third days after surgery. The indicators of coping were amount of ambulation, doses of analgesics received, length of postoperative hospitalization, and days between discharge from the hospital and venturing from home. Data on the last indicator were obtained by telephone interview.

Results ■ Significant effects were observed only in the sample of cholecystectomy patients. The first finding was that high levels of preoperative fear were significantly associated with stronger negative mood states postoperatively. The second finding was that preparation factors reduced negative postoperative moods only for those patients who were relatively fearful before surgery. For surgery, among patients who were relatively fearful before surgery, all three interventions (procedural information, sensory information, and instruction in exercises) reduced postoperative anger. Instruction in exercise enhanced postoperative happiness. While sensory information affected emotional responses as expected, instruction in exercise had the strongest effect on postoperative emotional response. Instructions in exercise seemed to affect two coping behaviors; compared to patients who did not receive exercise instructions, those who did used less analgesic and increased their ambulation. The key measures of speed of recovery, length of postoperative stay, and days after discharge before venturing from home were affected primarily by sensory information. The patients who received sensory information had shorter hospital stays and ventured from home sooner than those who received no experimental information, but it was the combination of instruction in exercise and sensory information that resulted in the shortest postoperative hospitalization.

Although we offered several plausible explanations for the absence of effects in the herniorrhaphy sample (Johnson et al., 1978a) the negative outcome was disappointing. We favor the notion that the indicators of the postoperative course were not sensitive enough to reflect differences in recovery in this sample.

Discussion ■ The notion that emotional and coping responses are parallel was supported by the evidence that specific interventions were to some extent selective as to type of response effected. Discrepant with the parallel response model was the finding that instruction in coping (exercise) did not have stronger effects on the coping indicators. Exercise had only marginal effects on the two indicators that the activities might directly affect: amount of analgesic used and ambulation. When patients have been instructed in ways to ambulate that minimize incisional pain it could be expected that they would require less pain medication and ambulate more than noninstructed patients. Therefore the assertion that instruction in a skill will result in the behavior was only weakly supported. The instruction in a coping activity had the strongest effect on emotional response. The reduction in negative moods and increase in positive moods associated with instruction in coping is consistent with the enthusiasm demonstrated by the young women receiving such instructions in the study of response to preparation for pelvic examinations.

The sensory information intervention, contrary to the predictions of the parallel response model, had strong effects on general indicators of coping with the experience. Not only did it facilitate early hospital discharge but its effects were still apparent after the patients returned to their homes. However, the combination of sensory information and instruction in coping activities had the strongest effect on length of postoperative hospitalization. Interventions consisting of both sensory information and skill training tended to have the greatest effects on outcome variables in each study where the two types of preparation were studied (that is, the gastroendoscopy Study 2, the pelvic examination study, and the surgical patient Study 1). In addition, this combination also had the greatest effects in the study of reactions to labor of childbirth described later in this chapter.

Our suspicion that sensory information did not act primarily by reducing emotional response in complex clinical situations was supported by the results of the cholecystectomy patient study. However, we had a strong commitment to the original predictions; and the results from the earlier studies, especially the studies of ischemic pain, seemed to be quite convincing. Perhaps the results of the cholecystectomy study occurred by chance and could not be replicated.

Surgical patient study 2

The second surgical patient study (Johnson et al., 1978b) was designed to replicate and to clarify a number of points raised in the first study. Thus the design was basically the same (three levels of information and two levels of coping instruction), but two important changes were made in the instructional protocols to follow-up on clues from the results of Study 1. These two changes illustrate the importance of theory in contributing to a "sharp eye" in examining data and the importance of precision in the statement of the protocol for an intervention.

For theoretical reasons, Study 1 had included questions to measure feelings of helplessness. We found that patients given the procedural message reported feeling less helpless than did patients given the sensory message or no message at all. A comparison of the content of the procedural and sensory interventions revealed that the temporal sequence of events was more explicit in the procedural message than in the sensory message. We reasoned that information about the onset and duration of a threatening event may make a significant contribution to the composition of the cognitive schema of the impending event. By adding more explicit temporally orienting information to the sensory message the patient could add to the schema information about the expected sensory experience along a time span. The second addition was that the sensory information was given to patients for the second time the first day after surgery. We thought that a second exposure would remind patients of what they could expect and thereby increase the effectiveness of the information.

The main results of the first study of cholecystectomy patients were replicated, and the temporally orienting information had the expected effect of reducing reports of feeling helpless, thus suggesting that information about onset and duration of sensations or events may be especially relevant to feelings about one's ability to cope. The second exposure to the sensory information resulted in a significant reduction in the number of doses of analgesics patients received during the postoperative period. That finding is consistent with Leventhal's interpretations, based on habituation processes that will be presented later.

Again there were no significant effects in the herniorrhaphy sample, but the trends were consistent with those observed in the cholecystectomy sample.

This strengthened our belief that the lack of effects observed for the herniorrhaphy patients was the result of methodological rather than theoretical problems. Thus we believe that the relationships between the variables agree with our theoretical analysis and that the measures used were not sufficiently sensitive to detect the effects. The treatment itself may not have been sufficiently relevant to produce changes in the recovery process; herniorrhaphy is a relatively minor surgical procedure.

REEXAMINATION OF THE EMPIRICAL AND THEORETICAL PICTURE

We have reviewed a large number of studies that included laboratory and field studies in health care settings. The studies provide convincing evidence of the effectiveness of preparatory information. Sensory information and behavioral instructions appear to effectively facilitate self-regulation, but the effectiveness of preparatory information in reducing distress is not the critical aspect of the findings. After all, other studies had shown that preparation can reduce distress and facilitate postoperative adaptation (Andrew, 1970; Egbert et al., 1964; Lindemann and Van Aernam, 1971; Schmitt and Wooldridge, 1973). The important features of our research are as follows:

1. The focus on separately manipulating the two components of preparation (sensory information and behavioral instruction
2. The measurement of both emotional and coping responses
3. Variation in the nature of the situational threat

This analytical approach to preparation also differentiates our approach from studies using films of models to prepare children for hospitalization. Melamed (1977) gives an excellent review of such studies as well as presenting several interesting studies of modeling that she and her students at Case Western Reserve University conducted. (See also Melamed and Siegel, 1975; Melamed et al., 1975a, 1975b. Mclamed et al.

The analytical approach taken in our program has helped rule out the fear-drive hypothesis (Janis, 1958). This is an important step as the fear-drive hypothesis suggests preparation procedures and nursing interventions oriented toward the stimulation of "optimal" levels of fear. As Vernon and Bigelow (1974) point out, preparation research provides virtually no support for this particular hypothesis and we believe it would be damaging to continue to use that theory to guide the development of nursing interventions. Rather than encouraging a type of global thinking that argues that fear or that active coping or control is uniformly better, as implied in drive models and models of learning helplessness (Seligman, 1975), our approach focuses on analysis of processes stimulated by preparatory activities. Our theoretical analysis and empirical findings point to the need to analyze further the mechanisms underlying the effectiveness of cognitive preparation procedures such as sensory information and behavioral instructions.

FURTHER ANALYSIS OF THE MECHANISMS
Background to the analysis

An exciting and at times exasperating aspect of research is the attempt to obtain a picture of the processes that underlie the behaviors we observe. We make inferences from means and standard deviations that are averages and/or estimates of what we are likely to see if we make repeated observations; the numbers do not describe any specific behavior nor do they directly picture the processes that underlie behavior. As we examine these values from one study to another, their fluctuations may generate the thought that we will not be able adequately to picture the underlying process. But try we must, and we each did from somewhat different data sets.

During the years that Johnson had been at Wayne State conducting the field experiments just described, the laboratory at Wisconsin continued to be active in exploring the various effects of sensation information on distress behaviors. The work conducted at each site implied a somewhat different perspective of the underlying process. The Wisconsin work emphasized the role of sensation information on fear-distress behaviors, giving less attention to coping behaviors. The Wayne State research, on the other hand, tended to emphasize coping behaviors; indeed, Johnson's data had suggested that sensation information has its primary effects on coping responses and not on distress. The two perspectives grew out of differences in the kinds of situations used to study distress and distress control. Most of the Wisconsin studies involved laboratory situations, such as exposure to cold pressor pain, which offered the participants in the experiments little opportunity for active coping. Most of the Wayne State studies were field experiments in treatment settings (for example, recovery from surgery, where distress waxes and wanes over a longer period of time and active coping is called for). Despite the differences, we shall see that the two views are complimentary rather than antagonistic.

Leventhal's interpretation

Our view of the problem in the early 1970s was that sensation information was most valuable as a means of reducing fear behaviors, and behavioral instructions were most valuable as a means of facilitating coping responses to danger. This perspective was suggested by the early studies of fear communications, where the threat components of the fear messages aroused fear and generated a clear conception of the danger, and the action instructions provided detailed opportunities to plan and rehearse behaviors such as seeking inoculations and quitting smoking. The endoscopy study also emphasized the independent contribution of two types of information with the combination of sensation information and action instructions leading to the most effective instrumental coping behaviors (little gagging and controlled swallowing of the fiber optic tube). A similar two-pronged effect was visible in the Wayne State studies of preparation for surgery with the combination of sensory information and exercise instruction leading to an advantage over sensory information alone (shortest postoperative hospitalization). In all of the studies where the combination of sensory information and action instructions were most effective, there was the possibility of active participation and active self-control. Thus behavioral instruction or skill training seemed most advantageous in settings calling for active participation, and sensory information, at least initially, appeared to function primarily as a means of reducing distress and minimizing interference between distress and coping behaviors.

This conclusion also seems consistent with some recent data showing that combinations of sensory information and behavioral control instructions are now always superior to the single treatments taken alone. For example, Mills and Krantz (1979) observed that blood donors were less pained, less discomforted, and less anxious when they were given sensory information and were *not* encouraged to cope by choosing the particular arm from which blood was drawn. Donors given both coping choice and sensation information were only slightly less pained and no less discomforted or anxious than control subjects given no information and no choice. The blood donor role provides relatively limited opportunity for active coping; the subject's best bet is to relax and remain passive and introducing behavioral instructions or choice may be counterproductive by encouraging an action orientation when a passive, acceptant set would be more desirable. These results appeared to reinforce the conclusion that sensation information functions primarily for distress control.

Given this view of the underlying processes, Leventhal and his colleagues proceeded to ask, "How does sensory information function to reduce distress?" They approached this question in a series of investigations of adaptation to pain and distress during exposure to cold pressor stimulation, a situation in which the subject's hand is immersed in ice water. The laboratory setting and the task permit little in the way of overt coping that can facilitate adaptation to the stressor. At the time, however, this seemed precisely what was desired, since the goal was to obtain insight into distress reduction rather than coping.

The mechanisms underlying pain and distress control

As a first step toward understanding how pain and distress may be controlled by sensory information we examined the literature on pain and pain control. Our review of this literature (Leventhal and Everhart, 1979) led to the conclusion that "everything but the kitchen sink" had been tried and found to be effective to some degree for the reduction of pain and distress. Indeed, the variety of effective procedures was so great as to defy absolutely drawing any conclusion about the processes that underlie pain reduction. Placebos in the form of inert pills, instructions to detach oneself from the stressor, relaxation training, generating pleasant images, attribution tricks (such as assuming the noxious experience comes from a neutral source), preparation within an attribution context, white noise, hypnosis, and many others have all been found to reduce distress. Table 6 presents a partial list of the procedures used for pain and distress control and a partial list of references to the studies used to evaluate these procedures.

If it seems difficult to infer the mechanisms underlying pain and distress reduction from the varied set of techniques mentioned in Table 6 it may seem

TABLE 6 ■ Methods of pain and distress reduction

Technique for distress reduction	Sample studies using technique
Placebo	Evans, 1976
Dissociative instructions (instruction to detach self)	Holmes and Houston, 1974
Models	Craig, Best, and Ward, 1975 Craig and Weiss, 1971
Relaxation training	Aiken and Henrichs, 1971 Bobey and Davidson, 1970 Meichenbaum and Turk, 1976
Attribution To neutral source To neutral source and to stressor (preparation)	Nisbett and Schachter, 1966 Ross, Rodin, and Zimbardo, 1969 Calvert-Boyanowsky and Leventhal, 1975
Decisions to expose oneself to stress (dissonance)	Zimbardo et al., 1966
White noise	Melzack, Weisz, and Sprague, 1963
Hypnosis	Hilgard, 1969, 1971 Sachs, 1970
Sensory information	Johnson, 1973 Leventhal, et al., 1979
Sensation monitoring	Blitz and Dinnerstein, 1971 Leventhal, et al., 1979 Reinhardt, 1979

impossible to do so when we recognize that some of the procedures seem to use opposite methods. For example, the blocking out of stimulation by white noise, and hypnotic analgesia instructions, seem completely opposite to procedures that require confrontation with or admission of the stimulus information into conscious awareness (such as sensory information and sensation monitoring). Yet more confusion is added by the fact that few if any of these techniques are consistently effective in achieving control of pain and distress. For example, in some studies hypnosis successfully reduces pain and distress only when it is combined with an analgesic suggestion, but it is effective in others without an analgesic suggestion (see Barber and Hahn, 1962; Hilgard, 1969, 1971).

We cannot work out all of the details of this problem in the present chapter, but we will lay out what seems to be a partial solution. First and foremost, it is essential to recognize that at least two kinds of reactions are involved in the reduction of stress reactions to noxious stimulation: (1) an informational response represented at the neurological level by a sensory conduction system that carries the basic informational properties of noxious stimulation (its pattern, temporal extent, and sensory properties of appearance, feel, and so forth) and (2) an emotional-distress response represented by an emotion-activating system. The neurology of the latter system includes the paramedial conduction system and the medial forebrain system, including structures in the reticular system, thalamus, and old forebrain (Casey, 1973). We cannot begin to make sense of the mechanisms underlying pain and distress control without this basic distinction. For example, Evans (1976) argues that to understand the impact of hypnosis on pain we must distinguish the suppression of sensory (information) pain experiences found only in the select group of subjects capable of deep hypnosis from the placebo component of hypnosis (reduction of emotional distress reactions) found in the majority of hypnotic subjects (McGlashan, Evans, and Orne, 1969). If we apply this distinction to the findings in the sensory information studies the questions become:

1. Does sensory information reduce distress by affecting the *information* component of pain and distress, or does it affect the *emotion-distress* component of pain and distress?
2. How does sensory information produce its effects?
3. Does sensory information act in the same way as other procedures such as dissociation, positive thinking, and hypnosis?

Blocking pain information ■ The studies we have discussed suggest that sensory information affects the emotional response component of pain and distress. By reducing the emotional reaction, it substantially reduces the degree to which we observe overt behavioral distress, reduces reports of subjective distress, and reduces interference with coping behavior. There is little evidence to suggest, however, that sensory information actually blocks the informational or sensory features of noxious stimulation. By contrast, deep hypnosis appears to achieve its very substantial reduction of pain and distress through an actual dissociation or blocking of information from consciousness (Evans, 1976; Hilgard, 1973). Thus deep hypnosis appears to literally dissociate the experience of the stimulus from consciousness (Hilgard, 1973).

It is not clear precisely how hypnosis achieves these blocking effects. One way could be by the activation of so-called gate mechanisms hypothesized by Melzack and Wall in the gate theory of pain (Melzack and Wall, 1965, 1970). The gate theory is basically a pattern theory of pain and distress. It assumes that both the informational and the emotional processes that make up pain are initiated simultaneously by any peripheral noxious stimulus such as a cut or burn (see Leventhal and Everhart, 1979). Gates exist because the activity in the information system appears to be able to block neural conduction in the emotion system. The blocking can occur both at the periphery (near the source of stimulation) and at the center (in the brain stem) of the nervous system. For example, transcutaneous stimulation such as applying a vibrating stimulus adjacent to a pain site (Higgins, Tursky, and Schwartz, 1971) appears to block the conduction of emotional information at the spinal cord, a relatively peripheral block. On the other hand, stimulation in the central grey matter, a more central portion of the nervous system in the brain stem, apparently blocks conduction from the source of stimulation (see Melzack, 1973).

It is not clear that hypnotic dissociation actually depends on such gate mechanisms, since the gate mechanisms seem most suited to stopping distress processes rather than completely shutting out awareness of the stimulus. Regardless of the eventual answer to this question it does seem clear that sensory information does not produce the same kind of effects as hypnotic blocking. Thus while studies of sensory information show some decline in the reported strength of noxious sensations, presumably the informational part of pain and distress, the reduction in stimulus awareness is quite small relative to the declines in reported distress, the emotional part of pain and distress (Johnson, 1973; Leventhal et al., 1979). It would seem, therefore, that sensory information acts primarily on the emotional component of the pain and distress response.

Reducing the emotional distress response ■ Our research suggests that sensory information acts not by shutting information out of consciousness but by reducing the intensity of the emotional distress reaction itself. The difference between these two processes can be clarified by thinking of the mind as made up of a conscious part and a preconscious part. Hypnosis would act to keep information from crossing from the preconscious to the conscious part of the mind. When exposed to a noxious stimulus the preconscious part of the mind would contain both the information about the stimulus and the emotional reactions to it. Thus both the informational and emotional processes are parallel in the preconscious portion of the mind, each generating information that can enter the conscious part of the mind (Leventhal and Everhart, 1979). Hypnosis, particularly deep hypnosis, acts as a barrier keeping both types of material from crossing into consciousness (Evans, 1976). A study by Hilgard, Morgan, and MacDonald (1975) illustrates the distinction. They trained subjects to become skilled in automatic key tapping so they could tap out how distressed they were feeling without paying any direct attention to either their tapping or to the noxious stimulus. When subjects trained in automatic key tapping were hypnotized and given an analgesic suggestion to a noxious stimulus they consciously reported no pain and distress though they automatically tapped out that they were experiencing considerable amounts of pain and distress. The automatic tapping was supposed to report the experience in the preconscious part of the mind. Many of the subjects reported very high levels of pain and distress in key tapping even though they reported virtually no awareness of pain or distress in their conscious verbal reports.

We believe that other procedures such as sensory information, thinking positive thoughts, and relaxation make use of a different mechanism. It is our guess that these procedures act directly on the emotional processes occurring in the preattentive part of the mind. Thus when less distress is experienced by subjects given sensory information or by subjects using relaxation we assume that the reduction in distress experienced occurs not because of a block between the preattentive and conscious attentive mind but because the distress in the preattentive mind has been weakened in some way. Relaxation seems likely to lessen distress by lowering the level of muscular tension, since the level of tension may raise the level of distress and other negative emotional reactions (Malmo, 1975) and muscular reactions play an important role in emotion (Leventhal, 1979). For example, the facial expressive system seems closely related to the kind of emotion one feels, and the tension of the postural muscular system seems important in intensifying emotions. Relaxation may also lower the level of activity in the autonomic nervous system (Lang, 1968). Relaxation procedures seem effective, therefore, for reducing the preconscious level of stimulation (from muscular and autonomic sources) that contributes to the intensity of emotional responses such as distress.

Another way of reducing distress emotion could be to remove connections between the noxious stimulus and the individual's emotional memory system. The theoretical basis for this procedure involves an assumption that noxious stimuli provoke severe emotional reactions because they are connected with memories in which pain information has been associated with emotional re-actions of distress, anxiety, anger, and so forth. Thus the noxious stimulus information (the sensations of coldness, aching, pins and needles, and so forth that make up the cold pressor pain stimulus) becomes more painful if this information can provoke emotion, and it is more likely to provoke emotion if it activates memories in which emotion was linked to noxious stimulus information. Johnson (1973, 1975) suggested quite early that the accuracy of sensory information was an important aspect of distress reduction, arguing that when subjects accurately anticipate the sensory (informational) features of the stimulus they become less alarmed while experiencing these sensa-tions.

The accuracy hypothesis, however, can be interpreted too simplistically. Common sense tends to read it as saying that when a person expects or is consciously aware of what is going to happen he is less frightened. This in-terpretation fails to distinguish between what happens preconsciously and what happens consciously. It is very possible that the effects of expectation occur at the preconscious level, that is, without the person's awareness. Thus whether the noxious stimulus information (such as coldness or pins and needles) contacts emotional memories that elicit strong distress or encoun-ters nonemotional memories that do not elicit distress may be determined by processes largely outside of the individual's conscious awareness (Leventhal, 1979; Leventhal and Everhart, 1979). The memory processes may act at an automatic perceptual level, that is, memories are automatically provoked by immediate experience and not deliberately recalled.

But why should preparatory sensory information be so important in reduc-ing the access of current noxious stimulation to emotional memories? Why don't other kinds of preparatory information, such as procedural information, work as well? This is an important question. It is similar to the question, why does drug A kill bacteria a, b, and c but not bacteria e, f, and g, and why does drug B do the opposite? In distinguishing between sensory and procedural information, we are generating a theory of information processing and hy-pothesizing that the relatively greater effectiveness of sensory information means this information is especially important in changing access to emo-tional memories; that is, its information content and structure are of special relevance to perceptual emotional memory. The special relevance emerges, we believe, because of the similarity of the sensation information (aching, pins and needles, numbness) to sensations that accompany most past nox-ious experiences. And we further suggest that a noxious stimulus will no longer be relevant to emotional memories for a person who has been given sensation information and is monitoring the objective stimulus sensations, because the individual will form a clear and precise template of the objective features of the stimulus sensations so the stimulus is now processed as an expected and certain event. Expected, certain, and clear events are much less likely to provoke emotional reactions than are uncertain unexpected events. Indeed uncertainty, particularly uncertainty surrounded by and interpreted as a threat (Bowlby, 1973; Sroufe and Waters, 1976), is likely to provoke all types of severe emotional and endocrine reactions (Mason, 1972). But if a clear template is formed of the stimulus the neural events generated by the stimulus habituate and the stimulus ceases to capture attention (Sokolov, 1963), though the habituation process can be disrupted by the presence of threat-induced anxiety (Froehlich, 1978).

What justification have we for the foregoing elaborate interpretation of the process underlying distress reduction by sensory information? One important source of information consists of data suggesting that individuals form very concrete perceptual memories of parts of the body that have been sources of pain and distress. Leventhal and Everhart (1979) suggest that disturbances such as phantom pain, an experience of an amputated limb or body part that recreates the image of the body part and of the pain and distress that was tied to it presurgically (Melzack, 1971; Simmel, 1962), provide one very vivid example of such a memory system. The presence of the painful phantom after the removal of the limb makes us acutely aware of the memory system. But this memory system exists even when no limb is removed. Fear memories also have a strong perceptual character. This is seen in the use of imagery and the relation of imagery change to change in autonomic reactions in systematic desensitization therapy for phobias (Grossberg and Wilson, 1968; Lang, Melamed, and Hart, 1970). It is also seen in the development of childhood fears (Bronson, 1968). Thus the role of sensory information in distress control fits well with theories of automatic emotion memory in that:

1. Sensory information is concrete and perceptual in nature (focusing on what a person feels, sees, or otherwise experiences through the senses).
2. Sensory information focuses on the body, a key component of the self system (Epstein, 1973) and the focus of threat in any setting where there is the potential of physical harm.
3. The bodily perceptions referred to in sensory information are likely to be connected with perceptual memories linked with past episodes of pain and distress (Engel, 1959; Leventhal and Everhart, 1979).

Studies of distress-reducing mechanisms

A series of studies has been conducted at the University of Wisconsin to explore whether sensory information reduces distress in ways consistent with the speculations just made. If the process of distress reduction depends on the formation of an accurate and precise perceptual memory of the objective features of the stimulus, and if this accurate (nonconscious) template automatically captures the incoming information from a noxious stimulus, avoiding contact with emotional memories, we should be able to vary the conditions of our studies to be sure that sensory information does or does not have the desired effects of distress reduction. If the subject is given sensory information and has no reason to feel threatened the incoming information will form an objective template of stimulus features and there will be little arousal and little distress. But if as Leventhal and Everhart (1979) suggest, the sensations discussed in the information are interpreted as threats and they come into contact with perceptual emotional memories, the subject will be highly distressed and the sensory information from the stimulus will arouse fear rather than reduce it. This reasoning implies that sensory information need not always be fear reducing. For example, if one believed that pins and needles during cold pressor meant one's flesh was being damaged, then pins and needles would evoke fear, distress, and intensified pain. But when the sensory information readies the subject or patient to accept and deal with cues as "natural events," as things that are happening but that have no additional meaning, no surplus threat, no suggestion of danger, the sensory information will reduce fear and distress.

In past studies sensory information was presented in a nonthreatening style; it was an objective detailing of the physical sensations that were explicitly interpreted as normal or typical. This explains why one investigation (Staub and Kellett, 1972) found that information on the sensations of electric shock increased tolerance for shock only when subjects were also given reassurance that the shock was harmless. Without reassurance about the danger, sensory information was ineffective.

Sensory information and threat: the cold pressor study ■ Leventhal et al. (1979) conducted an elaborate six-condition study wherein they recorded subjects' judgments of sensation strength and distress while their hands were immersed in ice water (2° C) for 6 minutes. Two groups of subjects received information on the sensations produced by the cold pressor stimulus (coldness, aching, tightness of the skin across the hand, pins and needles, numbness). In theory, these two groups should be less distressed than another pair of groups given information describing the cold pressor procedure but no mention of the sensations. A third pair of groups was given information about general bodily signs of arousal that occur during fear and distress (butterflies in the stomach, alertness, sweating on the nonimmersed hand, and so forth). This latter pair of groups was included to see if information on the fear response itself would be distress reducing. Finally, the instructions for one group in each pair of groups included a simple warning of pain inserted near the beginning of the instructions: " . . . you will notice the . . . sensation of pain, which will begin to get very strong about this time." This threat of strong pain could change the context and meaning of the sensation information that followed. Each sensation could be interpreted and responded to as a sign of impending severe pain and not merely as something to be experienced in itself. An extra anticipatory meaning is given to each symptom that can attach the symptom to memories of prior emotional distress.

The experimental design allowed us to test two alternative ways of looking at the impact of sensory information. The first interpretation makes the commonsense argument that the simple accuracy of the information is all that matters. It would predict that accurate sensory information should reduce distress, and this should not change with the inclusion of the pain warning because the pain warning is an additional accurate piece of information. The second interpretation, based on our theory of schema information and perceptual memory, argues that the automatic interpretation or meaning of the sensations is what matters. It predicts that processing the stimulus as a set of simple straightforward perceptual attributes (that is, a schema of the ice water experience) would reduce distress. But processing the perceptual attributes of the ice water as potential signs of pain and strong threat will connect the stimulus to emotional memories and block the distress reduction usually seen with sensory information.

The data on reported distress during the 6 minutes of immersion in ice water for the three preparation conditions given the strong pain warning showed an initial increase and then a decline in distress for all three groups, the magnitude of the decline being somewhat though not significantly greater in the sensory information group. By contrast, for the three preparation conditions given no strong pain warning the decline in the sensory information group was substantially and significantly greater than the decline in the other two groups. Indeed, the drop in distress in the sensory information group was so great that the final distress ratings for these subjects were actually lower than the initial rating made only 10 seconds after immersion in the cold water. The ratings of sensation strength showed a similar pattern, but there was much less reduction of sensations, as expected. Data on skin temperature confirmed these findings; the sensory information group without a warning of strong pain actually showed an increase in skin temperature from the fourth through the sixth minute and there was no increase in skin temperature for any of the other five groups.

The results clearly supported the interpretation that sensory information is effective when it leads to the processing of sensory experiences in a non-threatening manner. Other studies support this interpretation by showing that threat enhances pain and distress and *slows* adaptation to noxious stimulation (Teichner, 1965; Hall and Stride, 1954). The findings also support

Johnson and Rice's (1974) earlier observation that the accurate identification of at least some objective sensations, rather than the accurate identification of the entire set, is sufficient for distress reduction. It is not the accuracy of the sensory information per se that is critical for reducing distress to a noxious episode but the creation of an objective schema in a nonthreatening context. In such a context, each sensation is automatically identified as part of the objective schema, an event that is happening now, and the sensations do not lead to emotional memories. Nothing more is implied by a sensation than the sensation itself. Sensory information draws on the cognitive mechanisms that lead to the automatic reinterpretation of the key elements of the perceptual field and prevents these elements from recruiting pain and distress memories and creating the subjective, expressive, and autonomic reactions that make for a strong emotional pain and distress experience.

Habituation and schema formation: laboratory studies varying attention ■ The first of the studies by Leventhal et al. (1979) showed that including a pain cue that leads to an interpretation of the situation as threatening blocked distress reduction by sensory information. But the data did not provide clear evidence for the formation of objective schema of the noxious event that served automatically to interpret the stimulus cues as concrete events rather than as emotions. Can we obtain clearer evidence to show that the cold pressor sensations failed to arouse emotion because preparation led the subject to focus attention on the sensory features and form a memory schema or template of the stimulus features, thereby habituating their ability to arouse emotion? If the noxious event is perceived and coded in memory as a set of objective concrete features (a perceptible pattern) only this same memory structure and no other (for example, no memory of past pain and distress) will be activated while the subject's hand is immersed in the ice water. If we continue to activate a common stimulus memory, we can expect it to habituate. If the trace becomes less active the stimulus will have less power to attract attention and produce neural activation and autonomic arousal.

A suggestion for testing the habituation hypothesis came from Groves and Thompson's review (1970) of the habituation literature. They suggested that habituation occurs most readily in response to stimuli that are mild rather than strong and to stimuli that begin at initially low levels and gradually increase in strength. If we transfer the findings to cold pressor stimulation, we could expect to find that it is necessary to focus attention on the stimulus for template formation and habituation and that habituation will occur most readily if attention is paid to the stimulus during the first half of cold pressor exposure, that is, when the sensations are at a low level and increasing in strength though they have not yet reached maximal strength. If attention to the stimulus is delayed until it is at its peak intensity it will be difficult to code as a set of objective events; instead it will be coded as an emotionally provocative and distressing experience.

These notions were tested by Seya Shacham in the second and third experiments of this set (Leventhal et al., 1979). Experiment 2 compared three conditions:

1. An attention group instructed, "We would like you to pay attention to the sensations or feelings in your hand only, so that you will be able to describe each of the specific feelings and sensations that you experienced." None of the sensations of cold pressor were actually described.
2. A group instructed to attend to both their hand and their bodily reactions.
3. A control group.

The group instructed to attend to both hand and body is highly similar to the groups given arousal information in Experiment 1 and was included to see if attentional instructions per se would achieve distress reduction.

Experiment 2 showed that subjects attending only to their hand reported significantly less distress than did subjects in the other two conditions. However, while attention alone was sufficient to produce distress reduction, it did not reduce distress as much as did sensory information in Experiment 2. It would appear, therefore, that habituation may be taking place but that the effect caused by attention-induced habituation may not be as great as that caused by sensory information, which may build on both accurate knowledge in a secure context and habituation caused by schema formation.

The failure to reduce distress through attention to both hand and body suggests that attention to general body sensations interferes with the reduction of distress. It is interesting to note that preparation with information on bodily arousal (given in Experiment 1) was also unsuccessful in reducing distress reports. It may be that knowing about or monitoring bodily arousal (autonomic activity such as heartbeat, gastric distress, and so forth) enhances contact with emotional memories. This contrasts interestingly with the data showing that monitoring facial expressions dampens positive affective reactions (Cupchik and Leventhal, 1974; Leventhal and Cupchik, 1976). Monitoring smiles and laughter may be sufficient to bring these responses under a degree of voluntary control and eliminate their power to stimulate feelings (Leventhal, 1974). Monitoring autonomic reactions, however, may not be sufficient to bring them under voluntary control, since volitional control over autonomic responses may require both monitoring and the performance of a voluntary response that can in turn control the autonomic reaction. Control of an autonomic response would take more time and practice, and the observation of the response would be only a starting point (see Brenner, 1974; Kimble and Perlmutter, 1970). Other research in our laboratory has shown that preparation directing awareness at autonomic behaviors may substantially reduce efforts to escape from a threat even if it did not diminish the subjective feeling of threat or anxiety stimulated by the noxious event (Calvert-Boyanowsky and Leventhal, 1975).

Experiment 3 gave a more direct test of the hypothesis that attention leads to some form of habituation, since Shacham varied the time at which the subject monitored the cold pressor stimulation. Four different groups participated in the study. One group was instructed to pay attention through the entire 5-minute and 10-second period of immersion in 7° C ice water. Slightly warmer water was used than that in the earlier studies, since a pilot study showed reductions in distress by sensory information at both 2° C and 7° C so there was no need to use the colder water. This attention instruction was repeated exactly halfway through the procedure. A second group was told to attend to the sensations generated by the cold water during the first half of the immersion and was shown slides during the second period. To be sure subjects attended to sensations and to the slides they were told they would be questioned about each task at the close of the experiment.

Both of these groups should report similar levels of distress if the process of distress reduction depends on the development of a schema or template of the stimulus features during the early part of the exposure period, that is, both their reported distress levels should be low in the second half of the immersion. Two comparison groups were studied to interpret the outcomes. One saw slides for the entire 5-minute and 10-second immersion period (timing and repetition of instructions was identical to that for the continual attention group). The other was instructed to look at slides during the first period of the immersion and to monitor hand sensations during the second period. The timing of instructions was identical to that for the group instructed to attend first and distracted with slides second. If the habituation hypothesis is correct neither of these groups should show distress reduction, since one never pays attention to the stimulus and the other pays attention in the second half of the stimulus exposure, *after* the stimulus has contacted a host of past pain and distress memories. At this time the level of stimulation is too intense to reexperience the hand as a set of sensory features and to form an objective schema unconnected to memories of emotional distress.

All of the groups showed an initial rise and peaked to virtually identical levels of distress, after which followed a decline in distress. But the rate of decline in the second half was substantially greater for two of the groups: (1) that attending to the sensory features continually and (2) that attending to the sensory features from the beginning to the middle of the stimulus exposure. It appears that some kind of habituation process is at work and that it can be produced by early attention to stimulus features. Sensory information very likely includes, therefore, at least two component processes: (1) the reduction of arousal induced by surprise, uncertainty, and threatening interpretations, and (2) the reduction of distress by some kind of habituation process.

The attention study advanced our understanding of distress control by making clear the importance of attention to sensations in the early part of stimulus exposure. This attention seems to be important in building a schema that may then function to "capture" or interpret later various stimulus events within a highly limited meaning system. The schema *means* stimulus features, not threat, injury, or need for help. This benign interpretation may limit the rate at which arousal is generated and lower distress. On the other hand, the schema might also be an active inhibitor of distress. We do not know which process occurs, though more recent studies suggest that an active, lasting inhibition develops from monitoring sensations.

A study of childbirth: a field study of attention ■ Rather than explore the alternatives just outlined, we decided to conduct an experiment using attention to reduce distress in a real life setting. The setting chosen was childbirth. The questions were (1) Would attention to sensations from labor contractions reduce distress during childbirth? (2) Would the distress reduction resemble the habituation-like process seen in the laboratory studies of distress induced by cold pressor?

There were two reasons for conducting a study using attention to reduce distress during childbirth. The first was that most childbirths in teaching hospitals are performed by residents in obstetrics who have had no prior contact with the mothers. Instructions to monitor labor sensations seemed an easy way to disrupt the distress experience, especially when contractions have nearly always begun well before the patient is examined to be admitted.

The second reason for the choice of setting was the observation by one member of our team (Elaine Leventhal) that women who have attented Lamaze childbirth classes often put themselves at risk by hyperventilating during labor. After the delivery of their child, these women felt they had done a poor job as they failed to control their distress. Careful observation suggested these mothers-to-be were using the Lamaze breathing methods to distract themselves from the pain and distress of their contractions. Thus instead of monitoring their contractions so as to breathe in synchrony with them they became increasingly involved in the breathing and breathed more and more rapidly so as to block out awareness of their distress.

The phenomena posed a challenge: Could the obstetric resident intervene so as to ease distress and eliminate the risk of hyperventilation and do so at the time of admission for delivery? It appeared that an easy way of doing this would be to have the mother-to-be focus attention on her uterine contractions and carefully monitor their sensory features (timing, form at onset and end, location, sensory attributes, and so forth). When a mother came to be admitted she was first classified as a first-time mother or one who had given birth before and as having or never having attended childbirth classes. Patients within each of these four subgroups were then randomly assigned to one of two conditions: (1) attention to and monitoring features of contractions and (2) general contact and suggestions for requests for helpful distractors (such as, "Would you like to read?"). The attentional instructions and the contact to offer distractors were repeated at hourly intervals up until the time the mother was moved to the delivery room. This occurred toward the end of the second stage of labor.

The major dependent measures were responses to a multiple-item mood adjective checklist completed the day after delivery. The items were embedded in a longer interview (conducted by graduate students in psychology) on the labor experience. The mother used rating scales to report her level of fatigue and tiredness, her negative emotions (fear, anger, tension, anxiety, and so forth), and her positive emotions (joy, happiness, and so forth). She reported on each of the three aspects of her experiences at (1) the time of admission to the hospital, (2) a half hour before delivery, and (3) during the last half-hour of delivery (that is, in the active pushing phase). The nurses were asked to make ratings of muscle tension and to measure heart rate at hourly intervals, but they were often too busy to comply and the data were too incomplete for analysis.

The findings are relatively simple to report. First, mothers in both the attentive and nonattentive groups reported identically low levels of bodily fatigue at admission and identically high levels of bodily fatigue at both a half-hour prior to active delivery and during active delivery. Labor is hard work, and it becomes more fatiguing as it progresses. Mothers in both the attentive and nonattentive conditions agreed on this. The finding was important, as it suggested there was no simple reporting bias affecting these self-rating data.

Substantially higher levels of negative emotion were reported a half-hour before active delivery began than at admission. The attentive group was very slightly but not significantly less negative at this time (a half-hour before delivery). The two groups differed vastly, however, in negative emotions reported during active pushing and delivery. The nonattentive group showed only a small decline in negative emotions, while the reported negative emotions of the attentive group declined significantly more in both a statistical sense and an absolute sense; its ratings of negative emotions during pushing dropped to the level of negative emotions at admission. The positive emotions ratings showed the same pattern of differences between the groups as that for negative mood ratings, except that the direction of each difference was, of course, opposite in sign.

The findings show that mothers can be directed to monitor their contractions and that monitoring has a beneficial effect on emotional distress reduction. The result is consistent with Shacham's laboratory studies on attention (Leventhal et al., 1979, Experiments 2 and 3). There is, however, an important difference between the results in the laboratory and field studies. Attention had a noticeable impact for ratings of negative emotions only during the final half-hour of labor and delivery, the time when the mothers were actively engaged in coping with the delivery process (active pushing). It did not alter distress during the long period that preceeded delivery. Thus both attentional monitoring and coping were essential for reducing fear and distress in the field setting. It is our belief that monitoring allowed the mothers to coordinate more effectively volitional breathing and pushing to the automatic contractions of the uterus, and that the coordination of the volitional and automatic response functions established a sense of control and eliminated negative emotional states.

There is one final datum that is of interest. We also compared the emotional reports of women who had and who had not been through the Lamaze childbirth classes. Compared to those who had never attended classes, mothers who had attended classes reported significantly lower levels of negative emotion (fear, danger, tension, and so forth) at the time of admission. But the reports of negative emotions for the two groups were at the same high level a half-hour before delivery—during the active phase of delivery itself. Thus the preparation of childbirth classes had its major impact on the mother's ease and comfort when she first encountered the various examination procedures on admission to the labor suite. The knowledge gained in classes did not carry over to the active phase of labor. For the latter stages of labor the combination of monitoring and active pushing was essential for the reduction of negative moods.

The childbirth study suggests that attention facilitated patients' ability to actively participate and coordinate behaviors to cues. Sensory information and monitoring served to reduce fearful interpretations, to facilitate habituation to concrete bodily sensations, and to enhance the coordination of active coping to perceptual signals. If the perceptual signals (bodily sensations) are very strong and painful, the distress they generate will motivate avoidance behavior (distraction) to control awareness of fear (fear control in our parallel model) and interfere with attention to the very signals that provide important information for guiding coping behaviors. Further support for the hypothesis that sensory information and attention can facilitate habituation in a field setting was present in the second surgical study discussed earlier (Johnson et al., 1978b). It will be remembered that the patients who listened to the sensory information for the second time the day after surgery required fewer doses of analgesic than did those who did not have a second exposure. The second exposure to the sensory description during the time that some of the sensations were being experienced could have facilitated habituation processes by reestablishing a schema that included only the objective sensory features and reduced the pain and distress response. Thus the data supported the attention-habituation interpretation with evidence on the importance of monitoring and also provided insight into the value of the monitoring of body cues to ensure coordination with coping and effective distress control.

Habituation, coping, or both

While the field data support the hypothesis that attention will have favorable effects for adaptation to distress, we should be clear on the questions they raise about the mechanism underlying distress reduction. The habituation hypothesis (that sensory information and attention lead to the habituation of the fear response) would lead one to expect differences in distress to occur sooner than they did, and it would not lead one to expect that distress reduction would depend on coping. However, the mothers in the labor study did not show reductions in emotional upset till the final hour or half-hour of an experience that may have lasted 3 to 8 hours; and the decline in distress occurred only when the mothers had a specific coping response available to them, when they had been instructed to push during the intense phase two contractions. It appears, therefore, that sensory information operated primarily by enhancing the mother's ability to regulate her pushing reactions. A similar pattern of results was seen in our early field study of endoscopy— there, too, distress was at its lowest when patients were given both sensory information and practice in deliberate swallowing, which allowed them to control the rate the endoscopy tube moved through the gullet to the stomach. Habituation, that is, fear reduction through some inhibitory process set up by schema formation, may play only a minor role in these experiments. Sensory information and monitoring provide guidance for and improve the effectiveness of coping responses. This does not rule out habituation. It merely suggests that the degree to which sensory information and attention operate through the alternative underlying processes of fear reduction by habituation or fear reduction by facilitation of coping depends on various characteristics of the situation. The habituation process is likely to be most visible in the laboratory, where threat of pain is high, possibilities for immediate active coping minimal, and implications of long-term threat and need for long-term coping minimal. On the other hand, the displacement of fear by the facilitation of coping is likely to be most visible in a field setting where severe pain and fear at any given moment may not be particularly high but where the possibilities for short-term coping are maximal, as are the implications for long-term threat and the need for long-term coping. The perspective we have as to how distress reduction occurs may depend, therefore, on the kind of situation in which self-regulation is observed. Some situations may make both processes visible. Other situations may reflect primarily one process or the other. Johnson's interpretation is based largely on data from the field.

Johnson's interpretation

In our early research on the effects of sensory information, it was assumed that cognitive intervention directly affected emotional response to threatening events. The field data suggest an alternative assumption—that in many situations sensation information reduces emotional response indirectly through its effects on coping or self-regulation. The research conducted at Wayne State University suggests that this cognitive intervention had its primary effect on coping responses, that people may not be in a high state of emotional arousal when facing many health care procedures, and that the disruptive effects of high emotional arousal may not be as severe as is often assumed.

Emotional response to health care procedures

Are patients in a high state of emotional arousal before and during health care procedures? If not, the control of emotional responses may not be a critical factor for adaptation to those situations. In each of the clinical studies conducted by the Wayne State University group measures of emotional state were taken when the patient entered the threatening situation. In every sample, levels of fear *before* the experience were not high. Thus while a few people reported high fear, the average fear level was in the lower third of the scales used (the scales ranged from no fear to extremely high fear). On the average the cholecystectomy patients reported little fear or anger during the postoperative period. The predominate mood was feelings of helplessness. The children in the orthopedic cast removal study and the young women in the pelvic examination study, also on the average, reported little fear during their procedures.

It could be expected that subjects in these studies would have freely admitted fear because most of them were women or children and there is little social pressure for women and children to withhold expressions of feelings. The conclusion that for the most part subjects in those clinical settings are not very fearful seems valid. Since emotional arousal was low (moderate at the most) both before and during the experience, it seems unlikely that the effects observed on coping behaviors were achieved through a reduction in the disruptive effects of emotion. The level of fear may have been low because all patients had known about the impending experience for some time, and the fear that may have been first aroused had waned. It is also possible that persons whose fear remained high coped with it by avoiding the health care experience and never became subjects in our studies.

The subjects who come to a laboratory for an experiment that involves a threatening experience may be more emotionally aroused than patients facing a health care procedure. The laboratory subject may be similar to patients at the time they learn of the need for a threatening examination or treatment. In the laboratory the subjects' immediate emotional response has little time to wane. The emotional response is salient because there is little else to be concerned about. Even though a contrived experience in a laboratory is much less important than a health care procedure to the totality of a subject's life, the emotional reactions to the immediate experience may be strong and central to the subject's attention and concern. By contrast, fears and concerns of people who present themselves for health care may be less focused on the features of the immediate situation and more concerned with outcomes; that is, on what will be found and its implications for the direction, quality, and length of life. Thus the quality of the subject's emotional state may be different in the field setting than in the more circumscribed threatening experience of the laboratory. The laboratory is well suited for the arousal of emotion by a circumscribed event and for the study of ways of reducing that emotional state. The health care setting may involve more diffuse concerns about ability to cope with the future, and it may be appropriate for studies in this setting to focus on ability to cope with wide-ranging problems.

Restraints on response and complexity of stimuli ■ A second issue relevant to the interpretation of the empirical work is the influence of situational restraints on the responses observed. The subject's responses are greatly limited by constraints in the laboratory situation. The experimenter's goal is to arrange the situation to narrow the range of the subject's response alternatives—the subject chooses to do A or B. Such control is an essential part of laboratory experiments. In health care settings the experimenter has much less control over the subject's response. The researcher must rely on measuring the responses that occur. There are situational constraints on responses in health care settings, and they should not be overlooked. For example, if the setting demands passive coping the subject is pretty well limited to using passive coping techniques or to not coping at all; active coping may be difficult or impossible. The studies of orthopedic cast removal and pelvic examination demanded passivity from the patient. The study of endoscopy was somewhat less this way, but it too called for little more than controlled breathing and swallowing. Because these situations demanded passivity we may have confused passivity with the absence of hyperemotionality. Thus sensory information may have abetted passive coping rather more than it reduced emotional distress per se.

Another important difference between the laboratory and clinical settings is the number of stimuli to which the subject is exposed. In the laboratory studies pain was an isolated experience. There may be health care settings with similar characteristics but we have not studied them. In fact pain was a part of patients' experience only in the studies of surgical patients, and then it was only one aspect of a complex array of stimuli. It seems doubtful that surgical patients focused only on their pain in the same manner as the subjects who experienced pain in the laboratory. This suggests explanatory statements about responses to situations involving only painful stimuli may not be generalizable to the clinical setting.

Multiple responses ■ The studies of surgical patients provided the best opportunity to measure a variety of specific coping behaviors, such as amount of ambulation, in addition to measures of emotional response. The results of the cholecystectomy patient study suggest that the cognitive intervention did not foster coping by reducing the patient's emotional responses. Reported emotional disturbance was low for these patients both presurgically and postsurgically. For patients with some degree of preoperative fear all of the interventions tended to affect fear and anger during the postoperative period, which suggests that there was no one characteristic of the interventions that selectively affected emotional reactions. On the other hand, different interventions tended to have different effects on indicators of coping behaviors. The intervention that had the strongest effect on emotional response, instruction in specific coping activities, had a weak effect on the specific targeted behavior (amount of ambulation). The sensory information intervention had a weak effect on emotional response and the strongest effect on general indicators of coping (length of hospitalization and days after discharge before venturing from home). If the effect of sensory information on general indicators of coping operated through reduction in emotional response we would expect the greater effects to be on emotional response rather than on coping. The relatively great effect on length of postoperative stay by the combination of interventions could reflect the combined effect of (1) instruction in specific coping activities reducing emotional response and thus indirectly affecting coping and (2) sensory information directly increasing coping abilities.

The same pattern of effects was observed in the pelvic examination study. Only sensory information significantly affected cooperative behavior during the examination, but subjects identified the instruction in a coping activity as most helpful, suggesting that the instruction affected the subjective emotional state directly.

Sensory information and self-regulation ■ If the effects of sensory information on coping cannot be accounted for by reduction in emotional response, then what is the mechanism? To answer that question, we have to consider what is involved in self-regulation during a complex threatening event. According to White (1974), a threatened individual has to regulate his emotional reactions and coping behavior at the same time. Obtaining and processing information about the environment is essential for guiding behavior. We believe that the cognitive intervention we have called sensory information increases the person's ability to obtain and process information and thereby facilitates his use of his existing repertoire of coping strategies and behaviors. The composition of the person's cognitive representation of the event (schema) is the mechanism through which the cognitive intervention fosters self-regulation during threatening events. Information that reduces ambiguity about the impending event from the experiencing person's vantage point influences the structure and content of the schema formed. The composition of the schema can facilitate information processing and use of the subject's existing repertoire for coping. In Leventhal's interpretation, the schema is seen primarily as acting to facilitate the habituation of emotional response during threatening experiences. While habituation processes may be involved in the observed effects of sensory information on emotional response, and a high level of emotional arousal can disrupt information processing and coping behavior, the field study data imply that sensory information has effects that go beyond mere reduction of emotional responses. This argument rests on the assumption that a threatening event directly taxes a subject's ability to emit coping behaviors as well as the subject's ability to control emotional responses.

The cognitive intervention used in the clinical studies in which the situation was complex has consisted of several components. In addition to descriptions of sensations in objective terms, the intervention included contextual information about spatial properties of the environment and the experiencing person's position in the environment. It also identified the cause of the sensory experience and provided a temporal orientation giving the sequence in which items would be experienced and providing cues about when a particular event would begin and when it would terminate. These messages implicitly identified what would be excluded from the experience and described the experiences as typical or normal in the situation. The descriptions focused on the objective and concrete properties of the impending experience.

Information about an impending event that focuses on the objective and concrete properties of the various components of the experience fosters construction of the internal cognitive representation of the event (schema or template) that is composed of those properties. A schema serves to guide interpretations of incoming information and behavioral sequences (Miller, Galanter, and Pribram, 1960). A schema is composed of a description of the general properties of the experience, and it provides structure and organization to events, thereby reducing their ambiguity. In some ways it serves a purpose similar to a road map. It allows one to proceed toward a goal without necessarily focusing on each detail by providing landmarks along the way that are salient to most individuals.

Sensory information allows the person to determine which properties are and are not relevant to the experience. The information may confirm some previously formed expectations about the properties of the experience, add new properties, and cause other possible properties to be excluded by suggesting that those properties are not characteristic of the experience. What subjects are led to exclude from the schema may be as important as what they are led to include. The reports of subjects in one of the ischemic pain studies indicated that the sensory information added little new information to their expectations about objective properties of the experience, but it did lead them to give up expecting unlikely properties of the experience (Johnson, 1973). Also, the evidence from the pelvic examination study suggests that in some situations sensory information can lead to a restructuring of the subject's schema of the experience. All of the subjects had had the examination previously and therefore one would expect they had a schema of the experience in their memory system. Since the subjects who received sensory information behaved differently during the examination than those who did not receive it the intervention must have caused restructuring of the schema.

Sensory information may also be important in clarifying the patient's role in a setting. In health care settings some patients expect and desire to be passive participants. Those patients expect that their needs will be anticipated and that they will have no responsibility for their own well-being (Johnson, Dumas, and Johnson, 1967). Descriptions of unavoidable sensations indicate to the patients that caretakers cannot protect them from those experiences. The intervention may help such patients to form a more realistic notion about their role during the event. Those patients who wish to participate actively but expect that they may be forced to be passive may also form more realistic expectations about their role from the intervention.

As a person proceeds through an experience, the incoming information is compared with the schema and interpreted in that framework. Concentration on detail may not be as important as following the general form of the experience. As feedback consistent with the schema occurs, confidence that the schema is an accurate representation and can predict the experience increases. The objective-concrete properties of the experience that sensory information provides for construction of the schema could, as Leventhal has pointed out, reduce attention to emotional properties and tend to guide the subject to exclude those properties of the experience from the schema. Thus some effect on emotional response would be expected, especially in situations that have high potential for eliciting emotional response or for those people who are prone to react emotionally.

How does a schema constructed of the objective-concrete properties of the experience result in increased coping behaviors? Such a schema may bolster the person's ability to use coping strategies and behaviors that exist in their repertoire (Johnson et al., 1978b). To be an effective person it is essential to be able to secure and use information about one's environment (White, 1974). The cognitive intervention could stimulate the formation of a schema that provides a framework for organizing input as the experience progresses. A critical feature of schemata is that they allow behavior to be guided by specific situational cues without the subject having to concentrate on these cues. Langer, Blank, and Chanowitz (1978) found that people responded in habitual manner, without purposeful thought, when a message was structurally similar to what was usually encountered, regardless of the semantic content. The schemata constructed from interventions with sensory information may be structurally similar to schemata that would be formed from the vantage point of the person actually experiencing and attempting to cope with the situation. Such a schema would foster the use of existing coping strategies and behaviors and avoid the possibility that the situation would stimulate efforts to construct and execute new response patterns.

The interpretation that a schema that provides structure to the experience increases the person's ability to use existing repertoire is further supported by the effects of including information on the temporal sequence of experience in the sensory information message. Feelings of helplessness, as defined by the adjectives *unable*, *incapable*, and *helpless*, were significantly reduced by the additional information about temporal dimensions of the experience (Johnson et al., 1978b). Thus the information could have increased confidence about the adequacy of the repertoire.

Perhaps the strongest support for the interpretation that the sensory information intervention has its effect by construction of a schema that is structurally consistent with those usually used to guide complex behavioral sequences is the finding that major effects of the interventions were observed after the patient left the situation for which he was prepared! Little, if any, of the content of the sensory information message that was given to the cholecystectomy patients was applicable to the experiences after discharge from the hospital, but the patients gave indications of a rapid return to usual activities. The intervention must have stimulated the construction of a schema of the self as effective in managing illness. Positive feedback on the effectiveness of behavior based on such a schema during hospitalization could have encouraged the continuation of the same approach after discharge.

It may be difficult for people to reconstruct and report self-regulation processes that are habitual and do not require concentration (Nisbitt and Wilson, 1977). Nonawareness could be an indicator of a successful regulation process, a process that makes demands on the person. To overcome a specifically identified problem, coping instructions will focus attention on the new and difficult part of the experience. If there is feedback that a new technique was effective, the technique will be valued because it will be viewed as being effective in overcoming what was believed to be a difficult problem. On the other hand, instructions that support behavioral processes of which people are only partially aware and that demand little thought are unlikely to be identified as helpful. This theory explains why patients are much more enthusiastic about instruction in coping activities than they are about the provision of sensory information.

Summary

Johnson's and Leventhal's interpretations of the effects of sensory information emphasize two different causal sequences. Leventhal tends to focus on the intervention's direct effects on the subject's emotional response to threatening events, while Johnson tends to focus on the intervention's direct effects on coping behaviors. In Leventhal's interpretation, sensory information leads to the formation of a schema and the habituation of fear (emotional) behaviors. When fear behaviors are minimal, the individual can perform necessary coping reactions. Leventhal also suggests that sensory information may help guide the coping response. In Johnson's interpretation, sensory information leads to the formation of a schema whose primary purpose is to facilitate coping. More specifically, the schema operates at a relatively automatic level, making use of the individual's existant repertoire of responses. Under these conditions the individual need not struggle with the problem of acquiring new skills or be deliberately attentive to what he is doing. Sensory information will be successful in guiding coping as long as it generates an appropriate schema—one whose features match those of a person who has actually coped successfully with the situation described—since successful behaviors can help suppress or inhibit emotional upset.

Leventhal and Johnson agree on the role of behavioral instructions; they are important in constructing coping responses that may not exist in the individual's repertoire. Instructions of this sort are likely to be valued highly because they are a highly salient means of providing a skill to overcome a problem barrier. Sensory information, on the other hand, does not provide new, salient information; its function is to activate schemas that help existing responses function effectively. Because of this the individual will be less aware of the benefits he accrues from sensory information, and he will value it less highly.

The differences expressed by Leventhal and Johnson appear partially dependent on differences in the situations they have studied. The laboratory setting restricts the range of coping behaviors, and studies conducted under such conditions can readily emphasize a habituation process. On the other hand, the field setting permits a far wider range of coping behaviors, and studies in that setting can readily emphasize active coping. The difference in perspective applies primarily to the interpretation of the process underlying the cognitive preparation process of the giving of sensory information, and it is also clear that both perspectives may be true; that is, each may emphasize those characteristics of the process that are most salient in the setting under investigation. On the other hand, if we accept the idea that nonbehaving (that is, sitting and doing nothing) is a form of coping, particularly in the laboratory setting where there are no other coping options, one could argue that *all* of the studies show that sensory information serves to form a schema that facilitates coping, and that coping acts to suppress emotional behaviors. Indeed, one might argue that habituation is a form of active suppression of emotional behavior generated by alternative (active or passive coping) responses.

Two other areas of agreement should be stressed. First, both investigators believe it important to focus attention on the notion of self-regulatory systems. Adaptation to stress involves a complex regulatory system affected by a variety of preparatory inputs. The regulatory system must include a clear representation of the environment (the schema), and it must include an adequate set of coping responses. Finally, a good regulatory system, one that provides stable control over both the environment and one's own behavior, must include reasonable criteria for successful regulation. If one expects too much from coping or has no clear idea of what outcomes to expect, it is difficult indeed to evaluate the effectiveness of coping, to make reasonable coping choices, and to adapt.

The second point stressed by both authors is that self-regulation must be looked at from the perspective of the subject or patient. It is this person's perception and interpretation of the problem that guides coping, and it is this person's repertoire of responses that is being emitted and evaluated against his own criteria.

It cannot be assumed that health care providers know the typical experiences of people who have a chronic disease. The vantage point of the experiencing person is a critical factor. Careful observation and careful interviews to determine the parameters of the experience, from the experiencing person's vantage point, are required for the identification of the patient's typical experiences over time. The descriptions in the present medical and nursing literature are for the most part based on observations by health care providers. Such descriptions may not reflect typical experiences or may include subjective aspects of the experiences that can be known only to the patients. For example, people do not experience a chronic disease such as diabetes or hypertension as a specific entity; they experience it through bodily sensation. If there are no sensations, it is difficult for the person to identify that he is experiencing a threat to health, so when feedback that coping is successful is in the form of absence of sensations or symptoms, it may not serve to maintain the coping behaviors. Typically, a person's schema of his body leads him to interpret the absence of sensations as health. The position presented here suggests that people with chronic health problems require information that leads them to form schemata that include cues as to when the disease is under control as well as cues as to when the disease is not under control. Cues providing concrete feedback that the disease is under control may be as essential for maintaining the behavior that achieves that state as cues that the disease is not under control. The person may need to learn the skills necessary to perform behaviors essential to maintaining control of the disease (such as self-administration of medication) in addition to skills required for obtaining feedback about the state of the body (such as how to interpret tests and blood pressure readings).

Self-regulation when one has a chronic disease is complex and undoubtedly involves many factors. The approach suggested here has been tested previously in individuals with acute conditions. However, it provides an orientation that may also prove applicable to the systematic study of the process of becoming self-regulatory while living with chronic disease.

FURTHER DEVELOPMENT OF THE THEORY

In this section we will suggest directions for activities for further development of the theory of self-regulation. First, we will address some basic theoretical issues related to the differences in interpretation we have presented. Second, we will discuss the differences between individuals that predispose them to react in characteristic ways and to be more or less sensitive to interventions. Third, we will comment on the relationship of self-regulation theory to nursing practice theory.

Interventions, situational variables, and responses

The parallel response model proposed by Leventhal (1970) has proven to be useful in the study of reactions to threatening situations. The basic premise of the model, that emotional response and coping behaviors are to some degree independent of each other and are regulated by different mechanisms, stimulated new approaches to the analysis and study of the mechanisms underlying responses to threat. The research has provided consistent support of the basic premise of the model. While the model has been useful in theorizing about the mechanisms underlying each type of response, the development of a detailed theory of self-regulation has just begun.

Clarification of the relationships between interventions, emotional responses, and coping behaviors is necessary both for the advancement of psychological theory and for pragmatic reasons related to application of the theory to nursing practice. Establishing connections between the interventions and the outcomes will contribute to a better understanding of the processes that are involved. Detailed knowledge of the effects of different kinds of interventions on each kind of outcome is essential to the process of developing effective health care prescriptions. Experimentation is also required to detail further the process by which cognitive intervention affects emotional or coping behaviors. The study of this question should involve a situation in which emotional responses vary; coping behaviors are relevant and can be measured accurately and separately from the subject's degree of emotional response. The coping activities required must be available to all subjects either through their existing repertoire or through instruction.

Leventhal's suggestion that a schema that results in self-regulation can be constructed by attending to the objective sensory experience is of practical significance. It is time consuming to determine subjects' typical subjective experiences so that preparatory interventions can be constructed. Instructing subjects to attend to the sensations as they experience them would be a more efficient intervention. The relative effectiveness of each approach to schema formation and self-regulation as reflected in emotional response and coping behavior needs to be determined.

Answers to the specific questions raised by our different emphases in interpreting the research program will probably vary with the characteristics of the experiences or the situations studied. Understanding of self-regulation mechanisms will be advanced by more attention to the characteristics of threatening experiences. The mechanisms underlying emotional and coping behaviors may vary systematically with the type of demand imposed by the situation. Emotional response may dominate in some situations, demand for coping behaviors may dominate in others, or the situation may elicit both types of response with equal strength. Some threatening events are experienced repeatedly within a short time span, for example, painful dressing changes and radiation therapy. In some cases people are catapulted into a threatening experience without any forewarning. Other taxing experiences may last for years and may or may not include physical discomforts. Attention to the characteristics of threatening situations and the demands made on people attempting to cope with them is imperative to the further development of an understanding of the mechanisms involved in self-regulation. If the focus is on general characteristics of experiences instead of on specific situations, the knowledge will be more useful because it will be more broadly applicable.

Further studies have appeared that show how these ideas can be generalized to other areas wherein the individual's experience is critical for self-regulation. For example, series of studies have been conducted on the way patients respond during treatment for hypertension (Meyer et al., 1978) and during chemotherapy treatment for malignant neoplasms (Nerenz, Leventhal, and Love, 1982). These studies make clear that patients do not experience disease and treatment in medical, scientific terms; they experience it in personal, symptomatic terms. The studies also vividly illustrate the way schema formation affects the perception and interpretation of both the illness and treatment and how these perceptions and interpretations influence coping and emotional distress. For example, the studies of hypertensive patients show that they define their hypertension in terms of specific bodily symptoms (heart beating, face flushing, headaches, and so forth). The abstract label has little meaning to the patient; he must identify it with specific symptoms. Once the patient has identified the illness with a symptom, he observes the effects of different environmental events on that system. If his headaches become worse under work stress he will see work stress as a cause of hypertension; if his treatment does not alleviate his headaches, he will see it as failing to cure his hypertension. These perceptions have important implications for decisions and coping. They may lead the individual to cut back his work load, seek a less stressful job, or drop out of treatment. The decisions are direct expressions of the individual's schematic representation of his illness.

The same picture emerges in studies of cancer chemotherapy patients. In these studies the investigators found that patients identify their cancer with specific sets of symptoms and their treatment with other sets of symptoms. This differentiation of symptoms is crucial in determining the arousal of fear and the perception of appropriate coping alternatives. For example, a patient who understands cancer as a concrete, physical lump may become extremely frightened when he experiences a persistent, localized pain in the area near the excised tumor. He may well be indifferent, however, to pains that fluctuate and occur in other parts of the body. The emotional response depends on the schema or interpretation of the disease process and may have nothing to do with the actual physiological facts of the situation.

The cancer patients also show the same kind of behaviors seen in the hypertensive patients. For example, a patient with a lymphoma may see his disease as a specific set of symptoms (swellings, pains, and so forth). His symptoms may be more disturbing or noticeable during times of stress, since emotional arousal can increase the intensity of pain (Leventhal and Everhart, 1979). He may conclude, therefore, that his cancer is caused by stress. This schematization of the illness and its cause may direct the patient's perception of ways to cope with cancer. The patient in this example can cut back on stressful experiences by reducing his work day by half.

Underlying these examples are some very basic kinds of assumptions (schemata) used by people in responding to illness. The most important of these is the assumption that illness is symptomatic and wellness is not. Repeated experiences with gastrointestinal illness, upper respiratory disease and infections, and accidental injury have generated an implicit schema of illness that is highly concrete. Indeed, this schema does not seem particularly susceptible to change by verbal communication. Virtually 100% of the 200 or more hypertensive patients interviewed in the studies of Meyer et al. (1978) had been told by physicians that hypertension is asymptomatic. Yet in response to careful inquiries, questions that stressed interest in the patient's own, private experience, 90% of the patients told of specific symptoms by which they would tell when they were hypertensive, and a majority of these patients used these symptoms to schedule when and how much medication to take. It is amusing to note that the investigators encountered strenuous objections from nurses and physicians presented with the idea that patients used symptoms to dictate their medication. The medical audience insisted that patients could not use symptoms as a guide to hypertension even though the speakers had specifically said the symptoms were *seen* as a guide to hypertension and there was no physiological evidence of a true correlation between symptoms and blood pressure. More amusing yet were discussions in which the most vociferous objectors in the medical audience came up with examples of how they themselves had mistakenly associated headache or stress with hypertension but proved themselves wrong by taking their blood pressure. Health professionals have difficulty seeing the difference between their professional perspective on illness and the patient's perspective even when their own experience as patients shows the schema of a lifetime of experience with the body and illness is alive and active in their mind.

Another area that requires further study is the composition of the cognitive intervention central to the research discussed in this chapter. Further research is needed to tease out the effects of the several components that make up the interventions and their interactions on the response variables. The theoretical mechanisms of self-regulation we have discussed can serve as a base for systematic extension of the theory-research process both to determine the specific components that foster self-regulation in situations with identified characteristics and to elaborate the mechanisms that underlie the relationships. The discussion in this chapter illustrates the processes of identifying the characteristics of the situation, the components of interventions, and the mechanisms through which responses are affected.

Identifying the components of the cognitive interventions requires knowledge about the subjective experience of the subject. Some components, such as the sensory component, are more dependent on knowledge of the subjective experience than others, such as spatial orientation. Systematic documentation of the subject's experiences can make a contribution to the building of a theory of self-regulation. Nurses who have contact with subjects during threatening experiences are in an excellent position to document the components of the experience from the subject's vantage point.

Individual differences and underlying process

To this point we have focused on the effects of specific treatments on groups of subjects and patients randomly assigned to conditions. We have acted as if the treatments have common effects on all participants. But it is reasonable to assume that participants are affected equally?

The likelihood of individual differences in response to treatment is clear when we examine the data from nearly any one of the studies under discussion. First, it is clear that there are *very substantial* individual differences within any treatment condition. The treatments may differ from one another on the average, but they overlap substantially. Individual differences account for a substantial proportion of the variation in response, more variation than is accounted for by the differences between treatment conditions, even though these latter differences are statistically significant! This may be largely caused by measurement error and the effects of the randomized antecedent variables, but it may also be caused by differences between subjects in their responses to the experimental variables (that is, to statistical interaction).

It has not been a simple matter to identify the factors responsible for the differences in response between individuals. Cohen and Lazarus (1973) have suggested that people differ in their defensive preferences, with some subjects preferring avoidance and others preferring to confront stressful stimuli. They argue that avoiders do better when not given information about stressful settings or when they are allowed to reinterpret the setting as pleasant, while sensitizers do better when given preparatory information. In this instance, however, their argument is somewhat more persuasive than their data.

Wilson (1977), following the parallel model, argues that the perception of danger and the experience of fear are created in parallel, somewhat independent of one another. He suggests that individuals differ in the degree to which their coping mechanisms are oriented toward the control of objective, environmental danger versus the control of subjective, emotional states. His data show substantial differences, with sensory information resulting in reduced emotional response for patients low in the control of danger and relaxation training reducing negative reactions for patients low in fear control. The findings represent an interesting beginning for the development of insight into individual differences.

Our own data point to at least two sets of individual difference factors in pain and distress control. The first set is of individual difference variables that relate to the intensity of the emotional distress experience. Surgical patients high in trait anxiety and firstborns experienced particularly high levels of pain and distress (Johnson, Dabbs, and Leventhal, 1970). Those subjects who entered the situation with some level of fear were better able to control their emotional reactions when they received any relevant intervention (Johnson, Kirchoff, and Endress, 1975; Johnson et al., 1978a). Similar effects were also seen in our laboratory studies. For example, Shacham (1979) found that subjects sensitive to pain (a measure specific to the noxious stimulus) benefit most from creating images of the hand immersed in the stressful cold water. Similarly, Klemp and Leventhal (1974) and Brown, Klemp, and Leventhal (1975) found that pain-sensitive subjects behave as though the stressor task is one of escaping and avoiding pain and distress, while pain-tolerant subjects act as though the task is to tolerate and master the distress.

Individual differences do not just affect the definition or experience of the stressor; they also influence the ability to generate coping strategies and preference for one specific coping strategy over another. For example, Kornzweig (1967) found that low self-esteem is associated with feelings of helplessness and the inhibition of coping actions under highly stressful circumstances. High-esteem subjects, on the other hand, sought out action and appeared to be less likely to lose hope. We have found that the tendency for low-esteem persons to develop feelings of hopelessness in the face of high threat can be overcome if their self-esteem is bolstered before exposure to the threat situation. Perception that one is in control of a situation (Rotter, 1966) or that one has the ability to influence outcome (Meichenbaum, Butler, and Joseph, in press) is also likely to influence coping. For example, in the Johnson, Leventhal, and Dabbs (1971) study, patients who believed they controlled their fate were given more analgesics and stayed longer in the hospital, and Seeman and Evans (1962) have shown that tuberculosis patients scoring high on this factor are better informed about their condition and the hospital situation.

Scattered findings such as those just referred to should not be confused with the systematic scientific study of individual differences in response to stress. For the most part these studies, and there are many others like them, are illustrations that stress and coping reactions differ for participants who score high and low on different personality tests. Collections of facts of this sort do not generate a coherent theoretical understanding of the way individual differences contribute to stress and coping. Data on individual differences will make a scientific contribution when the measures are conceptualized as individual differences in the variables embodied in a stress response model, for example, as individual differences in the interpretation, elaboration, and organization of the stressor problem (goal definition and emotional response) and as individual differences in the organization and availability of specific coping skills and orientations to the evaluation of outcomes.

Reinhardt (1979) completed a pair of laboratory studies that provide an interesting example of research into individual differences based on these principles. In her initial study she exposed approximately 90 undergraduate subjects to cold pressor distress. After the subjects' exposure to the stimulus she carefully interviewed the subjects to find out how they perceived the situation, what they had expected to happen (interpretation), and how they coped with it. She uncovered a variety of strategies, including the strategy of self-monitoring and sensation watching discussed in this chapter. Interestingly fewer than 20% of the subjects spontaneously monitored the sensations from their hand; most used an avoidance strategy and regarded sensations monitoring as stress inducing. The group that did monitor could be divided into two subgroups: one that focused on how upset they were and wished the experience would end, and the other that focused more clearly on the sensations and waited for them to adapt. The latter group reported very low levels of distress during the cold pressor experience. They were also unusually low in measures of hypochondriases, that is, they did not focus on their bodies as sources of distress.

Reinhardt's first study suggested that monitoring was an effective means of distress regulation as long as the person observed the sensations of the stressor and did not combine them with a schema of expectations of distress and injury. To prove her point Reinhardt then constructed an experiment in which three groups of subjects were told to monitor sensations and then were compared to an uninstructed control. One of the monitoring groups was told to watch how the experience became increasingly severe and distressful and to look to the possibility that it would get worse. Another was given no outcome expectation. The third was told to watch how the sensations became stronger, peaked, and began to decline. The results were striking. All of the groups were initially low, rose to nearly identical peak levels of distress, and then diverged sharply. The group that expected sensations to peak and weaken reported drops in distress to levels lower than those reported 10 seconds after immersion in the cold water. Reported distress for the monitoring group that expected things to get worse stayed high; indeed it was slightly higher than for the unprepared control subjects. Reported distress for the group of subjects given monitoring instructions alone was in between the other two groups.

Careful interviewing to get at the subject-patient perspective can suggest new ways of generating preparatory interventions. But the interviewing must be based on a theoretical model. Reinhardt's questionnaire was constructed to cover the variables in the self-regulation model. The follow-up experimental test, using random assignment to conditions, demonstrated that sensory coping strategies were the antecedents and not simply consequences of distress. More importantly the experimental study demonstrated that the individual differences were not simply immutable characteristics of the subjects; the strategies could be clearly communicated to a group of people who then applied them effectively. In short individual difference research progresses in step with the analysis of the processing mechanism that underlies stress behavior. At this stage of knowledge we have a clearer idea of the areas in which individual differences should be measured than we have of specific individual difference variables.

Finally, the measurement of individual differences will take place at several levels (Epstein, 1973; Rotter, 1975), that is, variables that are fairly specific to particular situations will need to be identified (such as perception of physical threat, self, and physician competence), and more general variables that underlie entire domains of self-functioning will need to be identified (such as perception of vulnerability of the self to physical illness [Gochman, 1977] or perception of effectance in managing life situations [Bandura, 1977]). Developing a hierarchical view of individual differences that moves from deeper levels involving perception of body systems to more specific levels such as perception of specific symptoms or from deeper levels such as need for achievement or control to perceived ability to manipulate the health care setting poses a major challenge to our ingenuity.

SELF-REGULATION THEORY AND NURSING PRACTICE

We began our program of research because of our interest in helping patients cope with the various demands made on them by illness. We believed that our work would make the greatest contribution if it were directed at determining the mechanisms underlying the coping process. The work expanded from a focus primarily on the emotional component of the coping process to include the mechanisms underlying the behavioral component of the process; thus we have moved to the broader concept of self-regulation.

We believe our work is timely. Nurses are rapidly expanding their role in the health care delivered to the public. We believe that the development of theories about self-regulation is important to increasing the effectiveness of the services that nurses provide the public and that it is relevant to nursing practice regardless of the location of the patient, whether in the hospital, in an ambulatory setting, or at home. Although there is much discussion within the profession about the nature, role, function, and theoretical base for nursing, the notion that nursing is oriented toward assisting the patient to cope with his situation is generally accepted. Theories about how people cope with the demands made on them by health care activities could be as useful to nursing as theories about the causes and cures of diseases are to medicine. The practice of nursing requires more than the existence and application of a theory of self-regulation, just as the practice of medicine requires more than the application of theories about the cause and cure of disease. However, such theories provide a focus for the totality of the activities involved in the role of providing service to the public.

Even though self-regulation theory is only beginning to be developed it has direct implications for practice activities, which gives it the potential status of a practice theory such as described in Chapter one. The theoretical notions provide a structure for organizing various interventions to reduce stress and facilitate coping. Many of these interventions are currently being used in nursing practice, and their use is proliferating. If interventions can be organized according to the type of response they are intended to effect or the mechanism they are believed to activate, that alone will provide structure and clarity to a maze of unorganized facts. As such a structure is developed it can be refined with respect to situational characteristics, individual characteristics, and further detail as to the specific components of interventions likely to be most effective under various individual and situational conditions. As nurses attempt to use self-regulation theory in practice settings their experiences will provide feedback that will contribute to the elaboration, reformulation, and refinement of the theory. Self-regulation theory will be developed and evaluated with respect to usefulness as a practice theory through the combined efforts of behavioral and nursing scientists who test and elaborate the theory and practitioners who use the theory to guide the care process.

REFERENCES

Aiken, L.H., and Henrichs, T.F. 1971. Systematic relaxation as a nursing intervention technique with open heart surgery patients, Nursing Research 20:212-217.

Andrew, J.M. 1970. Recovery from surgery, with and without preparatory instruction, for three coping styles, Journal of Personality and Social Psychology. 15:223-226.

Averill, J.R. 1973. Personal control over aversive stimuli and its relationship to stress, Psychological Bulletin 80:286-303.

Averill, J.R., Opton, E.M. Jr., and Lazarus, R.S. 1971. Cross-cultural studies of psychophysiological responses during stress and emotion. In Levi, L., editor. Society stress and disease vol. 1. London, Oxford University Press, pp. 110-124.

Bandura, A. 1977. Self-efficacy: toward a unifying theory of behavioral change, Psychological Review 84:191-215.

Barber, T.X. 1963. The effects of hypnosis on pain: a critical review of experimental and clinical findings, Psychosomatic Medicine 25:303-333.

Barber, T.X., and Hahn, D.W. 1962. Physiological and subjective responses to pain producing stimulation under hypnotically-suggested and waking-imagined "analgesia," Journal Abnormal and Social Psychology 65:411-418.

Beecher, H.K. 1959. Measurement of subjective response, New York, Oxford University Press, Inc.

Blitz, B., and Dinnerstein, A.J. 1971. Role of attentional focus on pain perception: manipulation of response to noxious stimulation by instructions, Journal Abnormal Psychology 77:42-46.

Bobey, M.J., and Davidson, P.O. 1970. Psychological factors affecting pain tolerance, Journal of Psychosomatic Research 14:371-376.

Bowlby, J. 1973. Separation: anxiety and anger, New York, Basic Books, Inc., Publishers.

Brenner, J. 1974. A general model of voluntary control applied to the phenomena of learned cardiovascular change. In Obrist, P.A., et al., editor. Cardiovascular psychophysiology, Chicago, Aldine Publishing Co., pp. 365-391.

Bronson, G.W. 1968. The development of fear in man and other animals, Child Development 39:409-431.

Brown, D., Klemp, G.O., and Leventhal, H. 1975. Are evaluations inferred directly from overt actions? Journal of Experimental Social Psychology 11:112-126.

Butler, R. 1967. Aspects of survival and adaptation in human aging, American Journal of Psychiatry 123:1233-1243.

Calvert-Boyanowsky, J., and Leventhal, H. 1975. The role of information in attenuating behavioral responses to stress: a reinterpretation of the misattribution phenomenon, Journal of Personality and Social Psychology 32:241-221.

Casey, K.L. 1973. Pain: a current view of neural mechanisms, American Scientist 61:194-200.

Casey, K.L., and Melzack, R.: 1967. Neural mechanisms of pain: a conceptual model. In Leony Way, E., editor, New concepts in pain and its clinical management, Philadelphia, F.A. Davis Co.

Chamberlin, T.C. 1965. The method of multiple working hypotheses, Science 748:754-759.

Cohen, F., and Lazarus, R.S. 1973. Active coping processes, coping dispositions, and recovery from surgery, Psychosomatic Medicine 5:375-389.

Craig, K.D., Best, H., and Ward, L.M. 1975. Social modeling influences on psychophysical judgments of electrical stimulation, Journal of Abnormal Psychology 84:366-373.

Craig, K.D., and Weiss, S.M.: 1971. Vicarious influences on pain-threshold determinations, Journal of Personality and Social Psychology 19:53-59.

Croog, S. 1970. The family as a source of stress. In Levine, S., and Scotch, N.S., editors. Social stress, Chicago, Aldine Publishing Co., pp. 19-53.

Cupchik, G., and Leventhal, H. 1974. Consistency between expressive behavior and the evaluation of humorous stimuli: the role of sex and self-observation, Journal of Personality and Social Psychology 30:429-442.

Davison, G.C. 1968. Systematic desensitization as a counter-conditioning process, Journal of Abnormal Psychology 73:91-99.

Dohrenwend, B.S., and Dohrenwend, B.P. 1970. Class and race as status-related sources of stress. In Levine, S., and Scotch, N.A., editors. Social stress, Chicago, Aldine Publishing Co., pp. 111-140.

Dollard, J., and Miller, N.E. 1950. Personality and psychotherapy: an analysis in terms of learning, thinking and culture, New York, McGraw-Hill. Book Co.

Dumas, R.G., and Johnson, B.A.: 1972. Research in nursing practice: a review of five clinical experiments, International Journal of Nursing Studies 9:137-149.

Dumas, R.G., and Leonard, R.C. 1963. The effect of nursing on the incidence of postoperative vomiting, Nursing Research 12:12-15.

Egbert, L.D., et al. 1964. Reduction of postoperative pain by encouragement and instruction of patients, New England Journal of Medicine 270:825-827.

Engel, C.L. 1959. Psychogenic pain and the pain prone patient, American Journal of Medicine 26:899-918.

Epstein, S. 1973. The self-concept revisited: or a theory of a theory, American Psychologist 28:404-416.

Epstein, S. 1979. The stability of behavior: I. On predicting most of the people much of the time, Journal of Personality and Social Psychology 37:1079-1126

Evans, F.J. 1976. Hypnosis and the placebo response in pain control, Paper presented at American Psychological Association Convention, Washington, D.C.

Everhart, D.J. 1978. The strength and durability of distress reduction through sensation monitoring and positive thinking, doctoral thesis, Madison, University of Wisconsin.

Fordyce, W.E. 1976. Behavior methods for chronic pain and illness, St. Louis, The C.V. Mosby Co.

Fox, B.H. 1978. Premorbid psychological factors as related to cancer incidence, Journal of Behavioral Medicine 1:45-133.

Freud, S. 1961. Inhibition symptoms and anxiety, London, The Hogarth Press (reprint of 1926 ed.).

Froehlich, W.D. 1978. Stress, anxiety, and the control of attention: a psychophysiological approach. In Spielberger, C.D., and Sarason, I.G., editors. Stress and anxiety, vol. 5, Washington, D.C., Hemisphere Publishing Corp. 99-130.

Fuller, S.S., Endress, M.P., and Johnson, J.E. 1978. The effects of cognitive and behavioral control on coping with an aversive health examination, Journal of Human Stress 4(4):18-25.

Gochman, D.S. 1977. Perceived vulnerability and its psychosocial context, Social Science and Medicine 11:115-120.

Grossberg, J.M., and Wilson, H.K.: 1968. Psysiological changes accompanying the visualization of fearful and neutral situations, Journal of Personality and Social Psychology 10:124-133.

Groves, P.M., and Thompson, R.F. 1970. Habituation: a dual-process theory, Psychological Review 77:419-450.

Hall, K.R.L., and Stride, E. 1954. The varying response to pain in psychiatric disorders: a study in abnormal psychology, British Journal of Medical Psychology 27:48-60.

Hardy, J.D., Wolff, H.G., and Goodell, H. 1952. Pain sensations and reactions, Baltimore, The Williams & Wilkins Co.

Hempel, C.G. 1966. Philosophy of natural science, Englewood Cliffs, N.J., Prentice-Hall, Inc.

Higgins, J.D., Tursky, B.D., and Schwartz, G.E. 1971. Shock-elicited pain and its reduction by concurrent tactile stimulation, Science 172:866-867.

Hilgard, E.R. 1969. Pain as a puzzle for psychology and physiology, American Psychologist 24:103-113.

Hilgard, E.R. 1971. Hypnotic phenomena: the struggle for scientific acceptance, American Science 59:567-577.

Hilgard, E.R. 1973. A neodissociation interpretation of pain reduction in hypnosis, Psychological Review 80:396-411.

Hilgard, E.R., Morgan, A., and Macdonald, H. 1975. Pain and dissociation in the cold pressor test: a study of hypnotic analgesia with "Hidden Reports" through automatic key pressing and automatic talking, Journal of Abnormal Psychology 84:280-289.

Hinkle, L.E., Jr. 1974. The effect of exposure to culture change, social change, and changes in interpersonal relationships on health. In Dohrenwend, B.S., and Dohrenwend, B.P. (editors.) Stressful life events: their nature and effects, New York, John Wiley and Sons Inc., pp. 9-44.

Holmes, D.S., and Houston, B.K. 1974. Effectiveness of situation redefinition and affective isolation in coping with stress, Journal of Personality and Social Psychology 29:212-218.

Holmes, T.H., and Masuda, M. 1974. Life change and illness susceptibility. In Dohrenwend, B.S., and Dohrenwend, B.P., editors. Stressful life events: their nature and effects, New York, John Wiley & Sons Inc., pp. 45-72.

Horan, J.J., et al. 1977. Coping with pain: a component analysis of stress-inoculation, Cognitive Therapy Research 1:211-221.

Ickes, W., and Layden, M.A. 1978. Attributional styles. In Harvey, J., Ickes, W., and Kidd, R.F., editors. New directions in attribution research, (vol. 2), Hillsdale, N.J. Lawrence Erlbaum Associates, Inc., pp. 119-152.

Izard, C.E. 1971. The face of emotion, New York, Appleton-Century-Crofts.

Izard, C.E. 1977. Human emotions, New York, Plenum Publishing Corp.

Janis, I.L. 1958. Psychological stress, New York, John Wiley & Sons, Inc.

Janis, J.L. 1967. Effects of fear arousal on attitude change: recent developments in theory and experimental research. In Berkowitz, L. editor. Advances in experimental social psychology, 3, New York, Academic Press, Inc., pp. 167-222.

Janis, I.L., and Leventhal, H. 1968. Human reactions to stress. In Borgatta, E.F., and Lambert, W.W., editors. Handbook of personality theory and research, Chicago, Rand McNally & Co., pp. 1041-1085.

Johnson, J.E., Dabbs, J.M., and Leventhal, H. 1970. Psychosocial factors in the welfare of surgical patients, Nursing Research 19:18-29.

Johnson, J.E. 1973. Effects of accurate expectations about sensations on the sensory and distress components of pain, Journal of Personality and Social Psychology 27:261-275.

Johnson, J.E. 1975. Stress reduction through sensation information. In Sarason, I.G., and Speilberger, C.D., editors. Stress and anxiety, vol. 2, Washington, D.C., Hemisphere Publishing Corp.

Johnson, J.E., Dumas, R.G., and Johnson, B.A. 1967. Interpersonal relations: the essence of nursing care, Nursing Forum 6(3):324-334.

Johnson, J.E. Kirchoff, K.T., and Endress, M.P. 1975. Deterring children's distress behavior during orthopedic cast removal, Nursing Research 75:404-410.

Johnson, J.E., and Leventhal, H. 1974. Effects of accurate expectations and behavioral instructions on reactions during a noxious medical examination, Journal of Personality and Social Psychology 29:710-718.

Johnson, J.E., Leventhal, H., and Dabbs, J.M., Jr. 1971. Contributions of emotional and instrumental response processes in adaptation to surgery, Journal of Personality and Social Psychology 2:55-64.

Johnson, J.E., Morissey, J.F., and Leventhal, H. 1973. Psychological preparation for an endoscopic examination, Gastrointestinal Endoscopy 19:180-182.

Johnson, J.E., and Rice, V.H. 1974. Sensory and distress components of pain: implications for the study of clinical pain, Nursing Research 23(3):203-209.

Johnson, J.E., et al. 1978a. Sensory information, instruction in a coping strategy and recovery from surgery, Research in Nursing and Health. 1(1):4-17.

Johnson, J.E., et al. 1978b. Altering patients' responses to surgery: an extension and replication, Research in Nursing and Health. 1(3):111-121.

Kimble, G.A., and Perlmutter, L.C. 1970. The problem of volition, Psychological Review 77:361-383.

Klemp, G.O., and Leventhal, H. 1974. Self-persuasion and fear reduction from escape behavior. In London, H., and Nisbett, R., editors., Cognitive control of motivation, Chicago, Aldine Publishing Co.

Knox, V.J., Morgan, S.H., and Hilgard, E.R. 1974. Pain and suffering in ischemia: the paradox of hypnotically suggested anesthesia as contradicted by response. From the "hidden observer," Archives of General Psychiatry 30:840-847.

Kornetsky, C. 1954. Effects of anxiety and morphine on the anticipation and perception of painful radiant thermal stimuli, Journal of Comparative Physiology and Psychology 47:130-132.

Kornzweig, N.D. 1967. Behavior change as a function of fear arousal and personality, doctoral dissertation, New Haven, Conn., Yale University.

Kuhn, T.S. 1970. The structure of scientific revolution, Chicago, University of Chicago Press.

Lang, P.J. 1968. Fear reduction and fear behavior: problems in treating a construct, Research in Psychotherapy 3:90-102.

Lang, P.J., and Lazovik, A.D. 1963. Experimental desensitization of a phobia, Journal of Abnormal and Social Psychology 66:519-525.

Lang, P.J., Melamad, B.G., and Hart, J. 1970. A psychophysiological analysis of fear modification using an automated sesensitization procedure, Journal of Abnormal Psychology 76:220-234.

Langer, E., Blank, A., and Chanowitz, B. 1978. The mindlessness of ostensibly thoughtful action: the role of "placebic" information in interpersonal interaction, Journal of Personality and Social Psychology 36:635-642.

Langer, E.J., and Rodin, J. 1976. The effects of choice and enhanced personal responsibility for the aged: a field experiment in an institutional setting, Journal of Personality and Social Psychology 34:191-198.

Lazarus, A.A. 1961. Group therapy of phobic disorders by systematic desensitization, Journal of Abnormal Psychology 63:504-510.

Lazarus, R.S. 1966. Psychological stress and the coping process, New York, McGraw-Hill Book Co.

Lazarus, R.S. 1968. Emotions and adaptation: conceptual and empirical relations. In Arnold, W.S., editor. Nebraska symposium on motivation, Lincoln, University of Nebraska Press. pp. 175-266.

Leventhal, H. 1970. Findings and theory in the study of fear communications. In Berkowitz, L., editor. Advances in experimental social psychology, vol. 5, New York, Academic Press, Inc., pp. 119-186.

Leventhal, H.: 1974. A basic problem for social psychology. In Nemeth, C., editor. Social psychology: classic and contemporary integrations, Chicago, Rand McNally & Co.

Leventhal, H. 1975. The consequences of depersonalization during illness and treatment. In Howard, J., and Strauss, A., editors. Humanizing health care, New York, John Wiley & Sons, Inc.

Leventhal, H. 1979. A perceptual-motor processing model of emotion. In Pliner, P., Blankstein, K., and Spigel, I.M., editors. Advances in the study of communication and affect, vol. 5: perception of emotion in self and others, New York, Plenum Publishing Corp.

Leventhal, H., Ahles, T., and Rutter, T. 1977. The effects of verbalizing sensations and expressive sounds in the lateralized experience of pain and distress, University of Wisconsin (unpublished).

Leventhal, H., and Cleary, P. 1977. The smoking problem, The Sciences 17:12-18.

Leventhal, H., and Cleary, P. 1979. Behavioral modification of risk factors: technology or science. In Pollock, M.L., and Schmidt, D., editors. Heart disease and rehabilitation: state of the art, New York, Houghton-Mifflin Co.

Leventhal, H., and Cleary P. 1980. The smoking problem: a review of research and theory in behavioral risk modification, Psychological Bulletin 2:370-405.

Leventhal, H., and Cupchik, G.C. 1975. The informational and facilitative effects of an audience upon expression and evaluation of humorous stimuli, Journal of Experimental Social Psychology 11:363-380.

Leventhal, H., and Cupchik, G.C. 1976. A process model of humor judgment, Journal of Communication 26: 190-204.

Leventhal, H., and Everhart, D. 1979. Emotion, pain and physical illness. In Izard, C.E., editor. Emotion and psychopathology, New York, Pergamon Press Inc.

Leventhal, H., et al. 1960. Epidemic impact on the general population in two cities. In PHS Publication No. 766, The impact of Asian influenza in community life: a study in five cities, Washington, D.C., U.S. Government Printing Office.

Leventhal, H., et al. 1979a. Effects of preparatory information about sensations, threat of pain, and attention on cold pressor distress, Journal of Personality and Social Psychology.

Leventhal, H., et al. 1979b. Effects of attentional instructions on emotional response during labor and delivery, University of Wisconsin (mimeographed).

Leventhal, H., Singer, R., and Jones, S. 1965. Effects of fear and specificity of recommendation upon attitudes and behavior, Journal of Personality and Social Psychology 2:20-29.

Levy, D.M. 1945. Psychic trauma of operations in children, American Journal of Diseases of Children 69:7-25.

Ley, P. 1977. Psychological studies of doctor-patient communication. In Rachman, S., editor. Contributions to medical psychology, vol. 2, New York, Pergamon Press, Inc.

Lichtenstein, E., and Keutzer, C.S. 1971. Modification of smoking behavior: a later look. In Fensterheim, H., et al. editors. Advances in behavior therapy, New York, Academic Press, Inc.

Lieberman, M. 1965. Psychological correlates of impending death: some preliminary observations, Journal of Gerontology 20:181-190.

Lindeman, C.A., and Van Aernam, B. 1971. Nursing intervention with the presurgical patient: the effects of structured and unstructured preoperative teaching, Nursing Research 20:319-332.

Malmo, R.B. 1975. On emotions, needs, and our archaic brain, New York, Holt, Rinehart & Winston.

Mandler, G. 1975. Mind and emotion, New York, John Wiley & Sons, Inc.

Mason, J. 1972. Organization of psychoendocrine mechanisms. In Greenfield, N., and Sternbach, R., editors. Handbook of psychophysiology, New York, Holt, Rinehart & Winston.

May, R. 1950. The meaning of anxiety, New York, Ronald Press.

McClelland, D. 1978. Managing motivation to expand human freedom, American Psychologist 33:201-210.

McGlashan, T.H., Evans, F.J., and Orne, M.T. 1969. The nature of hypnotic analgesia and placebo response to experimental pain, Psychosomatic Medicine 31:227-246.

McKechnie, R.J. 1975. Relief from phantom limb pain by relaxation exercises, Journal of Behavioral Therapy and Experimental Psychiatry. 6:262-263.

Mechanic, D. 1974. Discussion of research programs on relations between stressful life events and episodes of physical illness. In Dohrenwend, B.S., and Dohrenwend, B.P., editors. Stressful life events: their nature and effects, New York, John Wiley & Sons, Inc., pp. 87-97.

Mechanic, D. 1969. Hypochondriasis: a sociological perspective, Psychiatric Opinion 6:17-26. Sociological Review 26:51-58.

Meichenbaum, D., Butler, L., and Joseph, L.G. In press. Toward a conceptual model of social competence. In Wine, J., and Smye, M., editors. The identification and enhancement of social competence, Washington, D.C., Hemisphere Publishing Corp.

Meichenbaum, D., and Turk, D. 1976. The cognitive-behavioral management of anxiety, anger, and pain. In Davidson, P.O., editor. The behavioral management of anxiety, depression and pain, New York, Brunner-Mazel.

Melamed, B. 1977. Psychological preparation for hospitalization. In Rachman, S., editor. Contributions to medical psychology, vol. 1, New York, Pergamon Press, pp. 43-74.

Melamed, B.G., and Seigel, L.J. 1975. Reduction of anxiety in children facing surgery by modeling, Journal of Consulting and Clinical Psychology 43:511-521.

Melamed, B.G., et al. 1975a. The use of filmed modeling to reduce uncooperative behavior of children during dental treatment, Journal of Dental Research 54:797-801.

Melamed, B.G., et al. 1975b. Reduction of fear-related dental management problems with use of filmed modeling, Journal of American Dental Association 90:822-826.

Melzack, R. 1971. Phantom limb pain: implications for treatment of pathologic pain, Anesthesiology 35:409-419.

Melzack, R. 1973. The puzzle of pain, New York, Basic Books, Inc., Publishers.

Melzack, R., and Casey, K.C. 1970. The affective dimension of pain. In Arnold, M.B., editor. Feelings and emotions, New York, Academic Press, Inc. 55-68.

Melzack, R., and Wall, P.D. 1965. Pain mechanisms: a new theory, Science 150:971-979.

Melzack, R., and Wall, P.D. 1970. Psychophysiology of pain, International Anesthesiology Clinics 8:3-34.

Melzack, R., Weisz, A.Z., and Sprague, L.T. 1963. Strategies for controlling pain: contributions of auditory stimulation and suggestion, Experimental Neurology 8:239-247.

Meyer, D., et al. 1978. Influence of sensory monitoring on adherence to anti-hypertensive treatment, Paper presented at National Conference on High Blood Pressure Control, Los Angeles.

Miller, G.A., Galanter, E., and Pribram, K.H. 1960. Plans and the structure of behavior, New York, Holt, Rinehart & Winston.

Miller, N.E. 1951. Learnable drives and rewards. In Stevens, S.S., editor. Handbook of experimental psychology, New York, John J. Wiley & Sons, Inc., pp. 435-472.

Miller, N.E. 1963. Some reflections on the law of effect produce a new alternative to drive reduction. In Jones, M.R., editor. Nebraska Symposium on Motivation, vol. XI, Lincoln, University of Nebraska Press, pp. 65-112.

Mills, R.T., and Krantz, D.S. 1979. Information, choice and reactions to stress: a field experiment in a blood bank with laboratory analogue, Journal of Personality and Social Psychology. 37(4):608-620.

Mortimer, E.A. 1978. Immunization against infectious disease, Science 200:902-907.

Nisbett, R.E., and Schachter, S. 1966. Cognitive manipulation of pain, Journal of Experimental Social Psychology 2:227-236.

Nisbett, R.E., and Wilson, T.D. 1977. Telling more than we can know: verbal reports of mental processes, Psychological Review 84:231-259.

Nerenz, D.R., Leventhal, H., and Love, R. 1982. Factors contributing to emotional distress during cancer chemotherapy, Cancer 5:1020-1027.

Reinhardt, L.C. 1979. Attention and interpretation in control of cold pressor pain distress, doctoral dissertation, Madison, University of Wisconsin.

Rogers, E.S. 1968. Public health asks of sociology, Science 159:506-508.

Ross, L., Rodin, J., and Zimbardo, P.G. 1969. Toward an attribution therapy: the reduction of fear through induced cognitive-emotional misattribution, Journal of Personality and Social Psychology 12:279-288.

Rotter, J.B. 1966. Generalized expectancies for internal versus external control of reinforcement, Psychological Monographs 80(609):1.

Rotter, J.B. 1975. Some problems related to the construct of internal versus external control of reinforcement, Journal of Consulting Clinical Psychology 43:56-67.

Sachs, L.B. 1970. Comparison of hypnotic analgesia and hyponotic relaxation during stimulation by a continuous pain source, Journal of Abnormal Psychology 76:206-210.

Sackett, D.L., and Haynes, R.B. 1976. Compliance with therapeutic regimens, Baltimore, The Johns Hopkins University Press.

Safer, M.A. 1978. Sex differences in hemisphere specialization for recognizing facial expressions of emotion, doctoral thesis, Madison, University of Wisconsin.

Safer, M.A., et al. 1979. Determinants of three stages of delay at a medical clinic, Medical Care 17(1):11-29.

Saward, E., and Sorenson, A. 1978. The current emphasis on preventive medicine, Science 200:889-894.

Schachter, S. 1959. The psychology of affiliation, Stanford, Calif., Stanford University Press.

Schacter, S. 1964. The interaction of cognitive and physiological determinants of emotional state. In Berkowitz, L., editor. Advances in experimental social psychology, vol. 1, New York, Academic Press, Inc.

Schachter, S., and Singer, J.E. 1962. Cognitive, social, and physiological determinants of emotional state, Psychological Review 69:379-399.

Schmitt, F.E., and Wooldridge, P.J. 1973. Psychological preparation of surgical patients, Nursing Research 22:108-115.

Seeman, M., and Evans, J.W. 1962. Alienation and learning in a hospital setting, American Sociological Review 27:772-783.

Seligman, M.E.P. 1975. Helplessness, San Francisco, W.H. Freeman and Co. Publishers.

Shacham, S. 1979. Imagery and pain sensitivity in distress reduction. doctoral thesis, Madison, University of Wisconsin.

Sime, A.M. 1976. Relationship of preoperative fear, type of coping and information received about surgery to recovery from surgery, Journal of Personality and Social Psychology 34:716-724.

Simmel, M.L. 1962. The reality of phantom sensations, Social Research 29:337-356.

Smith, G.M., et al. 1966. An experimental pain method sensitive to morphine in man: the sub-maximum effort tourniquet technique, Journal of Pharmacology and Experimental Therapy 154:324-332.

Snyder, S.H. 1977. Opiate receptors and internal opiates, Scientific American 236:44-56.

Sokolov, E.N. 1963. Perception and the conditioned reflex, Elmsford, N.Y. Pergamon Press, Inc.

Sroufe, L.A., and Waters, E. 1976. The ontogenesis of smiling and laughter: a perspective on the organization of development of infancy, Psychological Review 83:173-189.

Staub, E., and Kellett, O. 1972. Increasing pain tolerance by information about aversive stimulation, Journal of Personality and Social Psychology 21:198-203.

Taylor, J.A. 1953. A personality scale of manifest anxiety, Journal of Abnormal and Social Psychology 48:285-290.

Teichner, W.H. 1965. Delayed cold-induced vasodilation and behavior, Journal of Experimental Psychology 19:426-432.

Tomkins, S.S. 1962. Affect, imagery, consciousness, vol. 1. The positive affects, New York, Springer Publishing Co., Inc.

Vernon, D.T.A. 1967. The roles of anticipatory fear and information in tuberculosis patients' responses to hospitalization and illness. doctoral dissertation, Chicago, University of Chicago.

Vernon, D.T.A. and Bigelow, D.A. 1974. Effect of information about a potential stressful situation on responses to stress impact, Journal of Personality and Social Psychology 29:50-59.

White, R.W. 1974. Strategies of adaptation: an attempt at systematic description. In Coelho, G.V., Hamburg, D.A. and Adams, J.E., editors. Coping and adaptation, New York. Basic Books, Inc., Publishers.

Wilson, J.F. 1977. Determinants of recovery from surgery: preoperative instruction, relaxative training and defensive structures, doctoral dissertation, Ann Arbor, University of Michigan.

Winikoff, B. 1978. Nutrition, population, and health: some implications for policy, Science 200:895-902.

Withey, S. 1962. Reaction to uncertain threat. In Baker, G., and Chapman, D., editors. Man and society in disaster, New York, Basic Books, Inc., Publishers.

Wolfer, J.A., and Davis, C.C. 1970. Assessment of surgical patients' preoperative emotional conditions and post-operative welfare, Nursing Research 19:402-414.

Wolpe, J. 1958. Psychology by reciprocal inhibition, Stanford, Calif., Stanford University Press.

Wolpe, J., and Lazarus, A.A. 1966. Behavior therapy techniques, Elmsford, N.Y., Pergamon Press, Inc.

Zimbardo, P.G., et al. 1966. Control of pain motivation by cognitive dissonance, Science 151:217-219.

SECTION FOUR

Nursing theory, nursing research, and nursing practice

THIS FINAL SECTION analyzes the three chapters in Section III in terms of the metatheoretical and methodological considerations introduced in Section I. Since the intent is to address and articulate research and practice issues as well as theory issues the analysis is complex and multifaceted. This is a logical concomitant of defining the domain of nursing theory as scientific theory for improving practice effectiveness.

Research that directly describes the apparent success of a practice innovation is too often uncritically accepted without analysis of the extent to which the design of the research is adequate to establish the inferences that are drawn. Conversely, survey research on health-related issues that is methodologically sound and rigorous is too often uncritically accepted as relevant to nursing practice without analysis of the extent to which the empirical findings truly imply any specific nursing practice applications. A clear understanding of nursing theory as we defined it in Chapter 1 can help to phrase research questions so that they will simultaneously address behavioral science theory issues and nursing practice issues. A clear understanding of research design issues as we defined them in Chapter 2 and in *Methods of Clinical Experimentation to Improve Patient Care* (Wooldridge, Leonard, and Skipper, 1978) can help to design research procedures that will test these theory- and practice-relevant research questions as validly and directly as possible.

The reader should bear in mind during the following analyses that we deliberately selected scientists whom we respect and research that we believe to be worth the effort of critical analysis. In general, we believe that each study rates high on the criteria most relevant to the purposes for which it was designed. This does not, however, mean that the studies cannot be critically analyzed from additional perspectives relevant to establishing the theory as scientifically valid or applying it widely to improve the quality of nursing practice or both. In other words, it is the responsibility of the reader to examine nursing theory and research by whatever criteria are relevant to his or her own purposes and not just by the criteria relevant to the author's original purposes.

It is not inappropriate, for example, to take a study such as the Martinsons', which was not originally designed to test a general theory, and to propose one or more theories based on its findings. What would be inappropriate (or at least naive) would be to conclude that such a theoretical inference was proved or established by the Martinsons' research or if not that the research must have been poor. Researchers do speculate and should speculate about the meaning of their findings well beyond the limits of what they have actually established. It is up to the would-be scientific theorist to develop such a high level of skill in theoretical and methodological analysis that these speculations and inferences can be assessed and evaluated accurately with respect to whatever use the reader intends to make of them and that further research can be designed in a way that will be relevant to resolving the most salient ambiguities. In Chapter 7 the research reported in Chapters 4 through 6 is analyzed for the purpose of evaluating, developing, and validating general behavioral theories relevant to improving the effectiveness of nursing practice.

CHAPTER 7

EXAMINING RESEARCH FOR ITS CONTRIBUTIONS TO NURSING THEORY AND NURSING PRACTICE

Powhatan J. Wooldridge
Madeline H. Schmitt

In the first two chapters of this book a metatheoretical framework for defining social practice (nursing) theories and examining their relationship to behavioral science theories was presented. The third chapter applied this framework to an analysis of the work of five major nursing theorists. In the next three chapters of the book, three nationally known nurse-researchers and their colleagues wrote about research they conducted in response to a request from the senior author to "tell us how you used theory in your research and how you used your research to develop theory."

In this final chapter we would like to examine these research efforts, in light of what the investigators have to say about what they did, for their contributions to behavioral science theory and nursing practice theory. It is important to note at the outset that the selection was not intended to be representative in any strict sense. The request to the researchers resulted in very different types of contributions as you no doubt have already noticed. By design, the contributions reflect quite different substantive areas of nursing practice, different strategies of theory building, and different methods of research. On the other hand, there are some underlying theoretical commonalities that provide for interesting comparisons.

Martinson and Martinson present a thoughtful account of the development of practice guidelines and prescriptive theory by focusing on the impact of a home care mode of health care delivery for meeting the needs of terminally ill children and their families. Benoliel's chapter illustrates the development and application of theoretical typologies in her research on the impact of a chronic illness on the development of adolescent identity. Leventhal and Johnson give us a comprehensive account of the evolution and testing of a practice theory through a major program of research on informational interventions in preparation for health care events as reflected in their individual and collaborative efforts over the past decade.

Because of the major differences in approaches and stages of theory development reflected in these three chapters, it would be inappropriate to attempt to compare the *quality* of one contribution with another. That is not the purpose of the analysis in this chapter. We will, however, analyze the strengths and weaknesses of each approach for developing nursing practice guidelines, principles, and theory in terms of the metatheoretical framework and principles developed in Section I. One more word of caution is in order; since the metatheoretical approach that we have developed in this book is only one way of examining the growth and development of nursing knowledge, other frameworks applied to the same research contributions might well lead to different conclusions concerning their strengths and their weaknesses.

DEVELOPING A THEORY FOR HOME CARE OF THE DYING CHILD

The analysis in Chapter 3 began with nursing theories and the behavioral science theories they emerged from and moved toward an examination of the extent to which aspects of each theory had been tested empirically. By contrast, Martinson and her colleagues (see, in addition to this chapter, Martinson, 1979; Martinson et al., 1978a, 1978b) began where many practicing nurses do, that is, with a practice problem and an idea for an intervention believed effective in meeting patients' needs. More specifically, the initial question of *feasibility*—can the care required by a child dying with cancer be provided as effectively by parents and nurses at home (as in the hospital)—focused on questions of *framework* and *means*. Can the means of meeting the child's needs for terminal care, which are presently carried out in a hospital situation, be transferred with necessary modifications to the home situation? What variables influence this transferability, for example, what types of families might benefit or suffer; will physicians be willing to refer patients; will the community accept the idea?

Analyzing feasibility and nursing relevance

The descriptive information gathered by Martinson and her colleagues throughout the course of the study documented the feasibility of home care intervention in many respects. Several physicians were willing to try the alternative; many types of families received home care. Nurses could be located to provide care in every instance of referral, even in relatively isolated rural areas. Community response, though often not especially supportive, was not negative. Special equipment and other supplies could be obtained when needed. The home itself was not an unsuitable structure in which to provide care in terms of accessibility to the bathroom and so forth.

While home care might be demonstrated to be a feasible alternative mode of health care delivery for these patients, to what extent do the needs identified fall within the domain of nursing practice? Is this an area of care in which nursing might be said to have responsibility? In examining whether the research focused on a potential nursing intervention it is useful to look at whether the problems identified are situational. The Martinsons make it clear that their subjects become eligible for the intervention on termination of cure-oriented therapy, when the child's needs are for comfort and care in response to the illness' inevitable progression. The goal is palliation, and it falls clearly in the domain of nursing.

The means needed to achieve palliative outcomes and the extent to which these fall in the domain of nursing are not clear initially. The means hypothesized include some that are not entirely within the control of the nursing profession. Pain management is a case in point. Nurses and families must rely on the availability of a physician to prescribe analgesics and suggest modification as necessary to keep the child at home free from pain. Whether such pain as was manifested could be managed with oral medication was open to question.

Probably the most critical issue pertaining to means was whether parents could and would assume primary caretaking responsibilities for their children. The proposed home care program depended heavily for its implementation on the parents as caretakers rather than the nurse. While nurses did not have direct control over parental *desires* to provide home care for their children, they were able to manipulate parental ability. The nurses' role was defined as one of educating parents about what to expect, teaching them technical procedures, providing some direct care, acting as a liaison for consultation with the physician, and providing unlimited support to the child and the family. This role of nursing in motivating individuals and families toward self-care, especially through therapeutic communication, is at the heart of the social practice of nursing. Nurses have traditionally visited people in their homes for such purposes and are licensed to do so. While the nurse might have to learn some specific skills concerning certain needs of the dying child and his family, such as the counseling skills that Martinson (1979) explains, the type of nursing intervention proposed does not seem to require a new type of nursing education or special training.

The first objective of the Martinsons and their colleagues was gathering descriptive data that focused on the general feasibility of transferring the child to the home as well as on the specific means used to decide whether this type of intervention was feasible. As part of this objective they developed a new set of practice guidelines specific to home care, that is, a set of procedures that directs the nurse and family caretakers to perform in a given way certain treatment activities. They have offered these guidelines to others who might wish to start home care projects for dying children in other communities. From a research viewpoint, with what degree of confidence can we accept the conclusions of the Martinsons and their colleagues about the means necessary for caring for a child with terminal cancer at home and the likely outcomes for others using these means? The Martinsons' conclusions about the *outcomes* of the approach to home care for the dying child are based on family interviews and the clinical judgment of the professionals involved. Tentative conclusions about the program's positive outcomes, based on a sample of 32 families, are found in Martinson et al. (1978a). These include improved satisfaction of the child, better adjustment to the situation by the family, and reduced costs. Indicators of these outcomes included that all of the children preferred being at home; only one family member received any psychiatric help; there was no negative impact on siblings other than short-term disruptions; families returned to normal activities sooner; and home care costs were less by comparison with the costs for a similar group of children who remained hospitalized. Except for the cost variable, no comparison groups were used in the research design.

Evaluating the research evidence

In Chapter 2 there was a discussion about ways in which inferences about success drawn from clinical experience in the absence of adequate research design can be misleading. One way to be misled is to forget that the outcome might have been positive even without the intervention. Incorporating a control group that does not receive the intervention into the research design is a common means used for avoiding this error of inference. The Martinsons realize this but rely instead on the less reliable technique of comparing outcomes to general clinical expectations for this kind of situation. This results in a "one-shot case study" design that, as Campbell and Stanley (1963:6-7) point out, is subject to numerous threats to internal validity. Literature that Martinson and her colleagues have cited indicates that negative psychosocial outcomes, such as family crises, are a frequent concommitant of childhood cancer deaths. The absence of extremely negative outcomes in Martinson's sample suggests, therefore, that families who care for their children in the home do better than if they had cared for them in the hospital. Although Gehan and Freiriech (1974) have advocated the use of clinical expectations to replace control groups in certain kinds of clinical trials with cancer patients, it is doubtful that this technique is entirely adequate in this instance. The validity of such comparisons depends on the existence of accurate knowledge of the kinds of outcomes to be expected for the specific kinds of patients studied. In the Martinsons' research, it is hard to be sure that differences in outcome were not caused by differences in the kinds of families or patients involved, since the factors influencing negative psychosocial outcomes are not well known. This possibility threatens the internal validity of the inference that the home care approach led to more favorable treatment outcomes.

A second way that inferences drawn from clinical experiences may be misleading relates to the types of bias that can be introduced in evaluation of the patient's (or family's) condition before the intervention, after intervention, or both. In the Martinsons' study this is also a factor that may have significantly influenced the findings. A lack of standard and objective measures leaves room for error in the caregivers' and interviewers' judgments of outcomes. Such judgments might have been affected by the desire of the care-givers and interviewers to see the intervention work and reluctance to think that they may not have done what was best for the child. The family's desire to please staff members who have been warm and attentive may also have affected the nature of their statements about their experiences. The impact of such biases would be to make outcomes seem more positive than they really are. The possibility of such biases further reduces the study's internal validity.

A third way to be mislead is to assume that the means described as con-tributing to the outcomes of the intervention are in fact the major factors contributing to the outcomes. Other aspects of the intervention that escaped attention but that might explain a more favorable outcome include the greater motivation of the staff and the extra attention given to the home care families. Such factors might have led to unusually favorable outcomes even if the chil-dren had been treated in the hospital. This is also an issue of internal validity.

These and other factors affecting the internal validity of the study are not the only considerations in evaluating the extent to which the results could be obtained in other situations and with other caregivers. The matter of gener-alizability shifts our attention to additional issues of *external validity*. Even if we accept that the Martinsons and their colleagues were correct in believing that home care for the dying child led to more favorable outcomes in their setting, the results might not be generalizable to other geographic settings or to all kinds of children and families.

The Martinsons' results suggest a relatively high degree of empirical gen-eralizability, since the case load they served varied widely in family character-istics, child disease characteristics, geographic location, and primary nurse caregivers. However, the Martinsons' discussion suggests that there are some children for whom the home care alternative may not be appropriate or desir-able. Inability to distinguish between these two populations on the basis of the Martinsons' work raises the additional question of how clinicians who adopt this intervention will decide who can benefit most from home care.

The emphasis here is on distinguishing which children do better at home than in the hospital and vice versa. This question implies separate compari-sons of home and hospital care for different types of children that go well beyond the question of general feasibility in one setting. It would require comparison groups (control as well as experimental), quantitative outcome measures, and a substantial number of children of each type to address this question by means of statistical analysis. A more qualitative discussion, such as that of the Martinsons and colleagues, can be useful, however, in suggest-ing how to divide children into different groups for whom the results may be different. In other words, speculations about contraindications based on qualitative discussions of clinical experiences are valuable in suggesting hypotheses to be tested, but they should be regarded as only tentative until they have been validated by systematic research.

The Martinsons have not in general used quantitative statistical comparisons to test their conclusions. In further research, however, they have actually attempted such a comparison with reference to relative costs of the two programs. The costs for children in the home care program were compared with a group of 22 "similar" children who died of cancer in the hospital (Martinson et al., 1978a). While the reported reduced costs of the home care program are impressive, the possible lack of comparability of the two groups still leaves unresolved questions. In what respects were the 22 hospitalized children similar? Were they treated in the same hospital settings as the home care children had been? Were they cared for by physicians who did not refer children to the home care program, or were they a subgroup of children whom referring physicians consciously decided *not* to refer to the home care program for one reason or another? (See Edwardson, 1983).

Deciding on directions for further research

This attempt to provide comparative data on one outcome area sensitizes us to one of the key issues concerning comparison group research strategies. This is that differences between groups that existed prior to the comparison can produce misleading results. Undetected selection biases attributable to the referring physician or family create internal validity problems. As the Martinsons point out in the concluding section of their chapter, these may be decreased (and the probability that such biases led to differences quantitatively assessed) by the use of random assignment to treatment conditions. Since the researchers were interested in a variety of antecedent factors that might affect success of the home care, such as socioeconomic status of parents, rural or urban residence, and type of cancer the child had, these factors might be taken specifically into account through sampling restrictions, blocking, or matching as an adjunct to the randomizing procedure. This would improve the efficiency of the design by reducing the sample size required.

The systematic inclusion of these variables as part of the research design would also make it possible to study statistical interaction between them and the type of terminal care provided in influencing outcome measures. Instead of describing just the average difference in response to the interventions over all the patients studied, such an analysis would also describe variations in this difference for different kinds of patients. When the sample size is small, this might be done through dummy variable regression analysis rather than by a literal separation of the sample into a large number of homogenous subgroups (see, for example, Powers and Wooldridge, 1982). The study of such "statistical interaction" would enable the researcher to draw inferences about the empirical generalizability of the average effect and help the nursing theorist to specify the general conditions under which the family as care provider (the home care approach) is most superior to a hospital approach. Ultimately such research and theory building would help the practicing nurse to set up more effective guidelines for choosing between the home care and hospital approaches. In addition to outright contraindications to the home approach, if resources to implement the home care approach were limited, one might use it only in those cases where the benefits would be the greatest.

The Martinsons and colleagues are sensitive to the need for a randomized control group, but argue that "any limitations of the parents' and the children's freedom of choice would be viewed as untenable or unethical by the vast majority of referring physicians." While ethical issues should be attended to, it is not clear why use of random assignment for at least some of the subjects in such studies would be unethical or unacceptable to referring physicians. Complete freedom of choice is not permitted patients in choosing among biophysical care modalities, and although patients may have the right to insist on at-home treatment, they are usually discouraged by physicians from exercising that right, even for such "natural" processes as childbirth and dying. In point of fact, the Martinsons' discussion implies that some children or families were felt to be unsuitable for home care and were not given that choice. In areas where the home care option has not been previously available, it may be possible to arrange matters so that the new option is phased in gradually on a trial basis with random decision by each physician as to which patients to refer. To the extent that the risks and benefits of home care in comparison to hospital treatment have not been established, assignment of a terminally ill child to in-hospital care would not involve depriving the child and his family of a treatment known to be superior nor even to a treatment that had previously been available. The need for randomized trials is well-accepted in medical treatment of cancer and should thus be a familiar concept to physicians who are treating childhood cancer. While such physicians may not accord the same importance to rigorous testing of psychosocial innovations prior to widespread adoption that they would accord to testing a new chemotherapeutic agent, our experience does not suggest that the vast majority would refuse to cooperate with such a study.

In a randomized treatment, any unknown risks of the new treatment are distributed in such a way that everyone has an equal chance of exposure to such risks, and any benefits of the new treatment are also distributed in this fashion. It would seem to be premature to decide at the outset that a new treatment will prove so beneficial that it must be given to all patients who desire it from the first moment that it is available to anyone. It is also unlikely that the kinds of patients for whom the new treatment would be superior will be so apparent at the outset that the choice between treatment modalities must always be made according to the judgment of the physician. Even if some patients cannot be randomly assigned because they or their physicians refuse to accept one of the modalities, there will usually be a substantial number of patients for whom the appropriate modality will be in doubt. For these patients if for no others random assignment should be employed. Such a design will not provide data on the generalizability of treatment effects to the subgroups excluded before random assignment, but it will be internally valid for the "doubtful" subgroups for which random assignment was possible. By assumption, these will usually be the groups for whom the relative effectiveness of the two approaches is most in doubt, so the importance of obtaining valid and accurate data to guide future decisions would seem to outweigh other ethical considerations.

For a new treatment to be widely adopted before its strengths and limitations have been adequately tested poses ethical dilemmas that may be at least as serious as the supposed ethical problems of random assignment. On what base of knowledge do decisions about who is to receive the home care rest? In the absence of valid research data the quality of such decisions depends on the clinician's intuitive ability, which may be incorrect to an unknown degree. Overly conservative clinical judgments might deprive children and families of an alternative treatment from which they would benefit, whereas overly liberal judgments might result in inappropriate assignments to home care. Leaving the decision entirely up the family might seen to be the "right" thing to do, but it also might be viewed as an abrogation of the clinician's responsibility to counsel patients and their families. The Martinsons cite the rapid acceptance of the home care alternative. It is possible that some of the acceptance is based on issues such as reduced costs to the health care providers—both monetary and psychological—rather than on benefits to the child and family. Lacking a sound data base for the characteristics of children and families who benefit versus those who do not there is no way to be sure that the program's acceptance is not to some extent a "dumping" phenomenon. On the other hand, for circumstances in which the home care approach is actually superior as well as less costly is it ethical to permit some clinicians to continue to insist on in-hospital care?

Our position can be summed up as follows. For circumstances in which one care modality has clearly been established as superior to the other no research is needed. When the patient has an established right to a given modality and chooses to exercise that right random assignment is unethical. However, for circumstances in which the new modality is not generally available and its superiority is in doubt, alternative health care modalities should be tested against one another through randomized clinical trials. Methodological rigor is just as important when the differences between care modalities are mostly psychosocial as when the differences are biophysical. This is not however, to deny the potential contribution of one-shot case studies with a descriptive emphasis such as the Martinsons' in developing the modalities and principles to be tested.

Developing practice guidelines and principles

Articulating the theoretical principles on which new guidelines are based in such a way that the *means* employed will be useful to other practitioners in other places is a challenge. There is a need to conceptualize such principles of effective nursing at higher levels of generality. Theoretical principles have the virtue of summarizing a large number of specific practice guidelines in a way that relates them to one another. In addition, because of the concepts employed such principles may suggest links to other principles. The Martinsons explicitly propose one such principle: "Reducing parental uncertainty leads to an increase in perceived parental control, which promotes patient satisfaction, comfort, and security, and family adjustment to the death of a child." This principle is really a testable theoretical hypothesis, the parts of which have operational referents. "Reduction of parental uncertainty," for example, has three operational referents that have evolved from exploratory descriptive research. They are as follows:

1. Teach the parents how to give basic nursing care to the child.
2. Through cognitive structuring, help them anticipate what change to expect.
3. Assist them to obtain necessary resources at points of critical need.

These referents help to define a way that parental uncertainty can be manipulated. The hypothetical set of relationships may be diagrammed, as shown in Fig. 1.

Since the type of nursing service to be offered in this study had no precedent in theory or practice, such principles were not evident at the outset but were derived later on the basis of experience. In addition to the already dis-

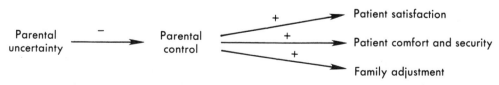
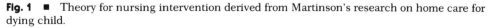

Fig. 1 ■ Theory for nursing intervention derived from Martinson's research on home care for dying child.

cussed additions to the research design, gathering data that specifically describes and measures the extent to which these means were employed would strengthen the ability to test whether the proposed means and the outcomes actually were related.

The examination of the "rightness" of the proposed principle involves empirically testing possible *interpretations* of why a particular nursing intervention works. Even at its present level of generalization, the Martinsons' theories suggest a link to a broader set of theoretical nursing relationships concerning the impact of interventions intended to promote self-understanding and self-care in the health care arena. (Note the similarity to Johnson and Leventhal's theory of self-regulation, for example.) Further, the attention to outcome variables such as family adjustment provides conceptual links to, for example, the "family crisis" literature in sociology, in which a broader array of family crises and adaptation to them is the focus of attention. This literature is in turn linked to nursing studies that have investigated the "crises" of childbirth, handicap, stroke, or chronic disease and have developed guidelines and theories related to the provision of home care by nurses to help families adapt to such situations. (Note Benoliel's research on one chronic disease, for example.)

In this chapter and in other published papers the Martinsons and their colleagues have described an interesting exploratory intervention. Others implementing similar programs in other parts of the country have the opportunity to recognize both the strengths and limitations of this study and to correct some of its limitations in their own research. Institution of new interventions should move slowly, and ideally each agency moving in the direction of a home care program for dying children will establish its own evaluation research program to gauge the efficacy of the program in general and for various patient subgroups in particular.

DEVELOPING A THEORY OF CHRONIC DISEASE IN ADOLESCENCE

Benoliel introduces us to a process for descriptive theory building that is quite different in key aspects from the Martinsons' process. Their starting point is the particular clinical situation, and their motive is explicitly practical. They want to demonstrate the effectiveness of a particular nursing means in caring for dying children. The nursing means is not derived from any specific set of theoretical ideas. The Martinsons' approach to descriptive theory building is inductive, and the theory-building goal is secondary to the practical clinical one. Benoliel, on the other hand, is involved in studying the clinical situation primarily for the purpose of descriptive theory building. In her initial exposure to the clinical situation she looks for variation in contingencies that affect identity formation in children who have been diagnosed as having one of a variety of chronic illnesses. These contingencies become the bases for designing a more systematic descriptive theory-building study. Benoliel's initial work is not so purely inductive as that of the Martinsons. She starts with a complex set of theoretical reference points taken from the behavioral sciences, which are used to help guide the observations she makes in the clinical situation.

The Martinsons' inquiry emphasizes the domain of practice theory in examining nursing means and their impact on clinical nursing goals, and only occasionally conceptualizes these variables in general behavioral science terms. Very little attention is paid to general contingencies that might affect the use of the proposed nursing means in different clinical contexts. This leads not only to a weakness from the general behavioral science theory viewpoint but also from the practice theory viewpoint. As we will see, Benoliel's work remains more within the domain of behavioral science theory. Benoliel focuses primarily on the analysis of contingencies and their relationship to various reactions to chronic illness and to the health and illness outcomes for children experiencing the chronic illness. The role of nursing means in effecting different, more desirable outcomes (goals) is alluded to, but not studied directly. The result of Benoliel's small-scale exploratory study is a descriptive typology of contingencies and hypothetically related effects. In this kind of study, use of general behavioral or social science theory or both from sociology and anthropology is most clearly pertinent, as discussed in Chapter 2. As in the Martinsons' study, the results demand further systematic documentation using a more quantitative research approach and a larger sample size.

Developing the conceptual framework

It is very difficult for a researcher to describe how a theory is built. Benoliel gives us good insight into this process through the detailed description of the stages of thought she went through. Initially she immersed herself in a pediatric clinic that cared for children with three different types of chronic, life-threatening illness. Her participant observation focused on the varying adaptation of the children and their families to the presence of these three diseases. While the specific disease was thought to be an important influence on adaptation, a more specific delineation of dimensions of disease, for example, visibility and prognosis, that would be most important resulted from the period of observation. Many other variables of potential importance in affecting adaptation also emerged from her observations and, to some extent, from suggestions in the literature, which was searched for relevant concepts and theories simultaneously. Many of the concepts and theories Benoliel uses in conceptualizing the process of adaptation were familiar to her as the result of prior study and research. The general theoretical perspective she uses is that of symbolic interaction, which describes the social process by which individuals form their identities and come to understand the meaning of their lives in terms of social role. She links many theoretical ideas to this overall framework: the developmental aspects of identity formation; the importance of different reference groups along the way (for example, peers and family); the ritualized aspects of key shifts in self and role-identity contained in the concept of "status passage"; and, in particular, the concept of the "sick role" as it applies to an identity-forming process altered by the presence of a chronic illness. This broad theoretical framework was used for its heuristic potential in directing Benoliel's attention to aspects of the situation she studied. In particular, it directs her attention to the *social meaning* of the diagnosis of chronic illness of a particular type for the patient and family.

In this theoretical framework such "meanings" are an important interacting variable in explaining why people behave in various ways toward a particular illness. It is Benoliel's belief that an understanding of the meanings attributed by patients and families to chronic illnesses of various types is essential to developing effective clinical care. The symbolic interactionist framework is one that was discussed earlier in this book as particularly productive of potential insights into the social practice of nursing because the patient's definition of the situation affects both his needs and his response to the nurse's attempt to help him and the nurse can ignore the patients' point of view only at the risk of professional ineffectiveness. This theoretical perspective is inherent in Orlando's emphasis on the social meaning of the illness situation to the patient, as discussed in Chapters 2 and 3.

Presumably a conceptual framework such as Benoliel constructs could be developed through a review of the literature only. Improper use of such a framework in research could result in a selective view of the world that would confirm the usefulness of such a framework regardless of its actual heuristic value. All observations would be "labelled" so as to be consistent with the framework whether or not they actually focused on those aspects of the situation most relevant to the process of adaptation. Little would be learned that is new. Proper use of such a framework in conjunction with observations made in empirical situations could result in the development of descriptive theory subject to empirical hypothesis testing. In using the symbolic interaction framework we would be led to a recognition that meanings of any "objective" situation (such as a diagnosis of chronic illness) to families and individuals vary. Understanding the nature of this variation as well as the reasons for it helps to identify the contexts that influence the differential success of specific clinical nursing interventions.

Using the theoretical model to guide research

The heurisitic potential of Benoliel's theoretical formulations can be established only by further research. Benoliel's initial exposure to a pediatric clinic situation, involving a variety of children being treated for different types of chronic illness and their families, led her to hypothesize that multiple variables were important in explaining the varying meanings given to illnesses such as diabetes, asthma, and cystic fibrosis by children, their families, and health providers. Using Benoliel's description as a guide, a general list of variables and their overall relationships to each other is shown in Fig. 2.

It is obvious that not all of these variables can be studied at once. At the end of the preliminary fieldwork phase, Benoliel made a decision on the basis of theory and observation that the meaning of diagnosis of various chronic diseases in children *to their families* was a key variable in patient outcomes and one that demanded closer attention. A variety of family background variables might be expected to be related to differences in the meaning of the illness to the families observed. Therefore to maximize descriptive theory building about the meaning of a chronic illness diagnosis to families Benoliel included families from varying backgrounds in her study sample. A key background variable related to a variety of family characteristics was the social

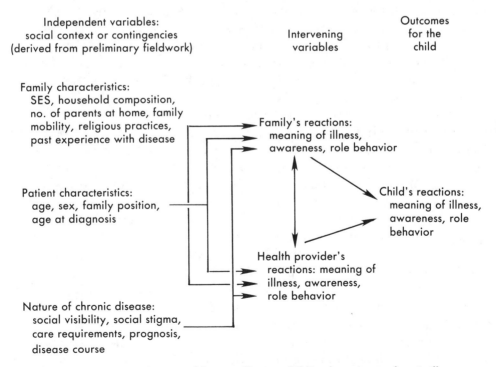

Fig. 2 ■ Conceptualization of factors affecting child's adaptation to chronic illness.

class of the family. The overall design that Benoliel created might be conceptualized as a kind of two-way analysis of variance design, as shown in Fig. 3. The two variables whose effects on family meaning were studied were type of chronic illness and social class of the family.

Many variables associated with these two key variables were hypothesized as relevant to explaining why there might be different meanings associated with family and, therefore, patient reactions to these diseases. For different types of chronic illness this included such variables as daily time and effort required to manage the disease, prognosis, and presence of observable symptoms—what Benoliel called the *social visibility* of the diseases. Differences in values, styles of living, child-rearing practices, and financial and social resources were variables of importance associated with social class. Other variables of importance indicated in Fig. 1, unrelated to either of these two important theoretical dimensions, included patient characteristics such as age of patient, age at onset, sex of patient, and duration of chronic illness at time of interview. Certain provider factors were also felt to be important in the patient's and family's reactions to the diagnosis but these were not singled out for attention in the study.

A final phase in designing the study led to a decision to focus only on one chronic disease initially and to expand consideration of the individual factors. This resulted in a new design, depicted as a modification of the two-way ANOVA-type design shown in Fig. 3. Fig. 4 is an N-way type design that takes into account the specific variables related to individual and family characteristics that were of interest to Benoliel.

The intent was to choose a sample for interview that would supply cases

Social class of family	Type of disease			
	Asthma	Cystic fibrosis	Diabetes	Chronic pyelonephritis
Middle class				
Working class				
Lower class				

"The logic of including different types of groups (in this case, families) made possible comparisons at different conceptual levels of analysis—families with the same type of chronic disease, families with different types of chronic disease, and finally, families with different types of chronic disease and from different social classes."
(Benoliel, Chapter 5, p. 145).

Fig. 3 ■ Two way ANOVA-Type design for studying family reactions to chronic disease in children.

Social class	Single parent	Diabetic parent	Individual characteristics Sex							
			Male				Female			
			Onset age							
			Younger		Older		Younger		Older	
			Current age							
			Younger	Older	Younger	Older	Younger	Older	Younger	Older
Middle	Yes	Y								
		N								
	No	Y								
		N								
Working	Yes	Y								
		N								
	No	Y								
		N								
Lower	Yes	Y								
		N								
	No	Y								
		N								

"The study now focused on (1) the *meaning of being diabetic* (sic) at different chronological points in the transition from preadolescence to adulthood, (2) meaning and management of diabetes by *different types of families* (sic), and (3) the effects . . . " (Benoliel, Chapter 5, p. 155).

Fig. 4 ■ N-way ANOVA-type design for studying reactions to diabetes in adolescence.

representing each of the theoretical combinations of the variables focused on. As Benoliel found, however, with so many variables at issue, it was not possible to obtain exact equivalences by age and sex in combination with the desired characteristics of the families. As can be seen from Fig. 4, to get even a single case representing each of the combinations, Benoliel would have needed a total of 96 cases, each with a different combination of characteristics. Her actual sample was only 9 subjects, all between 10 and 16 years old.

The scope of the exploratory theoretical task that Benoliel has undertaken can be appreciated even more if one realizes that quantitatively to test the insights she develops in this research a minimum of 960 cases (10 per cell) would be recommended to use N-way ANOVA. In addition, the practice implications of even such a large scale study would remain obscure, since the independent variables (sex, onset age, current age, socioeconomic class, single parent, and diabetic parent) would not be variables that the nurse could manipulate to affect the adolescent's reactions to diabetes. While such a study might help to identify risk factors related to negative reactions, it would not show how nurses can intervene to promote more favorable reactions. To have direct implications for nursing practice the research would have to add the type of nursing intervention strategy employed as an additional independent variable, further increasing the number of cells and the sample size needed. Even a data analysis using multiple regression with dummy variables would require a large number of cases to provide a reliable result. Finally, when we recall that Benoliel initially wanted to complete comparative analyses for *four* different diseases it becomes apparent that to study systematically all of the phenomena that she outlines, a full-scale research program containing many studies would be required. While this tends to be true of theory in general, the scope of the enterprise is likely to be particularly large for social science theories focusing on aspects of the framework.

Developing theory from qualitative data

The content of the interviews concerning the meaning of the diabetic child to families was developed from open-ended discussions with parents and children in the diabetes clinic. It was not possible to develop one interview that "fit" all family members. Consequently, three separate interview schedules were developed for parents, patients, and siblings. In scanning the content of the interview schedule and reading about the processes of data analysis Benoliel went through it is important to note a difference between quantitative descriptive research style and this more qualitatively oriented style. First, a quantitatively oriented researcher might give the family members standardized measures of one sort or another to assess their reactions to the disease, and the responses to these measures might well be reported descriptively without any additional theorizing about the meaning of the findings. A less direct relationship exists in Benoliel's analysis between the responses and the findings as Benoliel reports them. The data she gathers are reviewed in relation to theoretical concepts to describe the results in theoretical as well as empirical terms. Thus she reviews the data on three separate occasions to analyze three types of reactions: the stages of adjustment to the disease, the present meaning of the diabetes and its treatment to the family, and the personal meaning of the disease to the diabetic child.

The findings are summarized in typological format. The information on stages of adjustment and present meaning of the disease result in a typology of four overall family reactions to the diseases: protective, adaptive, manipulative, and abdicative. Similarly, a typology describing the response of the diabetic child to medical requirements of managing the disease is developed and the variation in these responses is linked to family reactions (Chapter 5, p. 179):

> The category of interaction that had the greatest impact on the character of the emerging diabetic role-identity was the pattern of day-to-day interaction that developed in the family for dealing with the regular events and untoward experiences that were part and parcel of living with diabetes

Benoliel's approach is related to analytic induction (Robinson, 1951) and to the "grounded theory" approach of Glaser and Strauss (1967) and of Shatzman (1975), but is different from any of them. For example, Benoliel relies much more directly on behavioral science theory to formulate her concepts than Glaser and Strauss recommend. (This is not necessarily undesirable, however, and it is in accord with the classical approach to such theorizing.) Despite her best efforts to inform us of her processes of moving between theory and data and back to theory and the complexities of doing so, Benoliel's discussion leaves a lot unsaid. It is important to note that the end result of this process is an empirically based set of typologies and hypotheses linking the variables in the typologies to each other. The variables comprising these typologies could be operationalized and the hypothesized relationship between them could be tested on a large representative sample of families and patients. The conclusions about the importance of these variables that Benoliel is tempted to draw at the end of the chapter, such as "the life style of working-class families makes them a high risk group," are highly speculative and cannot be firmly asserted unless they are confirmed by testing with a larger and more representative sample. Additional studies to look at the meanings of other types of chronic illness to children and their families would also need to be done (as we have discussed) to test the general heuristic potential of Benoliel's overall framework. Finally, studies of nursing interventions would have to test heuristic potential from a practice theory point of view.

Articulating the theory with nursing practice theory

Benoliel's theory building is not an example of an attempt to construct a broad *theory of nursing*, such as is characteristic of the theorists examined in Chapter 3. Rather, she relies on a variety of theories from psychology and sociology, her prior research experience, and a method of gathering empirical data for theory-generating purposes to construct her "social theory of chronic disease." Her primary goal in the overall research plan was to develop a theory of the impact of chronic disease in adolescence. Furthermore, in this study only the impact of a diagnosis of diabetes mellitus on a sample of adolescents is studied. Benoliel is interested in the social context of the family's and adolescent's reaction to a diagnosis of chronic illness (contingent conditions that broadly imply the framework for potential nursing interventions), and the nature of the reaction itself. To what extent are Benoliel's theory-building goals within the domain of nursing practice theory, behavioral science theory, or both?

We have argued that the domain of nursing practice theory addresses situationally derived needs relating to illness. These needs encompass a family's and patient's difficulties in adjusting to a diagnosis of disease and coping with its management. Nursing practice theory and research would examine the impact of nursing interventions on these difficulties in different contexts, and the specific type of difficulty and the context would be part of the framework specifying the means to be employed. Fig. 5 shows the relationship between

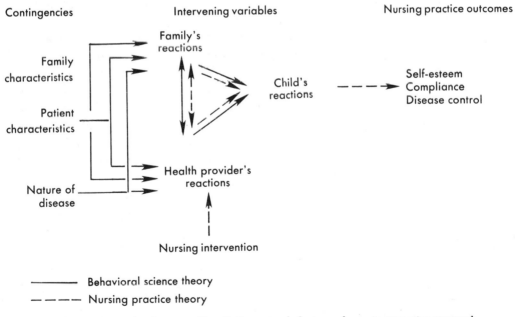

Fig. 5 ■ Relationship between Benoliel's research focus and nursing practice research.

the variables of interest to Benoliel in this research and those in a hypothetical nursing practice theory focusing on the same problem.

In comparing the placement of types of variables in Benoliel's framework with the location of certain types of variables in a nursing practice theory as discussed earlier in this book, we see many parallels. The physiological and psychological variables appear as contingencies and outcomes. The sociological variables also appear as contingencies. The psychosocial variable encompassing the social interactions that convey knowledge, awareness, and attitudes appears as the intervening variable or means by which the contingent conditions operate to effect outcomes. Some variables considered relevant to understanding relationships may not meet other, metatheoretical standards for building practice theory. For example, they may not be causes manipulable by the practitioner, the effects may not be relevant to nursing practice goals, the contingent conditions may not be present in practice situations, or the means for affecting goals may not fall within the prescriptive domain of nursing. On the other hand, some of the contingent variables identified as important in the family's and child's reaction to diagnosis and coping with the disease may define the context of nursing interventions and be part of nursing practice theory as variables to be controlled in a study. Their effects in a nursing practice study are sources of error variation.

Focusing on the development of practice theory directly would require selecting specific variables from Benoliel's theoretical framework that meet identified metatheoretical criteria. For example, in her concluding paragraphs Benoliel suggests that knowledge of valid facts about diabetes and its management were not provided systematically by the health care system. Even when knowledge was provided it was not the kind of knowledge needed but was "traditional teaching." She suggested several changes in the health care system, including modifying the type of patient education given by health care providers. In the past changes in the health care system have grown out of studies such as this. New services are introduced because they are implied by basic behavioral science research. However, research directed at the development of a practice theory would *begin* precisely where basic behavioral science research leaves off. Studies to examine systematically the kind of knowledge being given, the kind of knowledge needed by families, the most effective methods for delivering this knowledge, and the limitations of these types of interventions would fall into the domain of practice theory. Benoliel's research also offers some suggestions, which need to be researched further, about the limiting conditions (contingencies) to the effectiveness of adequate knowledge. She suggests that certain family characteristics and associated styles of adapting to a diabetic child may be limiting factors in effective use of knowledge-oriented interventions.

The goal of behavioral science theory has been defined as describing and explaining the causes of recurring patterns of human behavior. It can be seen that Benoliel's overall purpose in her research falls more in the domain of building behavioral science theory than in the social practice theory domain. Benoliel (Chapter 5, p. 183) indicates her belief about the importance of this type of research to nursing practice theory:

> The creation of social theory that clarifies the social impingements of critical changes and the conditions affecting how individuals and groups adapt to them can provide concrete direction for identifying circumstances of high risk structural defects in available health services, and needs for assistance not yet met by the system.

Indeed, good studies of contextual variables such as those Benoliel examines yield important information about which variables need to be controlled in studies in nursing practice. However, even though the substantive boundaries of Benoliel's interests overlap with the situationally derived concerns of nursing practice theory (perhaps as a result of her dual identity as a sociologist and a nurse), she does not focus on the development of guidelines and principles for effective practice directly.

DEVELOPING A THEORY OF SELF-REGULATION

The research of Leventhal and Johnson differs from the previous examples in a number of ways. First, it reports an entire program of research, including a variety of methodologies and approaches, rather than a single study with a single dominant approach. Second, their research is more operationally precise in its data collection and quantitative in its data analysis than either of the preceding examples. Third, the research is presented as a series of inductive (theory-generating) and deductive (theory-testing) steps, rather than focusing primarily on induction from experience (Martinson) or combined deductively derived typologies and inductive description (Benoliel). This research shows the tremendous effort involved in developing and testing explanatory theory, in which distinguishing between alternative theories that might account for research results ("the reasons for the relationship between the variables") becomes the central focus of inquiry. It is possible to lose sight of the nursing practice implications of this research in focusing so heavily on theory, but practice implications are always present, even when the authors do not make them explicit.

Defining the behavioral theory

The behavioral theory of self-regulation advanced by Leventhal and Johnson can be presented as a causal model. This model can be analyzed in terms of the *contingencies* or circumstances to which it applies, the independent variables whose effects are to be assessed, and the dependent variables that define the different kinds of outcomes to be assessed. (Note the parallel between such causal modeling and the definitions of practice guidelines and general principles of effective practice, Chapter 1, p. 23.) As a further complication, the dependent variables may also be causally related to one another, so that in addition to *direct effects* of the independent variable on a dependent variable there may also be *indirect effects*. An indirect effect on an outcome is caused by the effect of the independent variable on one of the other dependent variables in the model, which then affects the ultimate outcome. The dependent variable linking the independent variable to the ultimate outcome in such a cause-effect sequence is called an *intervening variable* when an indirect effect is being discussed. Finally, the effects of one independent variable may vary according to the value of the other independent variables and/or according to other contingencies not explicitly included in the model. These are called *interactive affects* or (as in Wooldridge et al., 1978) *specifications*.

The causal relationships between the variables in the basic theory that Leventhal and Johnson present are diagrammed in Fig. 6. This theory predicts that when a person faces a stressful situation about which the "preparatory input" of knowledge necessary for self-regulation is inaccurate or incomplete, the presentation of self-regulating information including:

1. "A clear representation of the environment" (the schema)
2. "An adequate set of coping responses"
3. "Reasonable criteria for successful regulation"

will reduce emotional distress and increase active (planned) or passive (automatic) coping behaviors. The positive effect of information on coping will be both direct and indirect through decreasing distress, and the negative ef-

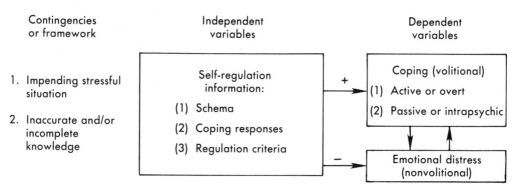

Fig. 6 ■ Causal model suggested by Leventhal and Johnson's theory of self-regulation.

fect of information on distress will be both direct and indirect through increasing coping. In Leventhal and Johnson's initial theoretical formulations, "sensory information" about what to expect was assumed to have direct effects on emotional distress, while "action information" about coping responses and when to employ them was assumed to have direct effects on active coping, thus constituting different processes in the "parallel response" model. This assumed differentiation was then used to test the two processes involved as separate entities by manipulating the two types of information separately. When the results in the "field" (that is, clinical) settings did not seem to support the assumed differentiation, Leventhal's and Johnson's emphases diverged in a complementary fashion.

Most of Johnson's theoretical interpretations focus on the reasons why both action information and sensory information have direct effects on coping. Coping is defined as consisting of "deliberate, volitional actions designed to regulate either the environmental agent causing the emotion or the emotional behavior itself," while emotional distress is defined as "automatic and involuntary reactions that are expressive of fear" (p. 197). Johnson implies that most of the effects of sensory information on distress are indirect (operating through direct effects on coping), while Leventhal implies that they are direct (operating automatically rather than volitionally through changes in the meaning assigned to the sensory input by the individual). In some places Leventhal even reverses Johnson's emphasis by discussing indirect effects of sensory information on coping through distress reduction.

One source of confusion in differentiating between these two theoretical processes is that the mental processes that intervene between sensory information and distress reduction may be thought of as a form of coping if the action (or lack of it) is considered to be a volitional attempt to reduce emotional distress. For example, Johnson and Leventhal suggest that "sitting and doing nothing" might be a form of passive coping (p. 246). Whether or not one is willing to think of sitting and doing nothing as a deliberate, volitional attempt to regulate emotional distress, the cognitive process of comparing sensory information to a schema while sitting may be such an attempt, and some subjects think of "self-monitoring and sensation watching" as a coping strategy (p. 253). The term *passive coping* might thus refer to the use of intrapsychic means in an attempt to control emotional distress, although such intraspsychic coping "behavior" cannot, of course, be observed directly.

Neither form of coping is *defined* by Johnson and Leventhal as actually reducing emotional distress, since the relationship would then be tautological, and the conceptual distinction between coping and distress required by the parallel response model would be lost. Similarly, if passive coping were inferred solely from emotional distress reduction the ability to separate these variables operationally would be lost. To maintain these variables as conceptually distinct, passive coping strategies (self-distraction, monitoring sensations, and comparing sensations to a schema) and active coping strategies (taking extra time in swallowing an endoscopy tube, coughing, ambulating, pushing in labor, and so on) must be defined as coping behaviors whether or not they actually reduce distress, reduce complications, or promote favorable outcomes. This suggests some possible additions to the contingencies.

Distress might be reduced by providing accurate information on which to base a schema only in those situations wherein an accurate schema and set of criteria will lead to nonthreatening interpretations of most of the events and sensations that the subject is likely to experience. (Note that on p. 253 Leventhal cites an example in which distress is not decreased when the subject is presented with a schema and regulation criteria that suggest prolonged pain will be experienced.) Further, while information about active coping responses may not promote more successful outcomes unless the coping responses suggested actually bear a direct relation to successful outcomes independent of the subject's belief in them, they may nevertheless tend to reduce emotional distress if the subject believes they are effective. In addition to these contingencies, Leventhal and Johnson suggest that information has a greater effect on reducing distress when distress is initially high and that the largest effects of information on emotional distress reduction and rapid recovery occur when all three kinds of information are provided and active coping is both possible and directly related to the clinical outcomes.

Articulating the behavioral theory with nursing practice theory

The application of a behavioral science theory to the formulation of specific guidelines for practice is closely related to the general considerations involved in putting into operation theoretical variables for research purposes, as discussed in the introduction to this section. In their clinical trials and discussions Leventhal and Johnson make implicit and explicit predictions about the kinds of practice circumstances, practitioners, and subjects to which the theory should be applied (the framework), the types of intervention techniques that should be used to manipulate the independent variable (the means), and the sorts of beneficial outcomes to be expected as a result of effects on the dependent variables (the goals). These considerations involve professional and practical criteria related to the role of nursing in health care settings that go beyond the considerations used to evaluate the theory from a behavioral science perspective alone. As Leventhal and Johnson note, their earlier research on such variables as birth order was valuable from a behavioral science theory perspective, but it had only limited implications for improving practice effectiveness, since nurses cannot manipulate the patient's birth order.

Framework

The contingencies in the behavioral theory seem highly relevant to a nursing framework. Most medical procedures (and many nursing procedures) are either unpleasant per se or contain an element of potential threat through their perceived risk or association with previous unpleasant experiences or both, as is illustrated in the wide variety of clinical trials that Johnson and Leventhal report. Although Johnson argues that the initial stress level is in many circumstances low for most patients, the effects on emotional distress, as well as coping, were great for most of the circumstances studied, particularly when all three aspects of the information needed for self-regulation were provided. Even patients who have encountered a procedure before may have major gaps in their knowledge of what to expect or what the phenomena they experience really mean, and most have little knowledge of the extent to which what they experienced was "typical" or "normal." Whether or not this lack of knowledge produces emotional distress, their evidence suggests that it usually retards coping and prolongs recovery.

In addition to the general contingencies just listed, other factors may affect the success of the techniques used by Leventhal and Johnson in their clinical trials. These include the patient's ability to learn what is communicated and motivation to do so and the extent to which the information is believed. With the exception of infants and adult patients who are comatose or otherwise incapacitated, almost all patients have some ability to understand and assimilate descriptions of impending events. Leventhal and Johnson's research suggests that even young children have this capacity, although the degree of communication actually achieved may depend on the extent to which the message is modified to take such factors as age, mental status, and educational status in account. With the possible exception of patients who use denial as their major defense mechanism, one might speculate that most patients want to know something about what is going to happen and what will be expected of them, although the degree and kind of knowledge desired may vary. Even patients who are fatalistic, excessively fearful, or preoccupied with some other aspect of their condition or life are unlikely to be totally unmotivated to develop a schema, but the degree of success achieved in helping the patient develop a schema may be contingent on the extent to which such factors are taken into account. While Leventhal and Johnson achieve substantial effects with standardized communications, it is still possible that the means employed could have been ineffective for some of their subjects (as they explicitly point out).

The nurse (or a tape-recorded message by a person identified as a nurse or physician) is likely to be perceived by the patient as an authoritative source of information on the kinds of issues mentioned, but the believability of the communication may also be increased when the information on sensations is based directly on the experiences of previous patients (as it is in most of Leventhal and Johnson's experiments). Contingencies such as these may be essential to create an effective schema, and some of the variation in the effectiveness of Leventhal and Johnson's manipulations may be the result of variation in such contingencies.

Nursing means

The independent variables in the behavioral theory seem highly relevant to nursing means. Nurses and the nursing profession as a whole have a considerable degree of autonomy in determining what information to convey to the patient about impending medical and nursing procedures in most of the practice situations covered by the contingencies. It would probably be necessary, however, to place some additional restrictions on the framework or practice guidelines derived from this theory to apply it to situations where physicians have a recognized authority to withhold certain kinds of information from the patient or to monitor its accuracy or both.

Most nurses would presumably have the educational background and basic communication skills to implement these means for most patients once the material to be communicated to the patient facing a given procedure had been determined. The determination of the specific material to be communicated is, however, likely to require special study for each type of situation, along the lines suggested by Leventhal and Johnson (p. 214). Developing this material may require research and theory skills beyond the ability of the average practitioner. The requirement that the content of the material focus on aspects of the experiences that are salient from the *patient's* viewpoint (p. 246) has much in common with the nursing approaches based on symbolic interaction previously discussed (pp. 45-51), although the focus is on the average patient instead of a single individual patient.

Special clinical skills may also be required effectively to communicate material to certain types of patients (as noted in the previous discussion and in Chapters 2 and 3). Eventually practice guidelines might add restrictions to the framework that would require certain kinds of specialty training for communicating self-regulating information to mentally disturbed patients, very young (or old) patients, mentally retarded patients, excessively fearful patients, and so forth. The success of Johnson and Leventhal in using prerecorded tapes in some of their experiments strongly suggests, however, that for typical groups of patients and practice conditions, no special skills in communicating and individualizing the information are necessary to have an effect that is beneficial *on the average* when contrasted with the amounts and kinds of information that are currently provided. If this generalization is correct, and if audiotapes can be used effectively in regular clinical practice, then the only important limitation concerning "agency" required in the framework might be the ability to determine and prepare the specific material to be communicated. Even this requirement might not be necessary if simply directing the patient to pay attention to sensations rather than attempting to ignore them would suffice, as some of Leventhal's research suggests.

These considerations may make Leventhal and Johnson's theory more widely and immediately applicable to the reduction of distress and enhancement of coping behaviors than Orlando's general theory (as discussed in Chapters 1 and 3), since a higher than usual level of training in communication skills is required to nurse in a truly "deliberative" manner. Seen in this light, Orlando's theory (which requires a separate nursing diagnosis and an individualized approach for each patient) might have more implications for the education of communication specialists than direct and immediate implications for the practice of the average staff nurse. The most successful research applications of Orlando's theory (a number of which are cited by Johnson and Leventhal) were implemented by psychiatric nurses, many of whom were trained either by Orlando herself or by Orlando's students. By way of contrast, any nurse (or even those who are not nurses) could play one of Johnson and Leventhal's tapes to a patient facing that specific procedure and presumably achieve comparable results. On the other hand, verbal communication is much more common than playing an audiotape in patient teaching by health care professionals, and even nurses without special training might increase their effectiveness by attempting to explore the patient's definition of the situation more fully. As Leventhal and Johnson point out, individualization of the information provided to take into account the unique aspects of the patient's situation is likely to be more effective than a standard package if the individualization is done well. If, in addition, emotional and other needs can be defined and attended to through a "deliberative" interaction, then the overall results may be still further enhanced, as is indicated by the large magnitudes of effects found in studies where all these factors were manipulated simultaneously.

The fact that a nonnurse might actually play the tape for the patient, or that the speaker in the audiotape is a physician, does not signify that we are no longer dealing with nursing theory or nursing guidelines. To the extent that the nursing profession has played the major role in developing the underlying practice theory behind an intervention, tested it through clinical research, and established the guidelines by which the theory is to be applied in clinical practice, the theory is nursing theory and the guidelines are nursing guidelines regardless of who actually implements them "at the bedside." It is important to note, however, that these issues are not yet resolved for applications of Leventhal and Johnson's theory. Guidelines based on their theory have not yet filtered down to everyday nursing practice in most hospitals, and not all of the development of the theory and guidelines have been by the nursing profession. In some cases physicians and dentists have set up the guidelines. The ultimate determination of the extent to which this area will come to be recognized as part of the specialized knowledge developed by the nursing profession lies in the future, although it is already apparent that nursing is playing a major role and thus establishing a strong claim.

Nursing goals

The dependent variables in the behavioral theory are relevant to nursing goals in different ways and to different degrees. Of the two types of coping, most nursing theories value active or planned coping over passive or automatic coping insofar as there is anything appropriate the patient can do to cope actively, but much of actual nursing practice tends to encourage passive rather than active coping. While it is widely believed by theorists that active and planned coping by the patient leads to better treatment outcomes and lower levels of psychological distress than does passive coping, the research evidence is far from clear on this point.

If coping is defined in terms of the behavior itself and the subject's intent rather than in terms of its actual effectiveness in reducing distress or promoting favorable outcomes, than neither type of coping is a goal of nursing per se. Direct measures of coping are often used as criteria for the evaluation of nursing practice outcomes when feedback on ultimate treatment outcomes is not available or only remotely related to the nursing means employed. The effectiveness of a patient education program may be evaluated by the patients' compliance with regimens, rather than by increased ability to function or reduced illness, for example. As Hochbaum (1979, p. 180) points out, such criteria are the most appropriate criteria for evaluation of the educational aspects of the program per se, but they are not the appropriate outcome criteria from the nursing theory perspective as we have defined it. (See also Diers, 1974, who makes this same point with respect to the evaluation of nurse-practitioner programs.) In some of Johnson and Leventhal's findings, greater effects were obtained for outcome variables that implied the patient had had a more rapid recovery or fewer treatment complications or both than were obtained for the coping behaviors themselves (in their surgery studies, for example). This may mean that not all of the active coping behaviors involved were defined and measured accurately or that passive coping contributed to the outcomes, or it may mean that some other process, such as the reduction of emotional distress, contributed to the effects.

Reduction of emotional distress would be regarded by most nurses as an important outcome goal in its own right, but it is also valued as a potential contributor to favorable treatment outcomes. In spite of Johnson's argument that distress reduction does not play a major role in interpreting the effects of information on treatment outcomes, the research results are not really conclusive on this point, as will be noted.

Evaluating the research evidence

Johnson and Leventhal's research includes nonexperimental survey research, laboratory experimentation, and clinical trials in a variety of settings. In addition, they cite a variety of results from the published research of other investigators. It is theory that links these apparently diverse studies and shows ways in which their findings can be generalized still further to a wide variety of clinical settings and circumstances.

In testing a general theory it is not necessary always to do the research in the actual clinical setting in which it will be applied. In Johnson and Leventhal's research the laboratory setting has advantages in that it permits better control of extraneous variables and permits the experimenter ethically (with the subject's consent) to introduce and control the painful stimulus to which the subject's response is monitored. The clinical setting has advantages in that there are "real-life" issues at stake and levels of pain and stress that go beyond the transient and relatively minor sources of discomfort introduced in the laboratory experiments. In the clinical trials the sources of pain and discomfort are not introduced by the experimenter, but are an inevitable part of the clinical situation. This permits the researcher to study response to much higher stress and pain levels than could ethically be produced in a laboratory setting. It also permits the study of "real-life" situations in which the potential outcomes include long-term, nontrivial risks to the patient. Such experiments are ethical if none of the treatment conditions of the experiment involve new and untried elements that would be likely to increase the patient's risk beyond the level that would prevail under normal clinical circumstances (if no research were in process). In Leventhal and Johnson's research none of the approaches depart from the routine practice in ways likely to increase risk or reduce benefits to patients. It is ethical to withhold detailed information about sensations from the control group patients, for example, because if the research were not being conducted such information would not be provided to any of the patients.

Spuriousness

As Johnson and Leventhal point out experimental studies with random-ized comparison groups have major advantages for ruling out the possibility that an association is spurious (the result of preexisting conditions or "ante-cedent variables" associated with the independent variable). Even experi-ments rule out such possibilities only within chance limits, however. This means that there is some possibility (equal to the level of significance) that the entire difference found between treatment groups may be caused by chance differences in antecedent variables and an even greater possibility that differ-ences in the magnitudes of the associations between treatment groups or between the various dependent variables in an experiment may be the result of chance. While further replication would be desirable, Leventhal and John-son's use of randomized comparison groups, replications of their own re-search, and extensive comparisons of their results to those of other studies provide an unusually firm basis for ruling out the possibility that their repli-cated results were caused by preexisting characteristics of the subjects or their preferences for different treatment conditions or both.

Since confounding by antecedent variables is unlikely to have seriously affected Leventhal and Johnson's results, and since, as Leventhal and John-son note, inverse causation (the possibility that variation in distress is causing the variation in the information provided) is ruled out entirely by the design, the major issues to be resolved in interpreting the findings are issues of alter-native theoretical interpretations of why their manipulations had the effects they found. Such alternative interpretations to a proposed theory are referred to as "operational biases" in Wooldridge et al. (1978:18).

Operational bias

There are two major kinds of operational biases and they can occur either singly or in combination. The first possibility is that in operationalizing the independent variable, additional elements that might affect distress but that are extraneous to information were inadvertently manipulated. This might be referred to as *bias in operationalizing the independent variable*. The second possibility is that a measure of the theoretically defined dependent variables (coping and distress) might be affected by extraneous variables, which in turn were affected by differences between the treatment groups. This might be referred to as *bias in operationalizing a dependent variable*. Bias in oper-ationalizing a dependent variable tends to vary from one measure to another, so the use of multiple measures in a single experiment can help to evaluate the possible impact of this kind of bias. Bias in operationalizing an indepen-dent variable is usually constant over any single study (unless a multiple treatment design is employed) but may vary from one experiment to another, so replications help to evaluate the possible impact of this kind of bias.

Leventhal and Johnson's use of highly structured preprepared scripts and tape recordings reduces the possibility that the subject's motivation or emotion or both were directly influenced without regard to the informational component. If the educational material had been presented by the investigator or had not been predetermined, it would have been more likely that extraneous differences between the experimental and control treatment might have led to differences in patient levels of distress. Much of the early nursing research on preoperative preparation confounded the provision of information with the provision of a wide variety of other kinds of input that might have affected outcomes. In experiments to prepare patients to face stressful situations through "deliberative" nursing, for example, the nurse was free to provide any sort of professionally appropriate service for the patient that she and the patient decided was needed. While informational components were often provided there was also a substantial emphasis on working directly on emotions through having the patient express feelings and fears and having the nurse support the patient with respect to his feelings. This might, of course, have had a direct cathartic or reassuring effect regardless of the informational component of the interchange. By avoiding the provision of the supportive component Leventhal and Johnson were able to focus more specifically on the effects of the cognitive, educational, and informational components. In addition, by separately manipulating different aspects of the informational component they were able to discriminate between the alternative cognitive processes that were confounded in the research of Egbert (1964), of Schmitt and Wooldridge (1973), and of others.

Leventhal and Johnson's discussions and disagreements concerning the appropriate theoretical interpretation of their findings is logically related to the possibility of operational bias in measuring the dependent variables. Research that finds a stronger relationship between knowledge and measures of coping than between knowledge and measures of distress would seem to support Johnson's point of view, and research that finds a stronger relationship between knowledge and measures of distress than between knowledge and measures of coping would seem to support Leventhal's point of view. There are several complications, however, in differentiating between these two interpretations. As Leventhal and Johnson note (p. 197), the same behaviors that are influenced by coping may be influenced by emotional distress. Even if the theoretical definitions of coping and distress are kept distinct it is difficult to find measures that clearly reflect only one of these variables and not the other. In the ischemic pain experiments, for example, it would be hard to devise questions that would measure the cognitive content of "passive coping" in such a way that the emotional content of "distress" was not also reflected in the subject's responses. Even physiological measures of emotional distress, such as might be obtained in the laboratory (through recording of blood pressure, respiration, galvanic skin response, and so forth) might also be directly affected by coping strategies such as relaxation. Even if separate and distinct measures of passive coping and emotional distress were available, however, the magnitude of the relationship of each to knowledge would depend on the relative sensitivities of each measure and the relative extent to which each relationship was attenuated by error variation from extraneous influences. Finally, in research employing relatively small sample sizes, differences in the relative magnitudes of correlations from one measure to another or from one experiment to another might be caused by chance.

In addition to measurement problems and random fluctuations the relative sizes of the direct effects would, even at the theoretical level, depend on the specific circumstances under which the research was conducted. (These are the interactive effects referred to by Leventhal and Johnson.) If subjects are not likely to be fearful, for example, then effects through emotional distress reduction would likely be small. When knowledge of "adequate criteria for self-regulation" makes the subject aware of a danger that would otherwise be overlooked, one direct effect might be to heighten emotional distress and thus (indirectly) to reduce coping, while another effect might be to increase coping to reduce the danger. (Fig. 7). Both these possibilities are referred to by Leventhal and Johnson but not the possibility that they might occur simultaneously within a given patient.

In such a set of circumstances the overall effect of knowledge would depend on whether or not its direct effects on coping were sufficiently great to produce an overall positive effect in spite of the negative indirect effects through emotional distress. For example, a hypertensive patient who knew enough to interpret correctly his large increase in blood pressure as extremely dangerous in spite of a lack of negative symptoms might be more likely to become emotionally distressed (with some impairment of the ability to cope) but

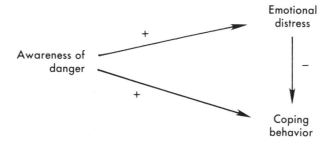

Fig. 7 ■ Model of possible offsetting causal processes in relating awareness of danger to coping behavior.

nevertheless more motivated to increase adherence to medical and nursing regimens (medicine, diet, exercise, and so forth). Whether the positive direct effect on coping would be greater than the negative indirect effect through emotional distress would depend on the relative sizes of each of the effects involved (knowledge on coping, knowledge on emotional distress, and emotional distress on coping). The relative sizes of the effects might in turn depend on the specific characteristics of the individual, the specific situation and coping behaviors involved, or both. Powers and Wooldridge (1982) found, for example, that providing the patient with additional knowledge of the dangers of uncontrolled high blood pressure reduced the tendency of recently diagnosed patients to assimilate additional information about hypertension but increased the tendency of patients with long-standing diagnoses to assimilate such information. (While learning additional information is not necessarily a coping behavior per se the basic theoretical processes involved in accounting for this result are essentially the same.) As Johnson and Leventhal also note (p. 248), the overall effect might also depend on whether the coping behavior is short term or long term or on the extent to which specific coping plans can be made at the time the patient becomes aware of the danger.

External validity

As Leventhal and Johnson point out, no one strategy of cognitive structuring may be optimal for every situation. Testing the generalizability of a theory to a variety of circumstances is much more difficult than testing the applicability of the theory to a particular set of circumstances. Leventhal and Johnson infer from the variation in the size of apparent effects between their experiments that sensory information alone is optimal in reducing emotional distress for situations in which active coping is not likely to have any direct effect in controlling the stressor or avoiding its negative consequences, but that instruction in active coping strategies is likely to be optimal in reducing emotional distress (perhaps in combination with sensory information) in situations that permit the patient to act constructively to control the stressor or its consequences.

To test this theory adequately for the interactive effects of self-regulation strategies a large number of clinical trials would have to be performed in circumstances dissimilar in the extent to which there is a constructive role for active coping but similar with respect to all other variables that might produce interactive effects. In addition to the difficulty of finding situations that meet these requirements, larger sample sizes would be required for each individual study to achieve reliable estimates of the interactive effects.

Even a considerable variation in the magnitude of an association from one small sample experiment to another may be caused by chance rather than by differences in the circumstances studied. This caveat should be kept in mind in evaluating those of Leventhal and Johnson's interpretations that present reasons for differences in the magnitudes of associations found. Whether or not an association is statistically significant in a given study is almost entirely a matter of its magnitude and the size of the sample, so discussions of whether or not a relationship was found to be significant are, when the sample sizes are similar, implicitly discussions of the relative magnitude of the associations found. It is not unlikely that some of the differences between individual studies for which Leventhal and Johnson propose explanations were caused simply by chance. On the other hand, those of Leventhal and Johnson's interpretations that are based on patterns of results found to be replicable over more than one study are far less likely to be caused by chance.

CONCLUSION

The three chapters in Section III show that different nursing investigators use theory in different ways and to different degrees in designing their research and interpreting their results. Theory is sometimes an afterthought in applied nursing research (as in the Martinsons' research) rather than an integral part of the design. When behavioral or social science theory is strongly involved in conceptualizing the research problem and designing the research, the links to nursing practice may be somewhat remote (as in Benoliel's research). Only in Leventhal and Johnson's research is there a clear and systematic effort to articulate research findings with basic behavioral science theory on the one hand and nursing practice on the other hand. It is perhaps no coincidence that their research is grounded both on laboratory experimentation and on randomized clinical trials and that nonexperimental research was used only at the outset, when they were initially probing their theoretical area of concern. In some of the seminal theoretical development in this area, however, general theoretical hypotheses were derived from a clinical case study of one patient (Janis, 1958, part 1), which were then tested nonexperimentally by means of a retrospective questionnaire survey (Janis, 1958, part 2). While we do not subscribe to the notion that theory necessarily develops in discrete stages, each with its accompanying research design, it is nevertheless obvious that the examples we chose for Section III typified different developmental stages of theory building, and that methodological rigor tended to increase in the later stages.

Although the extent to which the proposed theoretical interpretations had actually been tested varied widely, each of the studies we analyzed was excellent in its own way. In other words, each had the *potential* to contribute to the cumulative processes by which theoretical generalizations are developed and tested as part of a scientific endeavor. The points that we hope we have illustrated are that not all research contributes to theory in the same way and that the nursing theorist must exercise extreme care in evaluating research evidence in order not to be misled as to its practice implications.

For variables that are not manipulable by nurses, such as age and sex, effects on treatment outcomes do not *in themselves* suggest ways to improve nursing effectiveness. Theories about such effects are not, therefore, conceptualized from a practice theory viewpoint as we have defined it. On the other hand, such variables may:

1. Enter directly into practice theory as aspects of the framework that influence the relative effectiveness of different nursing means
2. Help to identify high-risk populations for which more effective nursing interventions need to be developed and employed
3. Serve as control variables whose effects should be reduced or eliminated in research designed to study the effects of other variables that can be manipulated by nurses

In addition, the theoretical interpretation of why such variables are related to treatment outcomes may serve to focus attention on intervening variables that nurses *can* attempt to influence. The point is not, therefore, that nurse-researchers should regard the relationship between demographic and historical variables and outcomes as irrelevant to practice; it is that they must go beyond the mere fact of such relationships to explore the precise way(s) in which the relationships may (or may not) have useful implications for nursing practice. It is this further exploration of theoretical issues in terms of their relevance to nursing practice that constitutes a nursing theory perspective, and it is the design of further research to resolve practice relevant ambiguities that constitutes a nursing research perspective.

Awareness of the existence of the metatheoretical and methodological issues that we have raised is only the first step on the road to acquiring judgment and skill in relating practice theory generalizations to behavioral science theory, to empirical research, and to actual practice. Now that you have read this chapter, you may want to go back through the studies in Section three to see if you can reproduce our analyses or, we hope, go beyond them. We selectively focused on some of the major theoretical issues raised by these studies, but a number of other issues could also be analyzed in a similar manner. We leave such further analysis as an exercise for the reader.

REFERENCES

Campbell, D.T., and Stanley, J.C. 1963. Experimental and quasi-experimental designs for research, Chicago, Rand McNally & Co.

Diers, D.K. 1974. Research and nurse practitioners: lessons from yesterday. Paper presented at Rochester Conference on Adult Ambulatory Care, Dec. 12, Rochester, N.Y.

Edwardson, S.R. 1983. The choice between hospital and home care for terminally ill children, Nursing Research 32:29-34.

Egbert, L.D. 1964. Reduction of post-operative pain by encouragement and instruction of patients: a study of doctor-patient rapport, New England Journal of Medicine 270:825-827.

Gehan, E., and Freireich, E.J. 1974. Non-randomized controls in cancer clinical trials, New England Journal of Medicine 290:198-203.

Glaser, B., and Strauss, A. 1967. Discovery of grounded theory, Chicago, Aldine Publishing Co.

Hochbaum, G.M. 1979. Comment on assessing effectiveness of health education, American Journal of Public Health 69:180-181.

Janis, I. 1958. Psychological stress, New York, John Wiley & Sons, Inc.

Martinson, I.M., et al. 1978a. Home care for children dying of cancer, Pediatrics 62:106-113.

Martinson, I.M., et al. 1978b. Facilitating home care for children dying of cancer, Cancer Nursing 1:41-45.

Martinson, I.M. 1979. Caring for the dying child, Nursing Clinics of North America 14:467-474.

Powers, M.J., and Wooldridge, P.J. 1982. Factors influencing knowledge, attitudes and compliance at hypertensive patients, Research in Nursing and Health 5:171-182.

Robinson, W.S. 1951. Logical structure of analytic induction, The American Sociological Review 16:812-818.

Schatzman, L., and Strauss, A. 1973. Field research: strategies for a natural sociology, Englewood Cliffs, N.J., Prentice-Hall, Inc.

Schmidt, F.E., and Wooldridge, P.J. 1973. Psychological preparation of surgical patients, Nursing Research 22:108-115.

Wooldridge, P.J., Leonard, R.C. and Skipper, J.K., Jr. 1978. Methods of clinical experimentation to improve patient care, St. Louis, The C.V. Mosby Co.

Index